Nursing: Communication Skills in Practice

Edited by Lucy Webb

Series editor Karen Holland

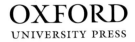

OXFORD
UNIVERSITY PRESS

OXFORD
UNIVERSITY PRESS

Great Clarendon Street, Oxford OX2 6DP

Oxford University Press is a department of the University of Oxford.
It furthers the University's objective of excellence in research, scholarship,
and education by publishing worldwide in

Oxford New York

Auckland Cape Town Dar es Salaam Hong Kong Karachi
Kuala Lumpur Madrid Melbourne Mexico City Nairobi
New Delhi Shanghai Taipei Toronto

With offices in

Argentina Austria Brazil Chile Czech Republic France Greece
Guatemala Hungary Italy Japan Poland Portugal
Singapore South Korea Switzerland Thailand Turkey Ukraine Vietnam

Published in the United States
by Oxford University Press Inc., New York

British Library Cataloguing in Publication Data
Data available

Library of Congress Cataloging in Publication Data
Data available

Typeset by Glyph International, Bangalore
Printed in Great Britain
on acid-free paper by
Ashford Colour Press Ltd, Gosport, Hampshire

ISBN 978–0–19–958272–3

3 5 7 9 10 8 6 4 2

Nursing: Communication Skills in Practice

This book is due for return on or before the last date shown below

2 3 APR 2013	3 0 JAN 2019	
2 3 JUL 2013	2 3 APR 2019	
	27/8/19.	
1 9 AUG 2013	12/4/23	
2 0 DEC 2013		
1 0 NOV 2014		
3 0 AUG 2016		
0 9 MAR 2016		
2 5 MAY 2017		
1 7 AUG 2017		
3 0 MAY 2018		

The Library (CGH)
Cheltenham General Hospital
Cheltenham
GL53 7AN
0300 422 3036

Series editor preface

Learning to be a nurse requires students to develop a set of skills and a knowledge base that will enable them to make the transition from learner to qualified nurse. As with any transition, this can often seem at times to be a daunting prospect, in the face of which the student may ask: 'How am I *ever* going to learn all that I need to know to get through this course and become a qualified nurse?'

For student nurses, this experience entails learning in 'two worlds': that of the university and that of the clinical environment. Although there is a physical distinction between the two, it is important that the learning that takes place in one is integrated with the learning in the other. This series of books has set out to do just that.

These 'two worlds' require that a student learns two sets of skills in order to qualify as a nurse and be ready to take on further sets of skills in whatever nursing environment he or she is employed. The skills that will be a core part of this series are numerous, and central to them is the idea of 'coping with the unknown'. Students face a new environment each time they start a new clinical placement, communicating with patients and a large number of health and social care professionals, dealing with difficult and often complex situations and sometimes stressful clinical experiences. In the university, there are also situations that may be unknown, such as learning new study skills, working with others, searching and finding information, and managing workloads. It is every student's goal to complete his or her course with the required foundation for the future and it is the essential goal of this series to enable the student to develop skills for a successful learning and nursing experience.

The central ethos to all of the books therefore is to facilitate and enhance the student learning experience and develop his or her skills, through engaging with a variety of reflective accounts, exercises, and web-based resources. We hope that you, as the reader and learner, enjoy reading these books and that the guidance within them supports your goal of successfully completing your course of study.

Karen Holland
Series editor

Preface

Communication and interpersonal skills are now recognized as essential skills for all nurses, regardless of the area of care; increasingly, communication skills are being used therapeutically by nurses to deliver improved quality care and expand the nursing role of health promoter. Communication skills are the bedrock of patient-centred care, individualized care, and patient-led care.

Nursing: Communication Skills in Practice has been written for student nurses developing communication and interpersonal skills in any field of care. The contributors are all nurses and experienced leaders in their different clinical fields, and have years of experience guiding nursing students through pre-registration education and training. The authors bring up-to-date knowledge and expertise to their topics, and demonstrate how theory and practice marry up in the different practice contexts.

There are many books on communication and interpersonal skills available to nursing students. What makes this book different is that it focuses on demonstrating how the theory is applied in practice. Student nurses are taught theory in the academic setting and practice in the clinical setting. This book helps the student to bridge that gap between the two. The skills and knowledge addressed in these chapters reflect the skills expected of all qualifying nurses as detailed in both the Nursing and Midwifery Council essential skills clusters (NMC, 2007) and the revised 2010 competency framework (NMC, 2010).

Many people have contributed in some way to this book. All of the authors have been assisted by all of our patients, colleagues, and students. Specifically, practitioners Hermione Montgomery, Honor Cann, and Guy Collins have contributed insights and practice examples, reviewers have offered invaluable guidance, and the staff at Oxford University Press have been diligent in keeping us to our task and encouraging us along the way. Colleagues at Manchester Metropolitan University, at the time of writing this, have yet to understand how much they will contribute to the online video material, although cameraman Mike MacKenzie already know that will be kept busy! Lastly, thanks must go to all of the students who have educated us about what student nurses need and how they want to learn it.

Lucy Webb (editor) and Soundman Neil Ormrod

Contents

Detailed contents

PART 3 **Advancing application of communication skills**

About the authors

Editor

Lucy Webb

Senior Lecturer, MMU Department of Nursing

Lucy is a mental health nurse and health psychologist specializing in child and adolescent psychiatry, and substance misuse in adults and young people. She has worked in general psychiatric and specialist areas of care, and led the Drug & Alcohol Liaison Team in St George's Hospital in London. Currently a senior lecturer at Manchester Metropolitan University, Lucy teaches mental health, communication, mentorship, and substance misuse across a range of vocational and academic healthcare courses, and has extensive research and publication outputs in her specialist care areas.

Contributors

Anne-Marie Bourneuf

Senior Lecturer, MMU Department of Nursing

Anne-Marie Bourneuf is a senior lecturer in nursing at Manchester Metropolitan University and specializes in A&E, acute/critical care nursing, teaching and learning in practice, management and leadership in health care, and telephone triage nursing. She is also engaged in healthcare research in Manchester and is a reviewer for *Nurse Education in Practice*.

Kathy Crew

Family Nurse, Stockport Primary Care Trust

Kathy Crew is a registered nurse, midwife, health visitor, and family planning nurse. Kathy is at present a family nurse working with the Family Nurse Partnership Programme, working with teenage parents to improve the health and development of children and their families. Kathy works within Stockport PCT and has been committed to work with teenage parents for many years.

Jacqui Gladwin

Principal Lecturer, MMU Department of Nursing

Jacqui Gladwin is principal lecturer at Manchester Metropolitan University. She specializes in emergency care and acute medicine, and practised as a senior nurse at Manchester Royal Infirmary before entering nursing education. She is a member of the Centre for Effective Emergency Care based at MMU, and interests include the development of technology to support and empower patients and healthcare professionals, and the effects of occupational stress on nurses in A&E and paramedics in pre-hospital care. She has been engaged in innovative developments in electronic patient record-keeping in Greater Manchester, helping to develop sensitive and patient-centred systems for primary care.

Val Helsby
Family Nurse, Stockport Primary Care Trust

Val Helsby, BSc(Hons) Nursing Practice, is a registered nurse (RN), sick children's nurse (RSCN), health visitor, and family planning nurse. Val is currently working as a family nurse within Stockport PCT Family Nurse Partnership Programme, working with teenage parents to improve the health and development of children and their families.

Maxine Holt
Senior Lecturer, MMU Department of Nursing

Maxine Holt is a senior lecturer in nursing at MMU, where her work is predominantly teaching public health within pre-registration nursing programmes. She is a registered nurse with experience expanding over thirty years across general nursing, with a particular focus on community and practice nursing. Her particular interests, publications, and research are in developing public health within nursing.

Eula Miller
Senior Lecturer, MMU Department of Nursing

Eula Miller is a senior lecturer in nursing at Manchester Metropolitan University. She has dual registration in general and mental health nursing, and is a qualified counsellor, community health specialist, and teacher/practice educator. She has researched and published around the subject of learning and developing self-awareness, and has recently contributed to the book *Exploring Self Awareness in Mental Health* (RCN Publishing, 2008).

Duncan Mitchell
Professor, MMU Department of Nursing & Manchester Learning Disability Partnership

Duncan Mitchell holds a joint appointment with Manchester Metropolitan University and Manchester Learning Disability Partnership, where he is Professor of Health and Disability. Duncan has been a learning disability nurse since 1986, and he has worked in both practice and education. Duncan has published research into the history of learning disability services, as well as health and learning disability. Duncan is currently editor of the *British Journal of Learning Disabilities*.

Gayatri Nambiar-Greenwood
Senior Lecturer, MMU Department of Nursing

Gayatri Nambiar-Greenwood is a senior lecturer in nursing at Manchester Metropolitan University. She has a Masters degree in Healthcare Law and Ethics. From a background of neurosciences nursing, Guy worked at the then regional Centre for Neurosciences at the Manchester Royal Infirmary, originally on the wards, then as a researcher coordinator, and finally as a specialist nurse in neurological diseases, for eleven years, before moving into education. She joined the Medical School at University of Manchester to set up clinical skills laboratories and as clinical skills tutor for medical undergraduates. Her main subjects of interest are inter-professional learning, reflective practice, mental and adult health co-morbidity, and law and ethics. She teaches these subjects at pre- and post-registration level for a variety of professional groups, and presents regularly at conferences in the UK and abroad.

Caroline Ridley
Senior Lecturer, MMU Department of Nursing
Caroline Ridley, MA Academic Practice; BSc(Hons) Nursing Practice, is a registered nurse, health visitor/family planning nurse, and a senior lecturer in nursing at Manchester Metropolitan University. Caroline's teaching commitment is predominately within pre-registration adult nursing and she has taught on childcare courses in further education. Caroline has a special interest in public health, child health, and young people's sexual health.

Gary Witham
Senior Lecturer, MMU Department of Nursing
Gary Witham, BA(Hons), RN, PG Cert Palliative care, PG Cert Academic Practice, is a registered nurse and senior lecturer at Manchester Metropolitan University. Gary's clinical background is in cancer care, with a research interest in rare cancers and communication skills. Gary's teaching commitment is predominantly within pre-registration adult nursing.

How to use this book

Communication Skills in Practice explains the theory of health care communication and outlines the communication skills required to be an effective nurse. This brief tour of the book shows you how to get the most out of this textbook and web package.

It's all new to me!

Find what you need fast! The detailed list of contents in the front of the book and the list of aims at the start of each chapter will help you find what you need quickly.

What does that mean? Each new term is highlighted in colour in the text and explained in the glossary at the back of the book - you can also revise these online.

> The **facilitative** styles help the patient find his or her
> self-care and self-healing. These styles are more in kee
> approach. The last facilitative style, **supportive**, is sugges
> to be always present in any communication transaction, w
> **prescriptive** or **confronting** approach. For Heron, this i
> between effective beneficial communication and '**degene**

Helping you to develop your skills

Learning points These activities will help you to acquire the knowledge and practical skills that are required for your academic assignments and nursing practice.

> **Learning point 1**
>
> Communication skills are often assessed in a practical
> (Objective Structured Clinical Examination). OSCEs are pop
> healthcare education as they can measure competency in p
> are likely to be required to demonstrate your active listen

Practice example Applying theory to practice can be difficult so concepts, issues and skills are illustrated and explored through scenarios from practice.

> **Practice example box 2: Egan's stages of help**
>
> Jane is a 16 year old with Down's Syndrome. She is offere
> college but her parents are worried that she will not cope
> uneasy because she wants to go, but doesn't want to leav

Nursing case studies Effective communication can enhance your interactions with patients and service users and these case studies highlight how you can achieve this.

> **Case study 3: Communicating with a 2 year o**
>
> Lucy is 2 years old. She has fallen, sustaining a cut to her
> arrival. She is accompanied by her mother who is also ups
> care at the time of the accident.

Cross references

The authors helpfully point out when an idea or issue is explored in more depth in a different chapter.

son's unhelpful thinking style which may lie at the roo[t] behaviour.

 You will find for an example of humanistic and beha[vioural] in Chapter 15 on motivational interviewing.

Conclusion and further information

Every chapter ends with a short summary useful for a quick recap and revising from later. You are also prompted to visit the Online Resource Centre where you'll find additional materials and tools. The authors also identify helpful books and websites at the end of each chapter which are highly useful for further study, assignments, and practice.

Conclusion

This chapter links to previous chapters in Part I on the[se] active listening, and further chapters in Part III, partic[ularly] earlier chapters outline the basic skills and theories of [c] illustrates some of the models or approaches which

Further reading

Bennett-Levy, J., Richards, D., Farrand, P., Christensen, H., [(]
Oxford Guide to Low Intensity CBT Interventions. Oxford:
Davies-Smith, L. (2006) 'An Introduction to Providing Cogni[tive]
Nursing Times, 102(26): 28–30.

Online Resource Centre

They key to developing communication skills is reflection and practice, practice, practice — this book has a dedicated website to help you get started. These resources are freely available but are password protected. To access the resources simply visit the website and enter the following username and password when instructed to in the book:

Username: **Communication Skills**

Password: **Flower**

www.oxfordtextbooks.co.uk/orc/webb

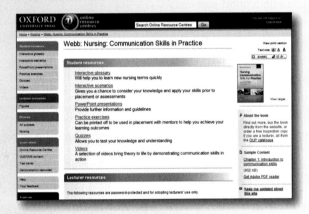

Students and lecturers can find:

At the end of each chapter the authors will guide you to the relevant **videos**.

Quizzes allow you to test your underlying knowledge and understanding.

Scenarios give you a chance to consider knowledge and apply skills prior to placement or assessments.

Practice exercises can be printed off to be used in placement with mentors to help you achieve your learning outcomes.

Interactive glossary will help you to learn new nursing terms quickly.

PowerPoint presentations provide further information and guidelines.

Lecturers can also download the figures for the book and use the above resources in your classes.

Theories of communication

PART 1

This part introduces essential knowledge and key models of communication before exploring fundamental aspects of nursing practice such as the nurse–patient relationship and therapeutic communication. It then goes on to outline and demonstrate essential skills such as active listening, attending, and working with groups of people. These skills form the foundation upon which other communication skills can be developed.

Chapter 1 introduces some key models for looking at communication and breaking it down into its component parts. Chapter 2 examines the nurse–patient relationship itself and the skills needed to ensure the safety of the patient and enhance the therapeutic process, and the management of the relationship from engagement to disengagement. Chapter 3 explains two key models of communication that underpin any person-to-person interaction and demonstrates how application of the theories enables the nurse–patient relationship to be therapeutic. Chapter 4 covers the basic skills and knowledge of communication and interpersonal skills in health care the aim of which is to engender healing and well-being. Chapter 5 extends the theory of communication to groups and examines what happens when we communicate in teams or with families, relatives, or cohorts of patients.

Introduction to communication skills

Lucy Webb

The aims of this chapter are to:

- ➔ outline the importance of communication skills in health care and nursing;
- ➔ explore the underpinning theories and definitions of communication;
- ➔ demonstrate theories of communication in the practice setting;
- ➔ provide a context for the rest of the book.

Introduction

Communication and interpersonal skills are essential components in delivering good-quality nursing care. Communication is identified as one of the essential skills that students must acquire in order to make progress through their education and training to become qualified nurses (NMC, 2010). This book has been designed and developed to help students to understand the underlying reasons why communication skills have become so important in nursing as well as the underpinning theories that attempt to define what communication is. In this chapter, as in all of the chapters in this book, you will find examples and explanations of how different aspects of communication are applied in the nursing context. In this way, this book will help you to develop your knowledge and skills so that you feel prepared for practice.

Why is communication important for nursing?

Important skills for the Nursing and Midwifery Council

The Nursing and Midwifery Council (NMC) standards for pre-registration nursing education (NMC, 2010) stipulate that, within the domain for communication and interpersonal skills, all nurses must do the following.

- Communicate safely and effectively.
- Build therapeutic relationships and take individual differences, capabilities, and needs into account.
- Be able to engage in, maintain, and disengage from therapeutic relationships.
- Use a range of communication skills and technologies.
- Use verbal, non-verbal, and written communication.
- Recognize the need for an interpreter.
- Address communication in diversity.
- Promote well-being and personal safety.
- Identify ways to communicate and promote healthy behaviour.
- Maintain accurate, clear, and complete written or electronic records.
- Respect and protect confidential information.

You will find all of these competencies addressed throughout this book.

Communication as an aspect of care

In attempting to answer the question, why is communication important in nursing, it becomes apparent that communication and 'nursing' are indivisible. But first, what do we mean by nursing? According to McMahon (2002), Florence Nightingale once complained that her concept of nursing had been turned into nothing more than the administration of medicines. McMahon expresses concern that nurses themselves perceive nursing as some form of comfort-giving, or providing assistance towards the patient's self-care, claiming that nurses themselves find it difficult to define what the nature of nursing is. Nursing proves as difficult to define as 'care', which means that the role of the nurse and how it is differentiated from that other health professions is often misunderstood. Perhaps nurses provide care and doctors provide treatment, but McMahon (2002) argues that this neither addresses the skills and knowledge needed in modern nursing to provide good-quality 'care', nor explains why students take three years to train before they become qualified nurses.

Since Florence Nightingale's time, nursing could be seen as having moved from a task-oriented practice towards a therapeutic process that encompasses a wide range of nursing roles, focused on the individual patient and his or her health and well-being. McMahon (2002: 7) attempts to define therapeutic nursing abilities as being characterized by six skills:

- developing the nurse–patient relationship;
- caring and comforting;
- using evidence-based physical interventions;
- teaching;
- manipulating the environment;
- adopting complementary health practices.

These are all skills developed by nurses during their pre-registration education; all of them demand good communication skills for effectiveness. It appears that this argument supports the notion that 'nursing', in addition to the applied knowledge and attitude, is underpinned essentially by communication skills.

The therapeutic effect of good communication delivered through good care is supported by evidence. Social support appears to have a role in providing reassurance and can even lower blood pressure (Kamarck et al., 1998). Health professionals who can communicate at an emotional level are seen as warm, caring, and empathetic, and engender trust in their patients, which encourages disclosure of worries and concerns that patients might otherwise not reveal (Bensing, 1991; Letvak, 1995). Additionally, informative and useful communication between the practitioner and the patient is shown to encourage patients to take more interest in their condition, ask questions, and develop greater understanding and self-care (Crow et al., 1999). This is particularly so when the patient is given time and encouragement to ask questions and be involved in treatment decisions. It is also shown that patients can experience measurable health benefits when nurses provide a good environment, use therapeutic communication, give accurate information, and encourage positive motivation in patients (Kwekkeboom, 1997).

So, good communication in the nurse–patient encounter is itself a beneficial and therapeutic intervention as well as the vehicle for good care, and can be regarded as important as other care or treatment. In brief, evidence suggests that health communication helps patients to:

- express their physical and emotional needs;
- ask questions and be more involved in their care;
- gain a sense of control over their condition and treatment;
- develop trust and confidence in the process and so comply with treatment;
- gain physical health benefits such as reduced pain and lowered blood pressure.

The changing nature of health care

Another key element that underlines the importance of good communication is the changing nature of health care itself. Improved medicine and treatment over the last century has moved health care away from a focus on acute illness to the management of chronic disease. More people are living with survivable chronic illness and need to be encouraged to be self-caring: for example, those with diabetes need to manage their blood sugar levels. Quality of life has become as important as survival now that people are living longer with chronic conditions such as cancer, bipolar disorder, and severe physical or learning disability.

Therefore treatment choice has become much more dependent on the individual patient's preference and what suits the patient's values and expectations. In many circumstances, the patient has become the expert in their own treatment and care management (DoH, 2001a).

A raft of government initiatives has driven health provision towards patient-centred care in the UK. The Patient's Charter (DoH, 1992) and the NHS Plan (DoH, 2000) initiated a shift of services to revolve around the patient rather than the patient needing to fit in with the services: for example, broader appointment times and access hours and waiting list reduction. Patients started to be acknowledged as the experts in their care, especially in managing chronic ill health (DoH, 2001a). Patients are viewed as active participants in their care and the provision of care services, with a focus on service users' rights and contributions to policy and service planning (DoH, 2001b; 2006a; 2006b). We have also entered an age of consumerism in which patients expect more from their healthcare providers and in which patients have access to information and are much better informed about health issues. This can be referred to as a shift from a medical model of health care to a bio-psychosocial model of health care whereby the biological, psychological, and social aspects of the patient's well-being are taken equally into consideration in a holistic manner to address the patient's quality of life (Ogden, 2004).

Overall, there has been a major shift in the relationship between patient and practitioner, which has turned the old paternal system of 'doctor knows best' into one of patient-centred care and the 'expert patient'. Bensing (2000) sums this up in a simple diagram of two dimensions that dictate the relationship between the patient and the practitioner (see Figure 1.1).

This model maps out the patient–practitioner encounter, with who has control on one dimension and how medicalized the communication is on the other dimension. For instance, a visit to the GP may involve the doctor informing the patient that he or she must take the medication in order to get better (a doctor-controlled, medical encounter), or the patient informing the doctor that the side effects are interfering with his or her work and social life and that another type needs to be tried (a patient-centred, bio-psychosocial encounter).

We can encapsulate the modern approach to the patient–practitioner encounter by outlining the three key factors seen in Table 1.1.

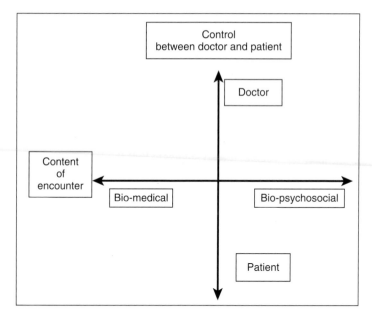

Figure 1.1 Bensing's dimensions of patient-centredness (repr. from Bensing, 'Bridging the Gap: The Separate Worlds of Evidence-based Medicine', *Patient Education and Counselling,* 39(1): 17–25; with permission from Elsevier)

What is communication?

There are a large number of models and definitions of communication, which in itself signifies that communication is a vast topic and difficult to pin down to simple explanation. Communication occurs whenever one person, in some way or another, transmits a message of some sort and someone else picks it up and interprets it. DeVito defines communication as 'the act, by one or more persons, of sending and receiving messages that are distorted by noise, occur within a context, have some effect, and provide

Table 1.1 Paradigm of patient-centred care: the three elements

	Consequence	Impact on nursing
Changes in morbidity	People surviving and needing chronic illness management	Shifts focus from biological need to quality of life and self-care
Availability of and access to medical information	Less trust in the 'paternal' system, rise in consumerism and higher patient expectations	Patients become 'experts' in their own care and treatment
Power balance toward the patient	Better educated patient has access to medical information	Patients become active participants in their care; need information and control over their own care

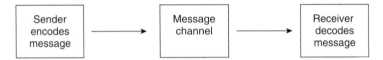

Figure 1.2 Linear model of communication

some opportunity for feedback' (1988: 4). This definition implies an interaction of some kind between at least two people. It also suggests that the interaction is two-way—that the person sending the message receives some sort of feedback, even if it is non-verbal, or even silence.

Basic models of communication have key factors in common. They usually represent a sender and a receiver of a message and some form of distortion of the message between the sender and receiver. These see communication as linear, which can be depicted in a simple flow chart (see Figure 1.2).

The sender needs to adapt the message in a way that can be received accurately and the receiver needs to share many aspects of the sender's context (cognitions, culture, language, and symbolism) in order to decode it correctly. For example, if a nurse tells a patient that the doctor is concerned about the patient's 'discharge' (meaning, in this case, their discharge home from hospital), the patient needs to understand the context of 'discharge' to know whether the nurse means that a physical bodily discharge is worrying the doctor or that the doctor is reluctant to send the patient home.

Linear models represent the single exchange of information quite well, but often struggle to represent the complexity of communication context and the interference, or 'noise', that is inherent in the communicating process. Circular models attempt this by representing the feedback to the sender and the adjustments that the sender can then make. An example is seen in Figure 1.3.

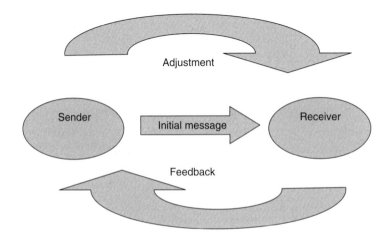

Figure 1.3 Circular model of communication

This type of model shows more than a two-way interaction. In this model, the sender is getting feedback on how the message has been received. In our example above, the patient hearing the doctor's concern about discharge asks the nurse where the discharge is coming from. The nurse then adjusts her message and explains that the doctor is worried that the patient might not cope well at home.

Still, the model does not include any explanation about what has caused the misunderstanding. This is often represented in models as 'noise', or interference. A systemic model would attempt to include this important element (see Figure 1.4).

A systemic model acknowledges that the messages to and from the sender are subject to interference, from the very way in which the message is encoded, through the environmental distortions, to the way in which the message is decoded. A simple example might be our nurse–patient scenario of misunderstanding the word 'discharge'. The nurse assumes that the patient is more aware of her condition than she is and will understand that there is no physical discharge present. The patient, however, has not taken much notice of explanations about her condition, but has been concerned about possible physical discharge after her operation; it has been on her mind, unspoken. Therefore, the patient immediately interprets the word 'discharge' to mean a physical process rather than her return home.

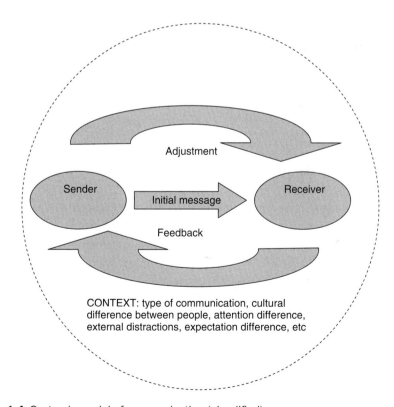

Figure 1.4 Systemic model of communication (simplified)

A more complex scenario might be where a nurse is giving information to worried relatives about the condition of a loved one. The relatives may be too worried to attend to the information objectively and may feel more anxious after hearing words that were meant to reassure, such as 'resuscitated successfully' and 'is in intensive care now'. This communication also relies on a quiet and undisturbed environment with no distractions for the family or the nurse. Also, the nurse needs interpersonal skills to understand that the family is likely to be distracted and worried, and requires simplified language and information in order to understand accurately what the nurse says. See the Practice example box 1.

Practice example box 1: Complex communication

A gentleman with moderate dementia was taken out on a trip to a steam railway. He got confused by the historical nature of the environment and refused to board the train without his wife (who had been dead some years). Rather than tell him bluntly that his wife was dead, the nurse chatted to him about events in his past, including attending a funeral with his daughter, an event he could often recall. The nurse asked him whose funeral it was and he said 'my wife's funeral'. The nurse had used a conversational approach to remind him that he was in the present and that his wife had died some time ago. To do this, the nurse needed time and space with the gentleman to construct a conversation, distract him from anxiously searching for his wife, and reorient him to the present.

The gentleman boarded the train and was appropriately sad at remembering his wife's funeral rather than distressed that she was being left behind.

Interpersonal skills

As we can see in the models and example, effective communication relies a great deal on the skills of the message sender and the ability of the receiver to interpret what is being communicated. These aspects of communication epitomize the interpersonal skills of a good communicator. The skilled communicator has information-presenting abilities and good listening skills. In addition, a skilled communicator is aware of and makes allowances for barriers to communication such as cultural differences, the emotional and cognitive states of others, and external distractions. Michael Argyle (1983) suggests that skilful interpersonal behaviour includes the following.

- *Perception of others' reactions:* The communicator is attuned to the other's behaviour and signs of understanding or misunderstanding.
- *Attention to feedback and corrective action:* The communicator has learnt what kind of response is needed according to the feedback from the other.

For instance, reticence from the other may prompt encouraging remarks or open questioning.

- *Timing of social responses:* This requires the communicator to know when to speak, when to listen, when to interrupt or prompt, or when to take the lead or be led.
- *Self-presentation:* A good communicator has self-awareness and is able to use this self-knowledge to present themselves to the other. This gives the other feedback about who the communicator is and therefore how to interpret and respond to them. For instance, sitting in a forward-leaning position assures the other that they are being listened to.
- *Rewardingness:* This is the ability to engage the other in the communication and know how to reward communication behaviour. For instance, using nods, smiles, and eye contact encourages someone to talk about themselves.
- *Taking the role of the other:* Here, the communicator can put themselves in the shoes of the other in order to understand how they are seen. For instance, if they realize that being dressed formally is offputting to a young teenager, they can respond by removing a tie or rolling up their sleeves.

Argyle breaks communication skills down into behavioural skills rather than skills of insight, understanding, and cognition. Another definition of good communication comes from Becker et al. (1987: 9), who suggest that a skilful communicator 'must be able to identify the emotions or intent expressed by the other person and make sophisticated judgements about the form and timing of the appropriate response'. In this definition, the skilled communicator uses accurate perception and good judgement to understand the interactions and know how to make appropriate adjustments. It may be that all of these factors are part of the skills of a good communicator—that skills are made up of a good sense of reality, awareness of self and others, accurate reading of situations, good timing, and ability to use the self to facilitate meaningful and positive communication. Many of these skills can be learnt and developed through practice and through personal development by improving self-awareness, and awareness and understanding of other people and their cognitive and emotional states.

Power

Phillips (1978) describes interpersonal skills as:

> The extent to which [a person] can communicate with others, in a manner that fulfils one's rights, requirements, satisfactions, or obligations to a reasonable degree without damaging the other person's similar rights, [. . .] in a free and open exchange.
>
> (Phillips 1978: 13)

By this, Phillips means that a good communicator is equitable; he or she does not need to sacrifice anything of himself or herself to be understood, or to manipulate or expect the other to make sacrifices to understand. This suggests that a good communication results in both parties being satisfied with the communication and neither being left feeling ignored, forgotten, or otherwise ill used. Therefore, Phillips's version of good communication may exclude communication with a goal to manipulate, such as that used by a salesman or perhaps a politician!

This brings us on to an important aspect of communication in health care: the power differential between a practitioner and a patient. Earlier, we looked at the changing nature of health care and used Bensing's dimensions of patient-centredness to identify the type of relationship between a practitioner and a patient. The history of medicine and medical practice shows how the practitioner–patient relationship was one of unequal power: the doctor was the expert, while the patient was merely a recipient of his authority and learning. This describes a type of 'paternalistic' relationship of father and child. The culture of medicine and healthcare practitioner–patient relations has, arguably, retained much of this paternal structure in that the power imbalance is often still very much in favour of the practitioner, be they a doctor, nurse, or other health professional. Ellis et al. (2003) suggest that power-distorted communication is common in health care and is embedded in the language, procedures, and organizational practice that ensures domination by care professionals. Thompson (1986) suggests that health professionals feel better able to obtain compliance and cooperation from patients if they are in control and, when the focus of treatment is to fight the illness, the patient becomes less important in a formalized medical encounter. In such a culture, people who become patients often adopt an inferior position to the healthcare professionals and become passive recipients of care and treatment. Szasz and Hollender (1987) looked at doctor–patient relationship patterns of relating and identified three styles, outlined in Table 1.2. These can apply as much to nurses in modern health care, especially where nurses take a clinical lead in many aspects of care.

The changing nature of health care demands more patient empowerment in self-care and acknowledgement that the patient is often the best person to understand the context of his or her own healthcare management. This suggests that many nurse–patient

Table 1.2 Styles of doctor–patient relationship

Relationship style	Description	Characteristics
Activity/passivity	Full exploitation of medical power and authority	Cross-examination: doctor asks questions; patient gives answers
Guidance/cooperation	Doctor allows patient some autonomy and participation	Doctor's agenda dominates. Patient allowed some involvement within doctor's remit
Mutual participation	Both parties accept responsibility to problem-solve	Patient encouraged to use doctor's expertise to solve his or her health problems

Source: Szasz and Hollender (1987).

interactions are best served by a mutual participation style of relating, if effective long-term health and well-being is the objective of the healthcare professional.

It is important that nurses acknowledge power differentials inherent in patient–practitioner relationships and make those contextual and personal adjustments outlined in Figure 1.4 to facilitate communication. Burnard (1997) recognizes other important power differentials between people that are also relevant to healthcare encounters and which may be superimposed on the already existing differentials of healthcare provision itself, such as between people of different sex and gender, ethnicity, culture, ability and disability, and social class. Also, for many cultures, age difference can be a source of power differential.

Nurses are expected to work in anti-oppressive and anti-discriminatory ways in accordance with NMC requirements to respect diversity and challenge inequality, discrimination, and exclusion from access to care (NMC, 2010). Colin Goble (2009) suggests that the nursing profession has been slower than professions such as social work to pick up on this professional requirement, perhaps because the shift from institutional to person-centred community-based care is relatively recent in nursing. However, for Goble, improved empowering care requires nurses to develop such practice through individual and collective reflection in order to ensure equal access to, and delivery of, quality care.

Application of communication in nursing

Methods of communication

The model in Figure 1.2 suggests that the message from one person to another is encoded in some form and transmitted to the other. This encoding can form many types of format of transmission, or several types combined. For example, a person who does not want to engage in a conversation formats the information to the other by giving short answers or mumbling (vocal channels), reduced eye contact, and folding their arms (body language). They might also try to change the conversation, look at their watch (behaviour), or simply bluntly state they do not want to talk (verbal). Additionally, they could write this down or use other, and more sophisticated, tools for communication, such as sign language, flash cards, or even text messaging! DeVito (1988) states that communication is inevitable: no matter what we do, even silence or not responding says something to the other person. All behaviour, whether verbal or non-verbal, intentional or unintentional, is a form of communication, including how we move, dress, walk, or use touch. As communicators, nurses need to be aware of their own intentional and unintentional messages and also be skilled in reading the messages of others.

Practice example box 2: A reluctant patient

'A shy teenage boy presenting with depression was proving to be difficult to engage in any conversation during a school visit. He had his arms and legs crossed, avoided eye contact, and only gave me 'yes', 'no' and 'don't know' answers. I found I was virtually talking to the wall.

'We sat in an office-cum-storage room for privacy, and the room contained stacked stage and MC equipment. He frequently looked away from me at the equipment, and I read this as reluctance and discomfort in talking to me about his feelings. After some silence, I changed my focus and asked him conversationally: 'What *is* all this stuff?'

'He said something like: 'It's MC stuff for school discos and so on.' He suddenly sounded confident and on surer ground, so I asked him to explain what it all was. At this, he became quite animated and it appeared that he had an ambition to do MC-ing as a hobby or career, but never got the chance with the equipment. The conversation turned back to him and his frustrations. A stroke of luck that we happened to sit in that room, but no accident that I read his communication and attempted a different tack. I call this *'going fishing'* when I'm with a reluctant interviewee—trying other avenues of conversation and topic to get the words flowing.'

(Mental health practitioner)

See the Practice example box 2 regarding a reluctant patient. This shows the unintentional communication of the boy and how it was picked up by the nurse. Notice that the nurse does not know the change of talk will work, but that attempting to 'go through the door' that he was opening made a breakthrough.

DeVito points out that communication is inevitable. When we send a message that is picked up by someone, it stays sent. We cannot unsay or negate the message, although we might need to modify its effect. Consider a heated argument as an example. We've all been there and said something that we later wish we hadn't. We might then try to reduce the damage by apologizing, or attempt to qualify and explain what we meant. What we are doing, in fact, is trying to change the message received. For nurses in a professional role, we need to maintain a professional standard of behaviour in our communications with patients, relatives, and colleagues in order to maintain effective working relationships.

 Chapter 4 looks at channels of interpersonal communication in more detail.

The nurse–patient relationship

The relationship between the nurse and the patient is often seen as a therapeutic relationship in itself that is based on partnership, intimacy, and reciprocity (McMahon, 2002).

Its purpose is different from a social relationship in that it has a focus on the patient's well-being as a priority, and the nurse and patient do not need to have anything in common or even like each other (Arnold and Boggs, 2006). This relationship can last only five minutes in an accident and emergency department or primary care practice, or can continue and develop for months or years during chronic illness management. It can be intensely personal when breaking bad news, or quite superficial such as when directing a patient to the appropriate clinic room. However, all of these scenarios are nurse–patient encounters that impart to the patient something of the support and meaningfulness of their engagement with health care. They tell the patient whether they are viewed as important and valued, and whether they will be listened to or discriminated against.

 Chapter 2 examines the nurse–patient relationship in depth.

The nurse as a member of the multidisciplinary team

Nurses do not work with their patients in isolation. Nurses are members of multidisciplinary teams that should be coordinating their roles and expertise to provide the best care for patients. The NMC stipulates a level of competence in working effectively across professional and agency boundaries in its standards for pre-registration education (NMC, 2010). To qualify as a nurse, therefore, students should be able to contribute to teamworking by understanding their own role in the team, respecting the role of others, and managing the resources available within the team for the benefit of their patients. Working with others from different professional backgrounds and often with different priorities can be challenging, but it is often the nurse who takes the lead in coordinating health-based care by using good communication and management skills to provide a holistic care package for the patient. Nurses working with children will need to understand their specific role in safeguarding children, and nurses working with patients and families with social and psychological needs will also need good skills to work collaboratively with other care professionals to deliver integrated patient care.

Health and social care teams offer particular challenges for a range of historical organizational reasons. Thompson (1986) suggested that, traditionally, healthcare teams have often been little more than a series of individuals with responsibilities for different 'parts' of the patient's care and treatment, and that each individual in the team is inclined to act in their own sphere of expertise, with little consultation or information-sharing with others. The transformation of healthcare delivery from institutions to community-based care, the ethos of holistic care for the whole patient and improved technology, for McCray (2009), has changed the focus toward multi-professional practice.

Goble (2009) suggests several existing challenges to multi-professional working:

- power relationships between different professions;
- competing roles between organizations;
- differences in traditions and cultures between service agencies and professions;
- defending professional identity.

Goble suggests that different professions have different priorities for care to fulfil their roles and different traditional ways of exercising power. For instance, psychiatrists may focus on a patient's symptom control, while mental health nurses may focus on the patient's quality of life; social services may prioritize an unwell schizophrenic person's rights to liberty, while the medical profession will be mindful of the need to protect the public. Additionally, Goble suggests that different professions can feel threatened by a loss of clear role and adopting a 'siege' mentality.

Thompson (1986) suggested barriers of traditional professional practices and identities over twenty years ago that may still stand in the way of integrated and coordinated multidisciplinary teamworking. Outlined below, they appear scarily similar to those of Goble in 2009.

Traditional professional practices

Different professions have different traditions and cultures of communication. Doctors, for instance, may prioritize and record physical information in medical notes, often using formalized language, symbols, and abbreviations that have highly medical meanings, not understood by other professions. Nurses, too, can exclude other professions from information through the nurse-only tradition of handovers between shifts.

Professional identities

Different professions may feel threatened by other professions bringing new methods or expertise in promoting patient care. Protective practices of professional identity may include information withholding, disengagement from the care role, or even a 'battle' for supremacy to be the key care coordinator, none of which will benefit the patient.

The dynamics of teams can often be complex and can take on a destructive and obstructive identity. The structure and processes of groups will be examined in Chapter 5 of this book, which will also illustrate how the communication and interpersonal skills of the individuals involved are essential in identifying and avoiding the types of destructive behaviour that limits the effectiveness of a team approach to patient-centred care.

Conclusion

This chapter presents an argument that communication between the nurse and the patient is therapeutic in itself. Additionally, good communication aids the process of healing and care, while poor communication can be a barrier to good care. The relationship between any health practitioner and the patient has changed over the years, as our understanding of health and the factors that impact on health have changed. No longer is health delivered in a patriarchal 'doctor knows best' approach, but the patient is considered to be an expert in their own health needs. This has led to an approach to care and treatment that is a partnership between practitioner and patient, which changes the approach to communication and interpersonal relating greatly between the nurse and his or her patient.

A note on the structure of the book and terminology

This book is intended for nurses in education and training and newly qualified nurses. The chapters in this book are organized so that they take the student through the process of understanding the theory of interpersonal communication in Part 1, appreciating how this theory is applied to practice in Part 2, and subsequently developing skills in practice in Part 3. At the beginning of each part, you will find a short overview outlining the scope and breadth of content in that section.

Chapters are written to apply to all fields of care and strive to address the needs of all or any nurse in a range of settings. Some practice examples given in the chapters may appear to be specific to one particular field of care: for example, a case study in A&E, or working with children. However, each scenario can be applied across a range of practice areas and the communication skills being addressed are applicable to all fields of care. Therefore, each chapter has something to offer nurse students pursuing any particular care area.

It is recognized that different fields of nursing care may use different terminology for patients, carers, service users, and so on. We have chosen to refer to recipients of direct care as 'patients' and family members or informal carers are referred to as 'carers'. We have also used the term 'young people' to differentiate younger children from adolescents, as the needs of these two age groups can often be very different according to their psychological and social developmental stages.

Also, we have attempted to make clear that references to patients, family members, and nurses in general that are not gender-specific by referring to these groups as 'he or she', or 'they'. However, some authors may refer to a nurse as gendered because the author is identifying with the nurse.

 To find more resources to aid your learning, please now go online to **www.oxfordtextbooks.co.uk/orc/webb** See the video 'Why is communication important in nursing.'

Further reading

Burnard, P. and Gill, P. (2008) *Culture, Communication and Nursing*. Harlow: Pearson Education.

McCray, J. (2009) *Nursing and Multi-professional Practice*. London: Sage.

References

Arnold, E. and Boggs, K. (2006) *Interpersonal Relationships: Professional Communication Skills for Nurses.* London: Elsevier.

Bateson, G. (1979) *Mind and Nature.* New York: Dutton.

Becker, R., Heimberg, R., and Bellack, A. (1987) *Social Skills Training for Treatment of Depression.* New York: Pergamon Press.

Bensing, J. (1991) *Doctor–Patient Communication and the Quality of Care: An Observation Study into Affective and Instrumental Behaviour in General Practice.* Utrecht: Nivel/Utrecht University.

—— (2000) 'Bridging the Gap: The Separate Worlds of Evidence-based Medicine and Patient-centred Medicine', *Patient Education and Counseling,* 39: 17–25.

Burnard, P. (1997) *Effective Communication Skills for Health Professionals* (2nd edn). Cheltenham: Stanley Thornes.

Crow, R., Gage, H., Hampson, S., Hart, J., Kimber, A., and Thomas, H. (1999) 'The Role of Expectancies in the Placebo Effect and Their Use in Delivery of Health Care: A Systematic Review', *Health Technology Assessment,* 3(3): 1–96.

DeVito, J. (1988) *Human Communication: The Basic Course.* New York: Harper & Row.

Department of Health (1992) *The Patients Charter.* London: DoH.

—— (2000) *The NHS Plan.* London: DoH.

—— (2001a) *The Expert Patient: A New Approach to Chronic Disease Management in the 21st Century.* London: DoH.

—— (2001b) *Valuing People: A New Strategy for Learning Disability for the 21st Century.* London: DoH.

—— (2003) *Essence of Care: Patient-focused Benchmarks for Health Care Practitioners.* London: DoH.

—— (2006a) *Our Health, Our Care, Our Say.* London: DoH.

—— (2006b) *The Care Service Improvement Partnership: Integrated Care Network— Strengthening Service User and Carer Involvement: A Guide for Partnerships.* Discussion Paper, London: DoH.

Ellis, R., Gates, B., and Kenworthy, N. (2003) *Interpersonal Communication in Nursing: Theory and Practice.* Edinburgh: Churchill Livingstone.

Goble, C. (2009) 'Multi-professional Working in the Community', in J. McCray (ed.) *Nursing and Multi-professional Practice.* London: Sage.

Kamarck, T., Peterman, A., and Raynor, D. (1998) 'The Effects of Social Environment on Stress-related Cardiovascular Activation: Current Findings, Prospects and Implications', *Annals of Behavioural Medicine,* 20: 247–56.

Kwekkeboom, K. (1997) 'The Placebo Effect in Symptom Management', *Oncological Nursing Forum,* 24(8): 1393–9.

Letvak, R. (1995) 'Putting the Placebo Effect into Practice', *Patient Care,* 29: 93–102.

McCray, J. (2009) 'Preparing for Multi-professional Practice', in J. McCray (ed.) *Nursing and Multi-professional Practice.* London: Sage.

McMahon, R. (2002) 'Therapeutic Nursing: Theory Issues and Practice', in R. McMahon and A. Pearson (eds) *Nursing as Therapy.* Cheltenham: Nelson Thornes.

Ogden, J. (2004) *Health Psychology: A Textbook*. Buckingham: Open University Press.

Phillips, E. (1978) *The Social Skills Basis of Psychopathology*. New York: Grune and Stratton.

Szasz, T. and Hollender, M. (1987) 'A Contribution to the Philosophy of Medicine: The Basic Models of the Doctor–Patient Relationship', in J. D. Stoeckle (ed.) *Encounters between Patients and Doctors: An Anthology*. Cambridge, MA: MIT Press.

Thompson, T. (1986) *Communication for Health Professionals*. New York: Harper & Row.

The nurse–patient relationship

Eula Miller and Gayatri Nambiar-Greenwood

This chapter will help you to achieve competencies in:

- ➔ engaging with people and building caring professional relationships;
- ➔ recognizing barriers in developing effective relationships with patients;
- ➔ initiating and maintaining close professional relationships with patients and carers;
- ➔ developing self-awareness and challenging your own prejudices.

Introduction

The nurse–patient relationship is central to meeting the patient's care needs and therefore communication between the nurse and patient is the foundation on which this relationship is built (Crawford et al., 1998; McCabe and Timmins, 2007). According to Williams and Jones (2006), patients value the uncomplicated style of interaction, continuity of care, and nurse–patient time, all of which are afforded by the nurse–patient relationship.

The Department of Health recommends that healthcare professionals should value, respect, and listen to service users as individuals (DoH, 2004). For the purposes of this chapter, the nurse–patient relationship is defined as a series of planned interactions that puts the patient's need at the core. These interventions focus on the feelings, priorities, challenges, and ideas of the patient, with the progressive aim of enhancing optimum physical, spiritual, and mental health. The nurse–patient relationship is, therefore, based on patient-centred nursing, which is only possible when there is solid and reliable communication between nurse and patient.

However, there are inherent inequalities in the nurse–patient relationship (Millard et al., 2006). Unlike social relationships, patients have little choice about the health professionals who will care for them. This powerlessness renders the patient vulnerable, reliant, and dependent on practitioners to intervene effectively in their care (Rowe, 1999). The nurse then has a responsibility to interact, educate, and share information, genuinely putting the patient's best interest at the centre of the delivery of care (NMC, 2008). The development and management of an effective nurse–patient relationship is therefore a key skill in nursing, in any field of care.

The foundation of therapeutic relationships

Self-awareness

We feel that the first step to being able to facilitate effective communication is self-awareness: an individual cannot understand others until they come to know themselves. This concept has been documented in nursing literature for a number of decades (Boud et al., 1985; Burnard 1992; Freshwater 2002; Jack and Smith, 2007). Self-awareness allows us to relate to the experience of others, while developing the important and essential skill of empathy. It commences from early childhood when we are first able to recognize ourselves in a mirror (around 18 months to 2 years old), and continues throughout our life.

Rungapadiachy (1999) suggests that a nurse requires the ability to think, feel, and act appropriately in order to develop skills of self-awareness. So, for example, if a nurse has not come to terms with a personal bereavement, he or she may cope less effectively with the needs of a dying patient because of the fears and discomforts that the episode can generate.

There are a number of useful tools that promote self-awareness, such as the Johari window (Figure 2.1).

The Johari window is a well-known model of the self that can be used as a tool for mapping development of self-awareness. It is named after its constructors, Joe Luft and Harry Ingham (Kagan and Evans, 1995). The model challenges us to reflect on and explore aspects of ourselves that we may rarely consider normally. To explore and expand our knowledge of each window, we can set ourselves tasks of self-reflection or obtaining feedback from others.

The open area is what we present to others and is observed by others. This can be dominated by 'false fronts', or 'masks', we present to the world and perhaps ourselves, or aspects of ourselves that we are comfortable to share with others—perhaps our confidence or shyness. The hidden area contains those aspects we know about but don't want to share—perhaps anger or jealousy. The blind area is those aspects that others detect about us but of which we are unaware. This area is often best explored

	Known to self	Not known to self
Known to others	Open area	Blind area
Not known others	Hidden area	Unknown area

Figure 2.1 The Johari window (Luft, 1969)

through feedback from other people. The unknown area is that which is hidden even from ourselves, and too painful to confront or bring to consciousness. Personal development in self-awareness will make the open and hidden windows bigger and the blind and unknown windows smaller.

⊕ Learning point 1

Think of at least five aspects of your self (what makes you *you*) that apply to the open and hidden areas. You could put a copy of this in your portfolio and add to it throughout your course of study. As you gain different experiences in practice settings, you will be able to demonstrate self-awareness development by entering what you discover about yourself as a nurse in the blind and unknown areas. You can even record in your portfolio how you discovered these things about yourself.

A more recent adaptation of this self-awareness tool, specifically developed for nurses, has been documented by Jack and Miller (2008). These authors refer to this as the self-development awareness tool (Practice example box 1). The tool is divided into three stages of interpersonal acquisition, which are the 'now' stage, followed by the 'transitional' stage, and finally the 're-group' stage. The model shows the intricacies and the cue questions set at each stage that potentially facilitate the nurse's journey to becoming more self-aware.

Practice example box 1: The self-development awareness tool (Jack and Miller 2008)

The *now* stage

- Who am I at this moment? (Take into account thoughts, feelings, and behaviour.)

- What do I know about myself and what do I show to others? (Past experiences may dictate how we behave. Contextual influences, such as the behaviour of others in the practice setting, may have an influence on this.)

- What is it I would like to be more aware of? (This can be difficult, but try to imagine how others see you. They may be aware of certain behaviours that you had not even thought about.)

- What has triggered this desire to change? (Consider what is it you feel uncomfortable about, or what it is you would like to develop. It may be that certain assumptions you have are holding you back. Your motivation may be a personal desire to be more assertive with others, for example.)

The *transition* stage

- What strengths/limitations do I have already? (This will require a certain amount of honesty.)
- What do I need to develop? (You may need to seek support from others. This is a proactive process as you actively engage in and develop new learning to inform practice.)
- What are the opportunities and threats to my development? (You may need to discard prior experiences if they are causing conflict and build on more positive experiences of which you have been part.)

The *regroup* stage (acceptance of self at this stage)

- Where am I now? (What new knowledge have I gained about myself and the situation?)
- What has changed about me and the way I am in this situation? (Do I now think, feel, and engage in a different way in these situations?)
- How do we grow?/Where do we go from here? (How can we develop this new learning and way of being?)

The experience of this journey should affect our delivery of practice, as we are able to recognize our strengths and limitations and appreciate own acts and omissions in the care of those who require our help.

Empathy

Burnard (2005: 103) suggests that empathy is 'the ability to enter the perceptual world of the other person'. It is easy for the new student nurse to confuse sympathy with empathy, but the difference is fundamental. Sympathy is relating to another as though they were us and we were experiencing their situation. Empathy can be differentiated as being able to relate to another directly and understand how *they* experience their situation.

> Sympathy: the ability to put ourselves in someone else's shoes
>
> Nurse: 'If that were me, I'd be very upset.'
>
> Empathy: the ability to be in someone else's shoes
>
> Nurse: 'I can sense you were very upset.'

Empathy in practice also needs to be demonstrated to the other person to convey support, understanding, and being able to share the other's experience. This is done by communication. See Box 2.1 for a definition from a trained hostage negotiator!

Box 2.1 The hostage negotiator's definition of empathy

A trained hostage negotiator claims that the key communication skill essential for gaining trust and engagement in the negotiation process is empathy. A good negotiator may be there for the hostages, but needs to understand the position of the hostage takers. So, a good negotiator has sympathy for the hostages, but empathy for the hostage-takers.

(BBC Radio 4, 2010).

Trust

A nurse–patient relationship needs to be based on trust. The patient needs to feel able to disclose personal and possibly painful information about themselves and ask questions that may take courage to say. If a patient cannot ask a nurse a question that begins with 'I know this is going to sound silly, but ...', who can they ask?

For this reason, the NMC's *The Code: Standards of Conduct, Performance and Ethics for Nurses and Midwives* (2008) insists that nurses demonstrate respect for patients, and ensure and protect the dignity and confidentiality of patients. A registered nurse must at all times uphold the public trust in the nursing profession.

Practice example box 2: Confidentiality

An off-duty registered nurse on a train overheard three young women, obviously student nurses, discussing a patient from their recent practice experience. They commented on his appearance, behaviour, and his family, in derogatory terms. They named the ward he was on and discussed how they would try to avoid him in future. This conversation could be overheard by all passengers in the vicinity. The registered nurse reminded the students of the Code of Conduct (as it was called then) and pointed out that the general public would not be happy to be nursed by people who would discuss them in such a way.

....

⊕ Learning point 2

Consider what essential qualities you would expect in someone nursing you or a loved one. Do you measure up to those expectations? What skills and personal qualities do you need to develop to become such a nurse? What qualities do you have already? Are they already recorded in your Johari window?

Your portfolio Johari window will now become historical: what you put in to your blind and unknown areas will be those things you didn't know about yourself, but have since discovered during your nursing practice. The Johari window in your portfolio will act as evidence of your personal and professional development in self-awareness and communication skills.

Non-judgemental relating

The NMC (2009a) demands that nurses offer fair and equal care to patients from diverse backgrounds and circumstances. While we are not expected to be saints or to have no values or opinions of our own, when we are acting as a person's nurse, in whatever circumstances, we can put those to one side in order to offer the best care we can. We do not have to agree with the values, opinions, or behaviour of our patients outside the health context. We do, however, have to be able to accept the person for who they are regardless of differences in morals or beliefs.

As a nurse, we could be caring for a patient transferred from prison with a history of some heinous crime, but such patients still have heart attacks, strokes, or get depressed. Equally, we might want to 'go the extra mile' for someone we particularly like, but need to be mindful of what is appropriate. The nurse–patient relationship is a professional one that respects the patient in his or her health context regardless of our personal views.

Genuineness and authenticity

It would be difficult to develop trust in our patients if, privately, we weren't trustworthy or interested in their welfare. Also, it is sometimes difficult to empathize with a person's situation when their behaviour or attitude is very different from our own. **Genuineness** refers to being the person we present to the patient: being kind because we are kind; being interested because we are interested. This is acting with **authenticity**. Genuineness is proposed by Rogers (1967) to be a core principle in a counselling relationship, but arguably this can be challenging to the nurse–patient relationship. A counsellor has more opportunity to accept their client's way of life, but a nurse is charged with improving a patient's way of life towards health. However, it could be argued that the more a nurse is able to act with authenticity in his or her professional relationships, while being able to empathize, be trustworthy, and be non-judgemental, the higher quality of care such a nurse is likely to achieve. Genuineness is perhaps the quality in nursing that defines the perfect personality for nursing. The rest of us just have to work at our professional development!

The nurse–patient relationship must commence, develop, and terminate with the patient being confident that their nurse understands their situation, respects them as an individual, and does not judge them, but can invest their time and interest in their well-being.

Boundaries

The NMC describes boundaries as defining 'the limits of behaviour which allow a nurse or midwife to have a professional relationship with the person in their care' (2008: 1). We can regard the nurse–patient relationship as a process that has goals. It aims to be therapeutic (good for the patient) and facilitative (enable nursing care). We could add **humanistic** in that it also aims to be positive and **beneficent** to all concerned, and non-harmful (**nonmaleficent**) to either the patient or the nurse. It is important to recognize here that the nurse is not expected to be wholly self-sacrificial in his or her relationships with patients. There is no room, for example, for nurses to be abused or exploited by patients outside the context of the illness. Nurses are not expected to suffer physical or verbal injury in their role, although patients can and often do express their hurt and anger to their nurses.

However, as noted in Chapter 1, the nurse–patient relationship involves a power differential in favour of the nurse. For the NMC, nurses carry the responsibility maintaining appropriate boundaries to the relationship with their patient and conducting personal relationships with vulnerable patients is never acceptable.

Box 2.2 Student boundaries

It's really important that you establish clear patient care boundaries and don't overstep them. If a student is looking after a patient, it's possible that sexual interest could arise from either party. They may get on really well together and the next thing you know, one is asking the other out. But limits must be drawn here. You are not in a normal social environment and when a person is vulnerable, their decision making may not be entirely valid. It's also safer for students too—otherwise they may unwittingly put themselves in a position from which it's hard to extract themselves!

(NMC, 2009c)

The practitioner example in Practice example box 3 was used by the UKCC (now the Nursing and Midwifery Council) to illustrate financial abuse. These principles still stand today.

Practice example box 3: UKCC example of a breach of boundaries

Chloe nursed Miss G in her own home. Miss G was paralysed following a bout of meningitis two years ago. Although she required total physical care, she could write her name. During the six months in which Chloe had cared for her, Miss G had loaned her a total of £200. Chloe had told Miss G that she could not cope on her salary as an agency staff nurse.

(UKCC, 1999: 6)

Learning point 3

Look at Practice example box 3. What professional issues do you think this example raises? Answers from the UKCC are outlined below.

Suggested answers to Learning point 3

The UKCC (1999) outlined the following professional issues raised by the example:

- the vulnerability and dependency of Miss G;
- the imbalance of power in the relationship;
- Miss G's fear of the withdrawal of care if she does not agree to lend the nurse, Chloe, money;
- intimidation and exploitation of the client, even if it is unintentional;
- the distortion of the boundaries to the professional practitioner–client relationship;
- moving the focus of care away from meeting the client's needs towards meeting the practitioner's own needs;
- financial abuse includes the inappropriate use of a client's funds, property, or resources, and this includes borrowing money from a client.

The UKCC's practice example illustrates how the blurring of the professional and personal boundaries can result in abuse of the patient. The professional relationship often necessarily involves intimacy between the nurse and the patient, but this involves personal and intimate information from the patient to the nurse, not the other way around. There is some place for sharing personal information—in order to convey empathy and understanding, for example. The nurse is required to know what is appropriate and can be guided by ensuring that their care relationship is based on public trust in the profession: 'Because of the special privilege and responsibility that nursing and midwifery students have in terms of being in contact with members of the public, they must ensure they justify the trust that the public places in them' (NMC 2009c).

 Learning point 4

Cover up the two right-hand columns in the list of behaviours (Table 2.2) and decide whether the behaviour would be acceptable in ANY nurse–patient relationship. Remember, this could apply to short- or long-term relationships with surgical, medical adult patients, children and their families, or adults/children with learning difficulties or mental illness. See if you agree with the advice given.

Table 2.1 Nursing boundaries

Behaviour	Answer	Rationale
Beginning a personal relationship with an ex-patient immediately after treatment/discharge	No	Not *immediately* after a relationship and certainly not if the person is in any way still in a dependent and vulnerable state. Also, the nurse's knowledge of the person has been gained from a privileged position.
Visiting a person's home unannounced and without an appointment	No	Unless in an emergency in which there are serious concerns about safety of patient or others in their care.
Seeing a person in your care outside your normal practice hours	No	There should be no need to work outside normal practice hours. If the patient needs this, he/she should be referred to the appropriate service.
Lending a patient money	No	Under no circumstances
Borrowing money from a patient	No	Under no circumstances
Commencing a sexual relationship with a patient's relative	No	The relative is also in a vulnerable position and the relationship will affect the nurse–patient relationship
Buying a car from a patient	No	This blurs the boundaries between professional and social/business relationship.
Telling 'dirty' jokes	No	There is a danger of this being interpreted as sexual harassment or flirtatious behaviour from the nurse, and is, by definition, overfamiliarity.
Discussing sexual matters not relevant to care or treatment	No	As above. This might apply to health promotion or aiding personal development, but this should have solely a care aim and be part of the care plan.
Allowing a patient to hit you repeatedly because they are frustrated/angry	No	Some might regard this as 'cathartic' in allowing the patient to express their feelings. However, it conveys that hitting the carer is appropriate. This might be 'tolerated' on occasion, but never 'allowed' or encouraged.
Referring a patient to a colleague because patient makes persistent sexual references about you	Yes	If the therapeutic relationship is in danger of breaking down because of a patient's behaviour or misunderstanding, it is appropriate to recognize your limitations and facilitate a safer professional relationship.

If you are unsure of any of the answers in Table 2.2, make it an action point for your next practice placement and discuss a range of scenarios with your mentor.

You will need to explore the scenarios in Table 2.1, and others that you experience in practice, with a qualified nurse mentor. There are very few exceptions to these general guidelines, but the skill of the qualified nurse is deciding how he or she can justify these exceptions in the context of a patient's care.

The NMC guidelines *Clear Sexual Boundaries* (2009b) (see Box 2.3) lists the safeguards that a nurse should employ in order to protect themselves from overstepping the professional/personal boundaries.

> ### Box 2.3 NMC guidelines, clear sexual boundaries (NMC, 2009*b*: 3)
>
> - Keep to relevant personal detail in history-taking.
> - Provide adequate information and explanation that helps to avoid misunderstandings and misinterpretation.
> - Honour confidentiality.
> - Maintain proper appointment systems.
> - Provide suitable facilities with screens for undressing.
> - Offer the choice for the presence of a trained chaperone during intimate examinations or treatment.
> - Be aware of what is culturally acceptable to individuals, especially those of a different race or religion.
> - Never use sexually demeaning words or actions or dirty jokes.
> - Refrain from undue familiarity.
> - Be cautious of the context and intent if accepting a gift from a person in your care (there may be trust policies on this).
> - Be aware that people may be vulnerable at times of crisis in their personal life.
> - Get help early for personal crises. (This refers to the nurse.)
> - Do not involve the people in your care, or members of their immediate family, or any other person involved with their care in your personal problems.
> - Consult with colleagues about difficult situations.

Remember, the nurse–patient relationship necessarily incorporates a power imbalance, rendering the patient vulnerable and dependent on their nurse. It is the responsibility of the nurse to maintain the professional division between patient and nurse, and resist attempts from the patient to blur these boundaries. In so doing, the nurse can optimize the delivery of effective care.

 There is more on therapeutic relationships in Chapter 4, 'Active listening and attending'.

The nurse–patient relationship process

The nurse–patient relationship can be described as a good story: it has a beginning, a middle, and an end. Even if a very short or long relationship, the basic pattern should be the same. We make contact with patients for the first time and commence the

Table 2.2 The four phases of the nurse–patient relationship

Phase	For the patient	For the nurse
1. Orientation	Seeks professional assistance	Patient's needs are unknown. Establish a rapport and assist patient in developing a working relationship.
2. Identification	Patient uses nurse to find out what the problems are	Encourage person to identify health problems and express feelings about these.
3. Exploitation	Patient makes use of nurse to problem-solve	Develop patient's competencies, facilitate recovery and development. Act as a healthcare resource and facilitate external resources.
4. Resolution	Person becomes freed of need for help from nurse	Goal-set for person's future. Facilitate independence and self-care. Withdraw when no longer needed.

Source: Peplau (1997).

relationship-building process, then we use the relationship in order to deliver care, and finally, we complete the relationship by ensuring that the patient is no longer dependent on us and is ready to 'move on'. This process is described variously in nursing and other therapeutic health professions, but frequently in the similar terms of a staged process. Below, we will look at two of these.

Peplau's developmental model: a nursing model of the nurse–patient relationship

Peplau (1997) suggested that the nurse–patient relationship can be divided into four phases, and that the nurse may have a range of roles to play within the relationship (see Table 2.2).

For Peplau, the nurse acts as a stranger (orientation phase), then a resource, leader, surrogate, and counsellor (other three phases). Peplau's model can be seen as patient-centred and the nurse takes on a facilitative role rather than sets the agenda. Perhaps unlike Roper's model (Holland et al., 2008), in which the patient's needs are determined by a pre-set list of factors (the ADLs), Peplau's model depends on the nurse and patient identifying the patient's needs together. Arguably, Peplau's model is therefore more patient-centred.

Burnard's eight-stage counselling map

Burnard (2005) suggests a similar process suitable for counselling but also reflects the patient-centred approach (see Table 2.3).

Burnard's stages consider the counselling aspect of the practitioner–client relationship, but can be seen to apply to the nurse's role as a 'counsellor' and as a hands-on carer. Whether the patient is depressed, has developed a chronic health problem such as diabetes or schizophrenia, or is having straightforward elective surgery, the nurse helps the patient in explore their health beliefs, attitudes, knowledge, or behaviour. In doing

Table 2.3 Summary of Burnard's eight-stage counselling map

Stage	Counselling goals	Possible nursing practice
1	Meeting and establishing 'boundaries'	Introduction and initial assessment; relationship commencement
2	Discussing surface issues, testing safety, engagement	Getting to know each other, discussing routine health issues and surface health context of personal issues
3	Deeper issues: disclosures on deeper levels and using trust	Exploring person's healthcare concerns, identifying holistic needs and gaps in self-care
4	Ownership of feelings—cathartic	Encouraging person to address his/her relationship with health issues, i.e. heart disease fears or medication side effects
5	Developing client's insight and problem identification	Seeking and encouraging person's response to health information and self-statements of hopes, fears, ideas for coping and barriers to health, i.e. 'I'm too stressed all the time, I shouldn't work so hard'
6	Exploration of problems and possible solutions	Discussion of identified problems, and encouraging person to find and 'own' solutions, i.e. 'I shall have to cut down my hours while I recover'
7	Client action and practitioner support	Giving attention and support to person's new health behaviour—motivating, educating, facilitating resources
8	Disengagement and management of 'letting go' anxieties	Empowering person to continue without you, find more appropriate support, considering future without nurse–patient relationship

Source: Burnard (2005: 119–26).

this, the nurse's role is using the nurse–patient relationship to enhance the patient's relationship with their health problem.

Conclusion

This chapter has focused on defining the nurse–patient relationship, rather than techniques to establish and manage an effective relationship. It has addressed some of the issues of managing boundaries, but mainly with the aim of helping to define a good relationship and what may constitute a breakdown in the professional therapeutic space between the patient and the nurse. Management of a good nurse–patient relationship relies on some key personal and professional skills. These skills are largely good self-awareness of our own motivations, values, and characteristics, together with personal qualities such as approachability and trustworthiness. These factors are underpinned by good skills in leading the relationship and understanding its objectives.

The nurse–patient relationship underpins all of our encounters with patients and other service users. Without a sound understanding of and ability to engage in a nurse–patient relationship, we cannot deliver patient-centred effective care.

 To find more resources to aid your learning, please now go online to **www.oxfordtextbooks.co.uk/orc/webb** See the video 'Active listening 2' for a demonstration of listening skills and body lanuguage.

References

BBC Radio 4 (2010) Podcast: *Thank You for My Freedom*. Broadcast, 28 April.

Boud, D., Keogh, R., and Walker, O. (1985) *Reflection: Turning Experience into Learning*. London: Kogan Page.

Burnard, P. (1992) *Know Yourself: Self Awareness Activities for Nurses*. London: Scutari.

—— (2005) *Counselling Skills for Health Professionals* (4th edn). Cheltenham: Nelson-Thornes.

Crawford, P., Brown, B., and Nolan, P. (1998) *Communicating Care*. Cheltenham: Stanley Thornes.

Department of Health (2004) *The NHS Improvement Plan: Putting People at the Heart of Public Services*. London: DoH.

Freshwater, D. (ed.) (2002) *Therapeutic Nursing*. London: Sage.

Holland, K., Jenkins, J., Solomon, J., and Whittam, S. (2008) *Applying the Roper, Logan and Tierney Model in Practice* (2nd edn). Edinburgh: Elsevier.

Jack, K. and Miller, E. (2008) 'Exploring Self-awareness in Mental Health Practice', *Mental Health Practice*, 12(3): 31–5.

—— and Smith, A. (2007) 'Promoting Self-awareness in Nurses to Improve Nursing Practice', *Nursing Standard*, 21: 32, 47–5.

Kagan, C. and Evans, J. (1995) *Professional Interpersonal Skills for Nurses*. Cheltenham: Nelson Thornes.

Luft, J. (1969) *Of Human Interaction*. Palo Alto, CA: National Press Books.

McCabe, C. and Timmins, F. (eds.) (2007) *Communication Skills for Nursing Practice*. Basingstoke: Palgrave Macmillan.

Millard, L., Hallett, C., and Luker, K. (2006) 'Nurse–Patient Interaction and Decision-making in Care: Patient Involvement in Community Nursing', *Journal of Advanced Nursing*, 55(2): 142–50.

Nursing and Midwifery Council (2008) *The Code: Standards of Conduct, Performance and Ethics for Nurses and Midwives*. London: NMC.

—— (2009a) *Guidance on Professional Conduct for Nursing and Midwifery Students*. London: Nursing and Midwifery Council

—— (2009b) *Clear Sexual Boundaries*. London: NMC

—— (2009c) *NMC and You: Helping You to Train to Become a Nurse or Midwife*. London: NMC.

Peplau, H. E. (1997) 'Peplau's Theory of Interpersonal Relations', *Nursing Science Quarterly* (Winter), 10(4): 162–7.

Rogers, C. (1967) *On Becoming a Person: A Therapist's View of Psychotherapy*. London: Constable.

Rowe, J. (1999) 'Self-awareness: Improving Nurse–Client Interactions', *Nursing Standard*, 14(8): 37–40.

Rungapadiachy, D. M. (1999) *Interpersonal Communication and Psychology for Health Care Professionals*. Edinburgh: Elsevier.

United Kingdom Central Council for Nursing, Midwifery and Health Visiting (1999) 'Nurses, Midwives and Health Visitors Must Maintain Proper Boundaries to Relationships with Patients and Clients', *Register* (Autumn), 29: 6–7.

Williams, A. and Jones, M. (2006) 'Patients' Assessment of Consulting a Nurse Practitioner: The Time Factor', *Journal of Advanced Nursing*, 53(2): 188–95.

How to relate to others effectively

Lucy Webb

This chapter will help you to achieve competencies in:

- ➔ engaging with people and building caring professional relationships;
- ➔ recognizing and overcoming barriers in developing with patients;
- ➔ developing self-awareness and challenging your own prejudices;
- ➔ using helpful and therapeutic strategies to enable people to understand treatments and give informed consent;
- ➔ working confidently as part of a team;
- ➔ working with people to provide clear and accurate information.

Introduction

In this chapter, we will explore two different ways of relating to others that help the nurse to establish trust, confidence, and cooperation from others. When we talk to friends and family, we relate to them on the basis of our prior knowledge of them, our roles and existing relationships. For instance, we can be relaxed and playful with brothers and sisters, dependent on parents and partners, trusting with friends, and perhaps authoritative with children. When we don't know someone very well, we make assumptions about how we should relate to them—for example: 'They seem shy, I'll do all of the talking!'

As a nurse, you will meet a lot of patients with different needs and personal characteristics. You must be able to relate to them in way that is professionally appropriate and which enables you to develop a good working relationship with each person you come across. This means that, for instance, a shy patient needs to be encouraged to talk so that you can find out something important about their health worries. Knowing when to 'do all of the talking' and when to 'do the listening' is a key skill in communication. This chapter will help you to develop skills in *when* to listen or talk, and *how* to listen and talk.

There are some useful models of communication and relationships that help us to understand how we need to present ourselves to others and how to understand 'where someone is coming from' by their way of communicating. In this chapter, we will look at two common models used in nursing. The first half of the chapter will look at **transactional analysis** (TA), and in the second half of the chapter, we'll look at **six-category intervention analysis**.

Transactional analysis (TA)

Transactional analysis is a model of communication developed by Eric Berne (1964) that helps professionals to understand their style of communication, what effect it has on others, and how to develop more effective communication. Transactional analysis is one of the most common communication skills models used in nursing and has several different components, which are outlined below.

Ego states

An **ego state** could be described as the self-concept, or attitude of mind, or 'role' that a person adopts when communicating with others. Berne (1964) divided them into three: parent, adult, and child ego states. In this example, a nurse is talking to an anxious patient about her operation.

> Nurse: Now, Jane, there's nothing to worry about. It's only a minor operation and you'll be awake and right as rain in no time.

What age difference is there between these two people, do you think? Is Jane an adult or a child? Does the nurse sound like an adult, a parent, or a child? Now look at the same scenario acted out differently.

> Nurse: I can see you're anxious about this operation. What can I do to reassure you?

What's the difference? Which do you think is better? We could say that the difference is the attitude of mind the nurse has taken with the patient. In the first example, the nurse is a parent figure taking an authoritative position over the patient. In the second, the nurse has taken a position of equality and spoken to the patient as one adult to another. Which is better can depend on the situation, the patient's needs, and the nursing outcome desired. Look at the next example of an exchange between a nurse tutor and a student nurse.

> Tutor: If you continue to turn up late for tutorials, I can't be expected to wait around for you. I will have to see someone else in your place.
>
> Student: But I live further away than most people and have to rely on the bus. It's not fair.

The tutor is adopting a parent ego state and has elicited a child ego state in response See Figure 3.1.

In TA, an ego state can be like a parent adult or child. A parent state can be caring (a **nurturing parent**) or judgemental or authoritarian (a **critical parent**). A child state can be happy and carefree (a **natural child**), or sulky, stubborn, compliant, or rebellious (an **adapted child**). See Box 3.1 for an example of each state.

Box 3.1 Ego states and sub-states

Nurturing parent:	It will all be better soon.
Critical parent:	You missed your appointment time. You'll just have to wait at the end.
Adapted child:	I don't see why I have to wait! There's no one else here!
Natural child:	I don't mind. I've nothing better to do!

Strokes

When we communicate with someone, we give them attention. Berne called these attention episodes **strokes**. Strokes can be either positive or negative depending on whether we mean to be encouraging or discouraging. Bullying would be a good example of negative stroking, while praise would be positive stroking.

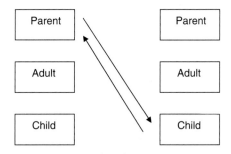

Figure 3.1 A classic ego state of parent and child

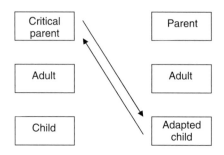

Figure 3.2 Critical parent and adapted child interaction

Positive strokes give approval, encouragement, praise, or affection, and improve another's self-esteem and confidence.

Negative strokes communicate disapproval and dislike and give rise to a person avoiding further contacts and communication, losing confidence, and developing low self-esteem.

Look at the transactions in the examples and note the negative or positive stroking and the ego states adopted.

Example 1: father to his child (see Figure 3.2)

> Father: You'll never do it that way. You've got it all wrong!
>
> Small child (*knocking over bricks deliberately*): It's stupid anyway.

Example 2: ward sister to student nurse (Figure 3.3)

> Sister: There, you see? You can give injections properly. It's just a matter of practice.
>
> Student nurse: Oh, it's easy isn't it! Now I've got the hang of it, I'll do them all now!

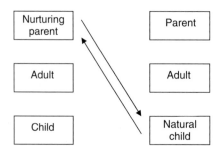

Figure 3.3 Nurturing parent and natural child

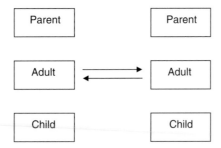

Figure 3.4 Adult-to-adult interaction

Example 3: student nurse to patient (Figure 3.4)

> Student nurse: I'm afraid there will be a bit of a wait. Would you like some tea or anything?
>
> Patient: That's alright, nurse. I've got a magazine to read. I'll just wait.

In Example 1, the father adopts a critical parent ego state and gives his child a negative stroke by criticizing the child's attempts to build something with bricks. The child is discouraged and responds by adopting a rebellious **adapted child** ego state. Imagine what a childhood spent in receiving a lot of negative strokes like this will do to the confidence and self-esteem of the person when he or she grows up!

In Example 2, the ward sister is behaving as a nurturing parent by giving praise for performing a skill successfully. This is accepted by the student who, feeling more confident about the skill, jokes about her enthusiasm. In this way, the student adopts a **natural child** ego state.

In Example 3, you may have spotted that the student nurse communicates information to the patient in a manner of equality and respect for the other's ability to make decisions. This is adult-to-adult relating and the patient responds in an appropriate adult way.

Transactions

The examples above also demonstrate that, in a communication **transaction**, one ego state can elicit a corresponding ego state. The critical parent state elicits an **adapted child**; the **nurturing parent** elicits a **natural child**; and the **adult** ego state of the student nurse elicits an **adult** ego state response from the patient. We respond to another's ego state by adopting what is appropriate, or what our egos need, for the situation.

We can also use a particular ego state to deliberately in order elicit a desired ego state. Look at the following examples.

Example 5

A ward sister comes into the laundry storeroom where a newly qualified staff nurse and a healthcare assistant are sorting out the fresh laundry. It is time for the handover and the sister wants the staff nurse to attend on time.

> Sister: Do hurry up with that laundry, nurse! Everyone is waiting for you!
>
> Nurse: I can't do it any faster!
>
> Nurse (*to HCA, after sister leaves*): She got out of the wrong side of bed this morning!
>
> HCA: Yeah, probably fell out!

The sister starts as a critical parent and the nurse responds as an adapted child. The sister may have felt annoyed and so gave out a negative stroke to make herself feel better and the nurse responded defensively to it. The nurse then adopted a natural child with the HCA in order to gain an ally (and gain a positive stroke). The HCA obliged by also adopting a natural child ego state and gave the desired positive stroke.

The dynamics of this team suggest a division between the leadership and others that is likely to lead to communication avoidance, lack of trust of the leader, and lack of responsibility from the team. The ward sister is seen as a critical parent, and the team become irresponsible children as they adopt child ego states with the sister and each other.

A better approach from the sister might be as follows

> Sister: Handover is about to start. It's important that you're present at the beginning for this one.
>
> Nurse: OK sister. I'll be there on time.
>
> Nurse to HCA (*when sister leaves*): I'd better do this later or I'll be late for handover.
>
> HCA: That's OK, I'll manage this myself. You go.

In this example, the sister adopts an adult ego state and the nurse responds with an adult ego state. The nurse does not need to be defensive or look for an ally elsewhere. The nurse can then relate to the HCA with an adult-to-adult transaction and elicits an adult ego state response.

This dynamic would suggest that this team respects each other's roles and can communicate unwelcome information effectively and without putting others down. This team treats each other as responsible adults and this probably works with patients too!

....

⊕ Learning point 1

When you are next on placement or in a social setting, observe the communications between people and try to identify the transactions taking place.

Check with your mentor by relating your observations and see if he or she agrees with you. This is also a skills development exercise in reflection and supervision.

....

Crossed transactions

When communication goes wrong, we can often see a crossed transaction where one person has misinterpreted the ego state of the other (see Box 3.2).

Box 3.2 A crossed transaction

In a pre-operation clinic, an anxious patient asks the doctor what the risks are. The doctor responds by giving a detailed description of the procedure. The patient gets more anxious and refuses to sign the consent form.

This patient was anxious and probably in an adapted child ego state, trying to elicit reassurance in a controlled way. The doctor, however, responded in an adult ego state and didn't give the needed reassurance (see Figure 3.5). A nurturing parent ego state from the doctor would have been more appropriate in the circumstances.

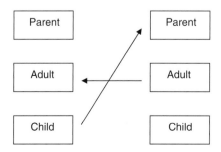

Figure 3.5 A crossed transaction

Table 3.1 Summary of transactional model

Ego state	Typical words and phrases	Typical behaviour	Typical attitudes
Critical parent	Disgraceful Ought, Should, Always	Furrowed brow, pointing, hands on hips	Condescending, judgemental
Nurturing parent	Well done There, there	Benevolent smile, pat on back	Caring, permissive, reassuring
Adult	How? When? Where?	Relaxed, attentive	Open-minded, inquiring, interested
Adapted child	Please can I? I'll try harder	Vigorous head nodding, whiny voice	Compliant, defiant, complaining
Natural child	I want I feel great! Wow!	Uninhibited, laughing	Curious, fun-loving, spontaneous

Source: Cork and Ferns (2008).

Non-verbal communication and TA

Transactional analysis is not about what people say only; it also includes body language, attitudes, and non-vocals such as tone of voice. Cork and Ferns (2008) give examples of each state, illustrating typical phrases, behaviour, and attitudes (see Table 3.1).

Positions

Harris (1973) summarized the states people tend to adopt as being 'OK' or 'Not OK'. Someone who has a positive self-concept, shaped by positive strokes from others from childhood, will be 'OK', and will treat others as 'OK'. In other words, they will take a positive responsibility for themselves and expect others to be able to do the same. This would be an adult–adult transaction.

However, a parent-to-child transaction would be 'I'm OK—You're not OK', because the 'parent' sees themselves as 'better' than the other.

Table 3.2 summarizes the typical positions people can take, often habitually, in certain circumstances.

A good rule of thumb for the nurse delivering the principles of self-care and empowerment is that every nurse–patient transaction is from the 'I'm OK—You're OK' position.

There are times, though, when it is therapeutic to adopt a different position. In the crossed transaction example above, we saw a patient in the 'I'm not OK—You're OK' position and in need of reassuring from an 'I'm OK—You're not OK' position from

Table 3.2 Positions in TA

I'm OK–You're OK	I am confident, capable, and have self-worth, and I presume you do too.
I'm OK–You're not OK	I am capable and powerful, but you are in need. (positive)
I'm OK–You're not OK	I am capable and powerful, but you are weak and worthless. (negative)
I'm not OK–You're OK	I can't cope, but you can and I need you.
I'm not OK–You're not OK	We are both (or all) worthless, so there is no point in anything.

the doctor. In health promotion, it is important to bring to patients' awareness that they would benefit from changing their behaviour. Consider alcohol misuse, for example. A patient with alcohol-related liver disease will need to stop drinking to maximize his or her recovery, or even to prevent death. It is very common for people addicted to alcohol to be in denial.

> Patient: It won't happen to me.
>
> Patient: I'd rather die young and happy than old and miserable.
>
> Patient: I can't stop drinking—it's no good trying.

The first two statements are 'I'm OK', and the third is 'I'm not OK'. To encourage someone to become aware of their problems, we might want to change their 'I'm OK' position to 'I'm not OK'. However, we don't want them to become hopeless and fall into the fifth position of 'I'm not OK—You're not OK'.

....

 Learning point 2

Can you think of any type of nursing circumstances in which you would use this approach to communication in health promotion?

....

Suggested answer to Learning point 2

Did you think of things such as encouraging smoking cessation, healthier eating and weight loss, compliance with medication regimes such as in self-care for diabetes or bipolar disorder, or in coming to terms with changed body image challenges following a stroke or acquired disability?

When someone needs to accept help, the ideal nurse–patient relationship would be 'I'm OK—you're not OK'. In this way the nurse becomes a source of hope for the patient. Look at the exchange in Box 3.3.

> ## Box 3.3 Changing 'positions'
>
> **Patient:** I like to drink. It's what makes life fun.
> **Nurse:** It's not fun when you get the shakes though, is it?
> **Patient:** No, but I just have another!
> **Nurse:** And how long do you think that can go on for?
> **Patient:** You're right, I know. But I don't like to think about it.

The patient has moved on from 'I'm OK' statements to 'I'm not OK—You're OK' position ('you're right', 'but I don't like . . .'—meaning, 'you can, but I can't'). Look at the next exchange in Box 3.4. The nurse adopts 'I'm OK—You're not OK' with this patient.

> ## Box 3.4 Changing 'positions'
>
> **Nurse:** I know it's hard for you right now. You can't see a way out.
> **Patient:** No, I can't. I don't see me being able to change.
> **Nurse:** I've heard many people like you say that. And they're now healthy and
>   enjoying life.
> **Patient:** Really?

The patient makes an 'I'm not OK' statement ('I can't change'), then responds to the nurse's 'I'm OK' position ('I know more than you') with recognition of the nurse's greater knowledge/power ('Really?').

This nurse–patient relationship has taken an 'I'm OK—You're not OK' position that provides some reality for the patient, but also some hope that his or her situation can change with the help of others.

While it is usually problematic to encourage dependence on the nurse, in this case it is important that the patient engages with the treatment process in order to tackle the health problem. This use of communication skills and knowledge tends to apply to specialist care areas, which we will look at in later chapters.

Games and ulterior transactions

Very often, we use our 'positions' to manipulate others and get some kind of 'pay-off'. Nurses and doctors are notorious for this, perhaps because they work in a stressful environment that relies on teamwork and dependence on others to solve problems. Families are also a rich source of game-playing, especially when there are teenagers around! Everyone plays games, but most people do not know that they're doing it, and don't really intend to manipulate or hurt others.

A 'game' is a series of habitual and unconscious interactions that attempt to manipulate other people. A 'game' consists of a series of **ulterior transactions**: where one position or ego state provides a subtle way of presenting another ego state. The clever put-down is a good example:

> Friend: I see you still have that dress from last year. So lucky the fashion now is 'anything goes'.

Here, an adult ego state supposedly giving a positive stroke actually delivers a critical parent message: 'You're out of fashion but I know better!' Game-playing involves a series of ulterior interactions that establish a fixed position for the player and manœuvre others into corresponding positions.

Games can be played from any ego state, but the transactions aim to put others in a desired position. A simple example from practice is in Practice example box 1.

Practice example box 1: Game-playing in a practice setting

The charge nurse (CN) of a day clinic called a meeting of all nursing staff at the end of the clinic. Everyone was waiting in the office for the meeting, but the CN was late. Two nurses (X and Y) popped next door to do some paperwork. The CN appeared in the office and said: 'Where's nurse X and Y? Why are they late?' Someone fetched the two nurses and, when they were in the office, the CN said to them (but really to everyone else in the room): 'Try not to be late in future. You've kept all your colleagues waiting.'

Practice example box 1 is an example of very typical game-playing. The CN felt guilty about being late and blamed the two missing nurses. The key here is that it was done in front of the team so that the CN could state: 'I am not keeping you waiting—it's them.' The two nurses blamed will be aware of the CN's real nature, but the rest of the team may not. The transaction puts the two nurses in the position of being at fault, while the charge nurse becomes the heroic defender of the other members of staff. This kind of game-playing is obviously bad for morale and teamwork, but in a team with an authoritarian (critical parent ego state) leader, if is all too common.

Box 3.5 Game-playing in patients' families

The mother of a young man with schizophrenia is very stressed by her carer role and is worried about how much longer she can care for her son. With the son present in the room, the mother tells the community psychiatric nurse that her son is becoming aggressive toward her and may do her some harm. He becomes annoyed at this accusation and forcefully denies this, saying he's fine but she winds him up. The mother then turns to the nurse and says: 'See, I can't say anything to him without him blowing up at me.'

Box 3.5 is an example of how patients and families may play games, either with each other or with staff. The community nurse in this example could make the mistake of becoming part of the mother's game by agreeing with her. The nurse will gain the mother's trust in the short term, but lose the trust and good relationship with the son. However, if the nurse is a good communicator, he or she will see the game as an expression of the mother's stress and recognize the threat to the son's stability due to this.

Games are not always destructive. Sometimes, someone likes to be in the role of 'nurse' and constantly put themselves out to be, or appear to be, helpful and caring. Patients may appropriately put themselves in a dependent role when they are ill. We all play social games when we pretend to be interested in someone's story, appear pleased to be visiting disliked in-laws, or pretend to be enjoying someone's birthday party!

In nursing, it is important to develop our self-awareness in order to recognize when we are game-playing and when it is destructive to patients or colleagues. We also need to be aware of games even if they are not harmful. Games still stop us communicating realistically with others and so allow others to play games.

Summary of TA

Transactional analysis is a very useful communication model because it helps to identify what roles people are adopting in a relationship. It helps the nurse to 'read' a person's emotional state and to respond appropriately. Transactional analysis has been recommended as a useful framework for students to develop communication skills through training and **reflective practice** (Bailey and Baillie, 1996; Rowe, 1999). Its emphasis on developing an adult ego state in patients is seen as a useful tool in the promotion of **self-care** (Parissopoulos and Kotzabassaki, 2004). It can also be used to monitor stress and coping among nurses by identifying the emotional ego states of *parent* and *child* (Florio et al., 1998). More recently, it has been identified as a tool with which to monitor and develop **clinical supervision** skills for supervisors and supervisees (Holyoake, 2000; McIntosh et al., 2006).

 You will see how important supervision and reflective practice are to continuing professional development in Chapter 16.

Heron's six-category intervention analysis

John Heron (1975) devised a simple system for professional development training in interpersonal skills. This system allows the practitioner to look at their practice and identify what areas of communication they are good at and where they need to develop. He proposed that there are six main styles of intervention, all of which are used to deliver professional interpersonal communication. Health-related communication could

Table 3.3 Heron's six categories of intervention

Category	Uses
AUTHORITATIVE	
Prescriptive: to give advice, be judgemental/critical/evaluative. Seeks to direct the behaviour of the other.	Advising patient on medications on discharge Demonstrating a procedure to a learner Stopping a child scratching a rash
Informative: giving instruction, information, interpretation. Aims to give new knowledge to another.	Orienting a new patient to the ward Presenting a patient at handover or MDT Writing up nursing notes
Confronting: being challenging, giving direct feedback. Aims to challenge or question restrictive attitudes, beliefs, or behaviour of others.	Mentor giving critical feedback on student's timekeeping Student questioning marks given for an assignment Nurse telling a relative that aggressive behaviour is unacceptable
FACILITATIVE	
Cathartic: release tension, encourage laughing, crying, expression of anger. Aims to enable others to get things off their chests ('abreaction' in Heron's description)	Providing a shoulder to cry on Telling a joke in an embarrassing situation Reassuring a child having a tantrum
Catalytic: facilitate problem-solving. Aims to enable self-learning in others.	Providing clinical supervision and reflective learning Listening to someone talk through a problem Providing play materials for children
Supportive: be approving, confirming, validating. Aims to show the other that they have worth and value.	All nursing situations All teaching situations All professional communications

be counselling, therapy, teaching, informing, or interviewing, and may involve patients, relatives, colleagues, groups, or multidisciplinary situations. Heron suggests that the different styles can be used for good when delivered with care and concern, but can be destructive when in a '**degenerate**' form that serves the self-interest of the practitioner. This idea shows that communication skills are very powerful and need to be used with care when put into practice in the caring professions.

Table 3.3 lists Heron's six styles, or categories, of intervention, with examples of typical uses.

The categories are divided into two main types: **authoritative** and **facilitative**. The authoritative styles of communication help the nurse to adopt a power role to deliver healing in some form, where the patient does as the nurse indicates. This is the **paternalistic** approach in health care, or the 'doctor knows best' stance. This is appropriate in situations in which the nurse needs to take the lead and adopt the more powerful position.

The **facilitative** styles help the patient to find his or her own solutions and encourage self-care and self-healing. These styles are more in keeping with the patient-centred approach. The last facilitative style, **supportive**, is suggested to be the style that needs to be always present in any communication transaction, whether accompanied by, say, a **prescriptive** or **confronting** approach. For Heron, this is what makes the difference between effective beneficial communication and degenerate communication.

Heron (1975) states that most professionals have the greatest difficulty in practising cathartic interventions—that is, encouraging people to express their emotions. This makes sense because we all find it difficult to deal with people who are crying or acting aggressively and we tend to steer clear of encouraging it for our own comfort. There will be occasions when you feel uncomfortable in certain nurse–patient situations: for example, when breaking bad news or broaching a sensitive subject such as death, sexual health, or abuse. We will look at such specific scenarios in later chapters, but this section outlines a key model for identifying and breaking down our communication skills to work on our strengths and weaknesses.

 Chapters 11 and 12 contain more information on breaking bad news and dealing with bereavement and loss.

In 1988, researchers Morrison and Burnard found that student nurses rated themselves most poor at cathartic and confronting styles of communication (Morrison and Burnard, 1989). But later, Ashmore and Banks (1997) found, on a training course that addressed communication skills, that students felt good about managing emotional styles such as being supportive and cathartic, but less good at informing and confronting due to their confidence levels and limited experience. Both sets of evidence suggest that the key to developing all of the skills is practice.

The skilful communicator, for Heron, is someone who:

- is proficient in all types of intervention;
- can move easily between different styles as the situation requires;
- is aware of what type of intervention he or she is using, and why.

Let's have a look at a real practice example by looking at the transcript in Practice example box 2 of a conversation between a female patient being admitted for a termination of pregnancy and a student nurse. The student has simply been instructed to carry out the admission procedure and is about to be landed with a bombshell! We come in during the orientation to the ward.

This student nurse questions the sister about this situation and finds out that the GP and the husband have persuaded her to have a termination. The patient is later offered counselling to help her to make up her own mind.

The student nurse demonstrates all of the styles of intervention during this episode. Her first approaches were **authoritative** and task-oriented—to inform and prescribe. She then had to adopt a **catalytic** style to help the patient to explore what the problem was. When needed, she facilitated **catharsis** by being with the patient while she cried. Later, she used a **confronting** style to find out what was going on with this patient and question the manner in which she had agreed to the termination. This led to a more satisfactory approach for this patient to make her decision.

Can you spot which statements from the nurse indicate the style that she is adopting? Remember, they can overlap.

Learning point 3

In Table 3.4 you will find a personal assessment sheet that can be used for skills assessment and reflection. Consider what categories you think you are particularly good at and which categories are you not so good at. Then make an action plan in order to seek opportunities in practice to develop these skills.

Note you can also download and print off this assessment sheet from the online resource centre.

To find more resources to aid your learning please now go online to www.oxford-textbooks.co.uk/orc/webb

Learning point 4

Now that you have identified your learning needs through self-assessment, below are some suggestions for you to develop your skills in TA and Intervention Analysis.

Choose a drama or soap opera on television that involves characters interacting verbally and non-verbally in typical social situations. Watch a dramatic scene where two people are interacting and take note of the styles of interaction each character adopts. Try to identify the ego states on display and note what it is about the words or behaviour that indicates which ego state is being used. Why do you think that character is adopting that style? What does the other person do in response? Are the styles used helpful to the situation or unhelpful? Why?

Obviously, the programme is fictional, but the script writers and actors will portray typical (if dramatic) communication behaviour. If you find this exercise easy, you are on the way to being able to 'read' others' communication styles and identify its effect on relationships.

You can also undertake Learning point 4 by observing others in real life. Take some time out of a social situation or while on the ward to observe the interaction of others. You can identify what ego states people are adopting and also what happens when they change. Check with your mentor by relating your observations and see if he or she agrees with you. This is also a skills development exercise in reflection and supervision.

Conclusion

The two models of communication we have looked at in this chapter have helped professionals structure their understanding of the skills and enabled assessment and development of skill deficits. **Transactional analysis** particularly aids the nurse in delivering patient-centred care and moving away from a more traditional patriarchal style of health care that existed in the past. **Heron's six-category intervention analysis** helps the professional, develop his or her skills in communicating, especially where a caring and concerned approach is required, such as in health and social care.

The first step to developing our communication skills is to identify what we already do, what we do well, and what we do less well. Models help us to identify what we are doing and give us guidelines for developing other areas of our practice. Both of these models are demonstrated to be useful for skills development in health and social care, and enable the student and qualified nurse to improve their communication skills in all areas of their professional practice.

 You will find examples of interviews and nursing interactions, plus more skills development exercises, on the Online Resource Centre: **www.oxfordtextbooks.co.uk/orc/webb**

See the video 'Active Listening 1,' to see the models of communication demonstrated in practice.

Further reading

Berne, E. (1964) *Games People Play*. Harmondsworth: Penguin Books.

Burnard, P. (2006) *Counselling Skills for Health Professionals* (4th edn). Cheltenham: Nelson Thornes.

Harris, T. (1973) *I'm OK—You're OK*. London: Pan Books.

Heron, J. (1975) *Six-category Intervention Analysis: The Human Potential Research Project*. Guildford: University of Surrey, Centre for Adult Education.

Rogers, C. (1957) 'The Necessary and Sufficient Conditions of Therapeutic Personality Change', *Journal of Consulting Psychology*, 21: 95–103.

References

Ashmore, R. and Banks, D. (1997) 'Student Perceptions of their Interpersonal Skills: A Re-examination of Burnard and Morrison's Findings', *International Journal of Nursing Studies*, 34(5): 335–45.

Bailey, J. and Baillie, L. (1996) 'Transactional Analysis: How to Improve Communication Skills', *Nursing Standard*, 10(35): 39–42.

Berne, E. (1964) *Games People Play*. Harmondsworth: Penguin Books .

Cork, A. and Ferns, T. (2008) 'Managing Alcohol-related Aggression in the Emergency Department (Part II)', *International Emergency Nursing*, 16: 88–93.

Florio, G., Donnelly, J., and Zevon, M. (1998) 'The Structure of Work-related Stress and Coping among Oncology Nurses in High-Stress Medical Settings: A Transactional Analysis', *Journal of Occupational Health Psychology*, 3(3): 227–42.

Harris. T. (1973) *I'm OK—You're OK*. London: Pan Books.

Heron, J. (1975) *Six-category Intervention Analysis: The Human Potential Research Project*. Guildford: University of Surrey, Centre for Adult Education.

Holyoake, D. (2000) 'Using Transactional Analysis to Understand the Supervisory Process', *Nursing Standard*, 14(33): 37–41.

McIntosh, N., Dircks, A., Fitzpatrick, J., and Shuman, C. (2006) 'Games in Clinical Genetic Counselling Supervision', *Journal of Genetic Counseling*, 15(4): 225–43.

Morrison, P. and Burnard, P. (1989) 'Students' and Trained Nurses' Perceptions of Their Own Interpersonal Skills: A Report and Comparison', *Journal of Advanced Nursing*, 14: 321–9.

Nursing and Midwifery Council (2004) *Standards of Proficiency for Pre-Registration Nursing Education*. London: NMC.

—— (2008) *Standards for Pre-registration Nursing Education: Draft for Consultation*. London: NMC.

—— (2010) *The Code: Standards of Conduct, Performance and Ethics in Nursing and Midwifery*. London: NMC.

Parissopoulos, S. and Kotzabassaki, S. (2004) 'Orem's Self-care Theory, Transactional Analysis and the Management of Elderly Rehabilitation', *ICUs and Nursing Web Journal*, 17: 11.

Rowe, J. (1999) 'Self-awareness: Improving Nurse–Client Interactions', *Nursing Standard*, 14(8): 37–40.

Sloan, G. and Watson, H. (2001) 'John Heron's Six-category Intervention Analysis: Towards Understanding Interpersonal Relations and Progressing the Delivery of Clinical Supervision for Mental Health Nursing in the United Kingdom', *Journal of Advanced Nursing*, 36(2): 206–14.

Active listening and attending: communication skills and the healthcare environment

Eula Miller and Lucy Webb

This chapter will help you to achieve competencies in:

- taking a person-centred, personalized approach to care;
- making appropriate use of the environment, self, and skills, and adopting an appropriate attitude;
- interacting with people in a manner that is interpreted as warm, sensitive, kind, and compassionate, making appropriate use of touch;
- anticipating how people might feel;
- listening to, watching for, and responding to verbal and non-verbal cues;
- having insight into your own values;
- using skills of active listening, questioning, paraphrasing, and reflection;
- being sensitive and empowering people to meet their own needs and make choices.

Introduction

In this chapter, we will describe and demonstrate how basic communication skills are applied in practice. We will explain the techniques used in conducting an effective assessment or therapeutic conversation in healthcare settings, using guidelines, tips, practice, and video examples to underline and demonstrate the techniques. The first half of this chapter will look at the basics of interpersonal communication and the second half will look at general approaches to conducting effective interviews, consultations, and patient assessments.

Core skills of effective communication

Whether we are conducting a formal interview or assessment, or taking the opportunity to converse with a patient to establish a good relationship, when we have any conversation, with anybody, there are some key basic skills that we can develop to improve our relationship-building, information-finding, or information-giving. All of these are essential to good nursing skills.

This chapter will look at active listening and questioning, attending, and use of the nurse–patient relationship for effective therapeutic change.

Active listening

Active listening is described as a form of communication that aids the nurse in listening attentively to the patient, but also *shows* the patient that they are being listened to (Adler and Rodman, 2009). Active listening encourages the patient to give information, express concerns, and generally communicate what is important to them in their care. In turn, the nurse can then structure care around the patient's holistic needs. Active listening can be effective in overcoming cultural divides between nurse and patient (Davidhizar, 2004), improving patients' sense of self-reliance (Engstrom and Fridlund, 2000) and empowerment and person-centred care (Gilmartin and Wright, 2008). Its absence can result in patients feeling abandoned psychologically, and not listened to (Barrere, 2007; Gilmartin and Wright, 2008). It is also recommended for multidisciplinary interactions: for example, handovers in accident and emergency (Jenkin et al., 2007).

Active listening is an important factor in a good nurse–patient relationship (Peterson, 2006). In order to develop an effective nurse–patient relationship, we need to employ essential communication skills (Barker and Watson, 2000) in:

- attending;
- hearing;
- understanding;
- remembering.

Active listening for the nurse also means facilitating active listening. The skills above rely on the nurse being able (Nelson-Jones, 2009) to:

- create a conducive environment;
- manage his or her time;
- provide authentic (genuine) non-judgemental support and concern.

Attending refers to the process of 'tuning in' or 'being there'—physically and psychologically. This process requires the health professional to use **active listening** skills.

Active listening encompasses appropriate eye contact (which shows that you are interested in what is being communicated) and appropriate response to cues. This response needs to be balanced with not interrupting before the patient has completed important statements, and hearing and detecting the meaning that the patient's statements have for them. Active listening could be described as 'hearing between the lines'.

 Learning point 1

Communication skills are often assessed in a practical examination called an OSCE (objective structured clinical examination). OSCEs are popular forms of assessment in healthcare education as they can measure competency in practical and clinical skills. You are likely to be required to demonstrate your active listening skills in practice within a communication skills OSCE. This will involve your reflection of key aspects of the listening skills you employ during a nurse–patient encounter. A key aspect of this conversation to note is how well you listened and heard what the patient said. We can often be distracted from attending to what the patient is saying because we are planning our next question! How well do you actually hear and understand what the patient is saying?

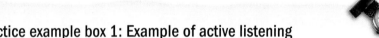

Practice example box 1: Example of active listening

A young man who had been admitted for accidental overdose of heroin was being assessed by a nurse for drug use. While giving the history of his heroin use, the young man said he was experienced in drug injecting and didn't have accidents. Because of the quietness of this statement, the lowered eyes and distracted fiddling with his sheets, this appeared to be a significant statement for this man to make. After sensitive exploring by the nurse, it was revealed that his overdose was actually an intentional suicide attempt and he still felt that he wanted to die. He stated later that no one during his admission had sat down with him and listened carefully enough for him to disclose this.

Practice example box 1 illustrates the core skills of active listening. The nurse *listened* to and *heard* what the patient was saying and assessed the situation in order to *understand* what he meant. The nurse was able to *remember* the details already gained from the patient to put what was said into context. Importantly, the nurse had facilitated the active listening encounter with this patient by giving time and attention, providing the appropriate environment, and gaining enough of his trust for him to confide this to someone. His statement was, to all intents and purposes, a plea for help.

Throughout this book, you will read more material on active listening and authors will put it into different practice contexts, as it is at the heart of professional communication and underpins all effective communication with patients, relatives, and colleagues. It is especially important in taking an accurate history and gaining insight into the patient's needs for delivering holistic care, and it is an essential skill in developing the nurse–patient relationship, through the establishment of an empathetic relationship and the conveyance of non-judgemental regard and interest from the nurse.

Asking questions

In support of active listening is asking the right questions. We can guide the other person through the encounter but turning the direction of the discussion through our questions. In this way, the nurse exercises a degree of power over the other person as the nurse sets and controls the agenda. How we do this depends on what types of questions we ask. First, however, we need to ensure the other person knows what we are asking.

Be clear

Questions to patients, relatives, or fellow professionals need to be clear and understandable. A question to a child is going to be put in simpler terms than a question to a consultant surgeon, but both the child and the consultant need to be clear about what information we want from them. To be clear, it is usually easier to ask one question at a time. This sounds obvious until you try to ask a complex question that has conditions and contingencies.

> Nurse: If you were to go home today, and you had support from your daughter, would that be easier for you than if we set up a home help for you?

Why not just ask,

> Nurse: Would you prefer to go home today and be looked after by your daughter, or wait till we can arrange a home help?

Closed questions

These elicit 'yes', 'no', or other single-word answers. These are great if you have a patient who is very easily distracted, i.e. a young child, an intoxicated or psychotic patient, or someone with major learning difficulties. An easy way to elicit these is to ask questions that can be answered with a single-word answer such as 'yes' or 'no', or either–or questions which give the person a single choice (Burnard, 2005).

> Nurse: Do you want a cup of tea?' Patient: Yes/No.
>
> Nurse: How many sugars do you want in your tea? Patient: [single word answer].
>
> Nurse: Is the pain worse in your leg or your foot?' [An either/or question.]

Open questions

These elicit more complex answers. They are much better at getting lots of information in an assessment, for example, or for encouraging a patient to talk about a topic in more detail (Burnard, 2005). People are often reluctant to talk about illness or their personal situations, but a string of open questions can let the person know that you are interested in the answers and that the patient is making a great contribution to their care by answering them.

In an assessment or interview, open questions are often started with inquiring words such as 'when', 'what', 'why', 'who', 'where', or 'how'. This is often referred to as the **5WH**, see Box 4.1.

Box 4.1 The 5WH of open questioning

What	what happened when you went to your GP?
Why	why did you go to your GP?
Who	who supports you when you feel stressed?
Where	where do you think you get your anxiety from?
When	when do feel like having a cigarette?
How	how does the asthma effect your child?

Exploring: sequential and circular questioning

Open questions help us to explore a topic with the service user, but sometimes the service user doesn't know the answers, or at least, has not really considered the issue in depth before. In this case, we need to adopt exploratory styles in our conversation. We can use various styles of questioning which have been shown to be particularly effective for exploring issues, particularly in family or group situations (Selvini Palazzoni et al., 1980). Two of these are called **sequential** and **circular questioning**.

Sequential questions aim to make visible patterns of behaviour, symptoms, effects, experiences, and so on. They are often direct and follow a sequence of events.

> Nurse: How did you feel when you were told you had cancer? How do you feel now? How will you feel when you start treatment?

Such questioning will make the person think about the topic specifically in relation to circumstances. The questions may help them come to terms with their feelings and anticipate the future.

> Nurse: When did you first experience the pain? What were you doing at the time? What makes the pain worse now?

This will give the nurse information about the symptoms and aid assessment and diagnosis.

Circular questions are even more exploratory. They assist in looking at the issue from a different viewpoint. Sometimes, this can give new insight into a problem that the interviewee didn't have before. The questions aim to make the interviewee consider or imagine the issue from someone else's perspective, or their own perspective in a different time or place.

> Interviewer: How do you think your husband views your behaviour when you are depressed? Before you were ill, how would you regard someone like you with your problems? What do you think most people would say about your behaviour? Why would they say that?

This type of questioning is very useful when dealing with groups or families (Selvini Palazzoni et al., 1980; Asen, 2002). The interviewer can ask members to give an opinion of another member's position. For example, in a family therapy session with parents of an anorexic teenager and the younger brother present, the interviewer could ask the younger brother the following question.

> Interviewer: In your opinion, what does Jane do when she feels angry?

As you will see in Chapter 5, the dynamics of groups are complex and very often people have fixed ways of thinking about themselves and others. By asking people to comment on others, people often let down their guard and say what they really feel. This affects not just them, but the other members of the group too. Group work and family therapy is a specialized form of therapeutic communication, but all nurses can adopt some of the techniques of questioning to assess or explore specific problems.

Socratic questioning

This is a very useful technique for establishing a mutual relationship between you and the interviewee, and helping the other to discover ideas for themselves. It uses a simple strategy of pursuing a line of questioning until all of the details are revealed. What the interviewer is aiming for, very often, is the underlying reason why a patient, relative, or colleague does or thinks the way they do. This is as much for the interviewee's learning as the interviewer's enlightenment.

Consider the following example.

> Interviewer: So why do you not like attending the self-help group?
>
> Interviewee: I am not sure.
>
> Interviewer: Why do you feel unsure?
>
> Interviewee: Sometimes it feels overcrowded.
>
> Interviewer: How does the overcrowding affect you?
>
> Interviewee: I think if I say something, everyone will think I am stupid.
>
> Interviewer: Why do you think they will think you are stupid?
>
> Interviewee: I don't know.
>
> Interviewer: Do you think the other members of the group are stupid when they say something?
>
> Interviewee: No, I don't, but I don't like making eye contact.
>
> Interviewer: So how do you think you could overcome this?
>
> Interviewee: By getting to know the individuals better and talking to them when we have a coffee break. Then I might not be so worried about talking to them when we are in a group situation.

The interviewer might well have a good idea of what the problem is, but needs the interviewee to explore it themselves. This way, the interviewee gets a sense of solving his or her own problem.

Focusing

Questions can be either broad and exploring, or narrowed and specific. Both have important roles. Often, broad questioning about a topic helps in the beginning of an interview, before we switch to more specific questions for more detailed information. Broad questions are often very open and focused questions can become almost closed questions.

Let's say that I want to know how the behaviour of a patient with dementia is affecting the informal carer. I may ask the following at first.

> Interviewer: What sort of behaviours do you find most difficult to cope with?

I find out that the main problem is wandering, so I focus on that aspect of the patient's safety management by using a closed question.

> Interviewer: What would happen if you put locks on all the external doors? Would you feel guilty about keeping him in?

Attending

Active listening and attending rely on being able to communicate to the other person that we are listening, understanding, remembering, and even interested in what they are communicating. We need to focus on what both the patient and ourselves are communicating in order to create a sense of 'mutuality' in the conversation. Mutuality will be addressed later in this chapter but, for now, let's focus on the basics. There are some simple rules and tips to adhere to in order to get the basics of attending right.

We can 'listen' to our patients in three key ways:

- **verbally**—what is said (or not said);
- **vocally**—how it is verbalized;
- **non-verbally**—what body language is being displayed.

We can also influence all of these by the questions that we ask, the way in which we ask and respond to them, and the body language that we use when talking and listening.

Verbal attending: paraphrasing

One really good way to show the person that we are listening is to use **paraphrasing**. This is simply repeating back to the person what you understand by what they've said, usually in your own words. This tells them that you are listening and that you understand them and helps you to check that you have understood what they are trying to say.

Vocal attending

This involves the vocal noises and responses we make and the way in which we use our voice, rather than just what we say, such as:

- **grunts**—such as 'ah-ha', 'yep', 'tut-tut', etc;
- **reflective responses**—such as 'I see', 'I know what you mean', 'no, really?';
- **tone, style, and pace of voice**—such as loud, excitable, fast paced, agitated, angry, or slow, deliberate, quiet, thoughtful, distracted.

Non-verbal attending

This can include body language, positioning/proximity, eye contact, and general appearance. Also, this relates to both the nurse and the patient or other person involved in communicating. We will look at non-verbal attending in the 'body language' section next.

Body language

This refers to the gestures, physical attitude and behaviour, and eye contact that we adopt when conversing. We can use these to convey different messages to our patients, but we need to be aware of what we are conveying as it is easy to give one message verbally, and another message accidentally through our body language. For instance, I tend to get very tired at the end of a long day, but am very aware I mustn't yawn too much when conducting an evening interview!

We can convey interest and concern by leaning forward slightly, using an open posture (not crossed arms or legs) with hand gestures and facial expressions to match the emotional message, such as surprise, shock, worry, support, joy. An underrated form of body language is *smiling*! If we smile with genuineness at patients, they may not smile back, but our warmth will register and make some small change in the contact between ourselves and our patient.

We can also 'read' the other person by their body language. Defensive postures such as folded arms, facing away, or poor eye contact tell us that the other person is feeling anxious or threatened in some way. Often, the body language accompanying what is said can speak volumes about that importance of a statement.

Proxemics and messages of appearance

Proxemics refers to the 'personal space', or proximity, of people to each other and the body zones that are acceptable for touching—or even viewing—both of which vary greatly between cultures and the type of relationship between people. Hall (1966) suggested that people have a psychological spatial safety zone around them and violation of that zone makes people feel uncomfortable. These may vary from person to person, influenced by personality and culture. However, it is important that two people sharing a space 'read' and respond to the other person's signals that signify the boundary of their comfort zone. How much a person is seen as a threat or a welcome contact depends on how they regard the other person. For instance, a 'motherly' stranger may be seen as less threatening and given more access than a stranger who comes across as authoritarian. Someone who reminds us of someone close and loved will not be as likely to 'violate' our space as someone who reminds us of a disliked figure. Behaviour that can violate personal space can be closeness, or proximity, touching, and even eye contact. Looking at someone too intensely can be a violation of their comfort zone.

Nurses delivering hands-on care frequently have to 'violate' someone's spatial comfort zone. It is important that nurses recognize how the other person is reacting to our physical presence and approach. This is particularly important with people who can't move away or communicate their anxiety or discomfort: for example, a person with a brain injury or people with severe learning difficulties (see the next Practice example box 2).

Practice example box 2: Awareness of patient proxemics

An elderly gentleman in a nursing home needed anti-Parkinsonian medication very early in the morning, often while he was still asleep. He had been in a Japanese prisoner of war camp where he experienced very cruel treatment. This gentleman had frequent flashbacks of his time in the prison camp when waking, often panicking when people were too close to him. The nurse waking him to give the medication needed to approach very slowly and make it clear that she was a nurse and that he was safe in bed, so that he wouldn't be alarmed and try to get away.

Any message that we can use as nurses to communicate 'safety' or 'non-threatening', which helps the other person to feel comfortable with necessary nursing intimacy, is worth considering. For example, a disoriented elderly patient is likely to feel threatened when being bathed by a stranger, unless the stranger is clearly in a nurses' uniform and behaving as the elderly patient would expect a nurse to behave. Very often, the nurses' uniform gives a reassuring message to patients that it's OK to let us bathe them, toilet them, discuss intimate details with them, and hold their hand when they are upset or frightened. For some, however, the uniform can be authoritarian and intimidating. With each patient, we need to consider carefully how we come across in appearance. There are a whole host of factors to consider, and many will be particular to individual patients. However, there are some general factors to which it is worth giving thought. First we could consider our sex, age, and general appearance (tall, bearded, petite, youthful, mature, and experienced). For instance, I know sometimes I come across as a bit scary—super-efficient, but brusque and matter of fact—and have found that timid patients will often feel more at ease initially with my more 'mumsy' colleagues! This is something that nurses tend to gain insight into with more practice experience and feedback from patients and colleagues alike. It is no bad thing to learn what your limitations are, as it helps you understand how and what you are communicating.

Eye contact and line of sight

Eye contact is a form of body language, but a very important one. It is a very primitive form of communication and contact with others. It usually comes naturally to people who are normally sociable and not anxious. When we are anxious or distracted, however, our eye contact can send a message that we would prefer not to disclose something. For example, a nurse who is concerned for his or her own safety with an angry patient can express anxiety through evasive eye contact or staring. A nurse who is anxious about the time or being interrupted will look around the room or at their watch. The patient will easily pick up on our true state of interest or arousal by our eye contact. Likewise, we can assess the state and even honesty of our patient by noting their eye contact.

Eye contact and line of sight can represent the balance of power between two people. Imagine two people conversing when one is in a wheelchair and one is crouching down to have a level-eye-line contact. How much more difficult would it be for the person in the wheelchair to converse if the other person were standing up? What if the other person were pushing the wheelchair from behind? Maintaining an equal eye line is often challenging in nursing where a patient may be in bed or sitting while the nurse is standing. Some little thought, and often a simple action, can go a long way to help the patient to feel empowered. How easy is it to sit or squat by the patient to gain an equal line of sight?

 Learning point 2

Next time you are in a public place with people around sitting or standing in conversations with each other, note how two people use their body language to convey meaning to the other. Even if you can't hear what they're saying, see if you can guess what they are talking about. Most importantly, when you've made a guess, identify what it was about their body language that gave you that impression.

 You can view the interview on Active Listening 3 on the Online Resource Centre (**www.oxfordtextbooks.co.uk/orc/webb**) and follow the instructions. This exercise will help you to observe a patient's communication and identify the techniques that the interviewer is using to elicit the patient's information. Note the power of eye contact in this example!

Communicating for the assessment of needs

Very often, we have a formal conversation with a patient or relative in order to assess their care needs. This is often called a 'consultation' or an 'assessment interview'. The key definition, however, is that the nurse needs to structure the conversation in order to gain specific information. Sometimes, this is already stipulated in an assessment form. However, the nurse should also gather more personal information from the patient or relative that will help to personalize care. Where the information needed is likely to be highly personal or individual—for example, assessing a patient's stress—the assessment will need to be quite flexible and the nurse will need to 'think on her feet'. We will call this formal conversation an interview, although different specialties and fields of care have a range of terminology for a formal assessment of needs.

Before you begin

Have a clear goal in mind for a formal assessment. What do you want to know? How are you going to approach the patient? What barriers are likely to be in place?

Think about the setting. Where will this interview take place? Can you cut out communication barriers, such as noise, interruptions, distraction, and discomfort? Ensure that you and your patient are dressed appropriately to put the patient at ease, and choose a time that is convenient to both parties. Arrange furniture, lighting, and other environmental factors for comfort and ease for both of you (see Practice example box 3). Be aware of who else might be in the room—another professional, a relative, or other patients within earshot. Ensure that you have everything you need for the interview beforehand, such as pen and paper, any assessment forms, and information sheets for the patient or notes.

Practice example box 3: The importance of environment

A sexual health nurse was asked to see a patient with a sexually transmitted disease on a general medical ward. The purpose of the interview was to take a history with the aim of referring the patient to the genito-urinary medicine clinic.

The patient was in an eight-bedded bay on a very busy medical ward. On arrival and following initial introductions, it was clear that there would be no privacy at the bedside to elicit the patient's history. So the nurse found the only empty space on the ward—which was the linen cupboard! The interview was conducted there very successfully. The unusual setting helped the patient to feel his needs were taken seriously and this built a good working relationship with the nurse from then on.

Starting the interview

Start by putting the patient at ease as soon as possible. Introduce yourself in a mutually respectful way and ensure that the patient is immediately aware that you respect them as an equal, but that this is a professional interview (see 'Setting boundaries', in Chapter 2).

The first sentences should be introductory, and reveal your human side. Seek to get the patient to relax and talk to you and don't be dominating. Set down the rules for the meeting with the patient. You must have their agreement (consent!), cooperation, and achieve mutual respect. You need to inform the patient:

- how long the interview is likely to take;
- the purpose of the interview;
- what is to be discussed.

Ending the interview

Finishing an interview well is as important as starting. If you have told the patient or relative when you will finish, you need to keep to that agreement, or check that it is OK if you finish at a different time. It is important to keep the patient informed of how the interview is progressing toward the end. The person will feel a little more in control of the process and also know when they will get the opportunity to disclose important information or ask questions. Throughout the interview, tell the person how the process is going and how much further there is to go! Near the end, it is helpful to 'telegraph' the ending in some way. This helps the patient to anticipate the end. It is surprising how often people will disclose something important at the last minute as they know this will be their last chance! To telegraph the end, the nurse can use phrases such as the following.

> Nurse: I only have a couple of questions left.
>
> Nurse: We will have to finish in about five minutes.
>
> Nurse: I must leave you soon, as your lunch will be here any minute.

 See Chapter 6 for more information on how to structure an interview or consultation.

Therapeutic use of self

The 'therapeutic use of self' refers to the nurse using personal strengths, experiences, understanding of human behaviour, and communication skills to interact purposefully with the patient (Videbeck, 2009). Therapeutic use of self in nursing is a phrase adapted from counselling that describes how the nurse can facilitate some form of healthy change in the patient through the nurse–patient relationship. The therapeutic use of self, and the building of this therapeutic alliance, is essential because it directly focuses on the needs, feelings, experiences, and ideas of the patient only.

We will look at some key examples below, but first we need to look at how the nurse ensures that his or her relationship and communications with patients generally benefit the patient's health rather than detract from it.

 This section adds to the introduction to the nurse–patient relationship covered in Chapter 2. Look back and remind yourself of the basic elements of the nurse–patient relationship.

Self-awareness

Key to the effective delivery of care through communication skills is the nurse's self-understanding and the use of self to communicate ideas to others. It is essential in marking the amount of sharing in the nurse–patient encounter and aids the depth of the material addressed by the nurse and patient. Chapter 2 introduced the notion of the nurse–patient relationship and the importance of self-awareness on the part of the nurse. In order to understand the patient, the nurse needs to understand how the patient is receiving the communication from the nurse. That requires the nurse to have good self-awareness about how they present to others and what messages they may consciously and unconsciously be giving out. See Practice example box 4 for a simple example of where this might be important.

Practice example box 4: The importance of appearance

A nurse dressed in surgical theatre scrubs approaches a 90-year-old lady on a surgical ward. The nurse asks her if she would like tea or coffee. The patient replies that she doesn't want either as she has a train to catch. The nurse then asks the lady if she would like to go to the toilet. The lady replies, annoyed, that she has a cheek asking such personal questions and that she is a very silly girl because, obviously, if she went to the toilet now, she might miss her train. The lady dismisses the nurse in an abrupt manner with a wave of her hand.

The nurse presumes this lady is senile, and is disoriented to time and place. It does not occur to the nurse that the uniform she wears bears no resemblance to a nurses' uniform to the elderly lady, but rather she appears as someone in overalls. The manner of her dress simply adds disorientation to person to the lady's confused state.

How would you handle this situation?

By understanding how we are seen, both physically and psychologically, we can understand the responses that people make to us, and then anticipate how we should present ourselves to enhance good relating. In the practice example scenario, the nurse could have introduced herself to the lady and helped to orient her to the hospital environment before asking her questions.

Empathy and self-disclosure

In order to develop a good nurse–patient relationship, even in a short interaction, it helps to 'get on the right wavelength' as quickly as possible and show the patient that you are 'with' them. This is often referred to as '**mutuality**' (Cox, 1978): the degree of relating between the nurse and the patient relies on the two sharing in some way. The nurse needs to be able to relate to all sorts of patients and have at least some understanding of their point of view. This does not mean agreement, but does allow the nurse to relate to the other's experience. The nurse also needs to show the patient that they have empathy, and this can be where a degree of self-disclosure is useful.

Self-disclosure is a tricky technique to use as it can overstep the mutuality boundary in the nurse–patient relationship. However, it can be useful to show a patient that you have experienced something similar or you can check if your experiences give you better insight into the patient. For example, a patient expressing fear of an operation may be reassured by a student nurse who discloses that he or she was also afraid of operations until they saw what happens and realized that it was OK. A more tricky disclosure might be where a patient expresses annoyance at a particularly brusque doctor and the nurse replies that, actually, everyone has trouble with his manner!

Self-disclosure can be useful, but must be carefully applied. It would be easy for the patient to assume that we are, in effect, saying 'I know how you feel', when we only know how we felt in similar circumstances. Or we could be taking away the personal uniqueness of the patient's experience by giving the message: 'I had that too and I didn't make a fuss.' We need to be aware (self-aware!) of why we are using self-disclosure and what kind of message the patient will receive from it. Is it to gain sympathy from the patient, or are we aiding the patient to recognize our empathy and therefore trust us a bit more? Are we using it solely to benefit the patient? Cox's work with mutuality and disclosure is well detailed in Burnard (2005).

Informing

Communication is used heavily for assessment and therapeutic engagement, as seen above. It is also, and particularly routinely, used to give information to patients, relatives, and other service users, and to pass on relevant information to our colleagues. Chapters 11–13 will look at information-giving in greater detail, but we can be aware here that how we give information to others needs to be styled in accordance with how the other person can best understand the information. When giving information to other health professionals, we tend to give it in a formalized manner, using certain phrases and adopting medical-style language. We know that what we are saying will be understood. When informing laypeople (people not medically trained), we need to use active listening skills to assess how to give the information and whether it has been understood.

Matching information styles

Let's say our patient is a plumber. He is due to have a hernia operation. In order to give information, we could first explore what he already knows, and, crucially, how he understands it.

> Interviewer: Tell me what you know about your problem.
>
> Interviewee: Well, I have a burst wall in my gut which is causing part of my insides to seep out.
>
> Interviewer: OK, do you know why it has to be fixed and how?
>
> Interviewee: I think so. It could get trapped, the doctor said, and cause that bit of gut to die. He said he has to stuff it back in and sew it up again to seal the hole.

So, the interviewer has gained a good idea of both what the patient knows, and how he knows it. For good communication, the interviewer needs to put the information into the patient's own terminology. So, the practitioner now knows how to explain any further procedures and recovery in similar terms.

Styles and levels of understanding become particularly important when dealing with children and people with cognitive difficulties. It is important to assess their understanding first or we could make assumptions about their inability to understand—and so patronize them—or assume too much ability and give them information that goes over their heads. With young children or people with cognitive difficulties, it is often useful to use pictures, diagrams, or even play or role-modelling to give information. Pictures are useful because they work at a concrete level of understanding. Concrete thinking helps us to understand something particularly complex. It is easier to set it out on paper, in diagrams, or use metaphors and similes. For example, I don't understand quantum physics and black holes, but I can picture a black hole in my mind as a giant whirlpool that sucks everything in!

See Chapters 5, 9, 11, and 12 for communication with colleagues.

⊕ Learning point 3

Have you ever noticed that doctors often refer to the abdomen as the 'tummy' when talking to patients? Why do you think this is? Do you think that its patronizing?

Suggested answer to Learning point 3

Doctors are trained in communication skills particularly to give information at the patient's level of understanding. In the past, doctors were renowned for talking medical language to patients, who then needed the nurse to explain when the doctor had gone! However, they don't have time to assess the patient's own style or level of understanding, so the best approach is for them to use simplified language with patients all of the time. This has become stylized to some degree, so that certain medical words are converted into specific lay language, such as 'abdomen' = 'tummy'.

Motivating

Another important use of communication is to promote healthier behaviour and attitudes. We need to consider how active listening aids the application of motivational communication.

Motivational communication is very important when we need to change someone's health behaviour or attitude to their health status. For instance, if someone is obese and at risk of type II diabetes, a nurse's health promotion role would be to encourage them to eat healthily and to take exercise. Also, if someone develops an illness that needs self-care, the person may need encouragement to regard coping with the illness as a challenge rather than the end of their quality of life. Good skills in motivating are like clever advertising: they aim to persuade someone to change something about themselves—to eat more salad or to buy X brand of soap powder! Motivational interviewing is becoming an important and effective communication strategy in nursing, particularly in health promotion and changing unhealthy behaviour (Holloway, 2006; Green et al., 2007; Morris and White, 2007; Kim and Kols, 2008).

The secret of active listening in motivational communication is, like informing, understanding how the person already regards the issue and their capability or desire to change. In short, we need to assess the person for changeable points. See Table 4.1 for verbal examples of a changeable point.

....

➕ Learning point 4

Look at the patient statements in Table 4.1. See if you can construct any questions from the examples in this chapter that challenge those statements. Remember you can use Socratic, circular, sequential, open, or closed questions.

....

Suggested question styles

- 'Once you've got cancer, that's it.'

    Do you think everyone thinks that? (Circular questioning)

Table 4.1 Motivational changeable points

Changeable points	Verbal example
Current health beliefs	Once you've got cancer, that's it.
Current view of ability to change	I'm too fat to take exercise.
Current desire (motivation) to change	But I need a cigarette when I'm stressed.
What barriers the person perceives	I would eat salads more often if it weren't for the kids. They like their chips!
What key factor will motivate them to change	I worry about how the family would cope if I weren't here any more.

- 'I am too fat to take exercise.'
  So what about people who lose weight by exercising? Weren't they fat when they started? (Closed, one-word answer)

- 'But I need a cigarette when I'm stressed.'
  What do you mean by 'need'? (Socratic questioning—pursue until the person defines need and realizes they won't die if they don't have a cigarette)

- 'I would eat salads more often if it weren't for the kids. They like their chips.'
  So, what would happen if you had a salad and they had chips? (Sequential questioning aimed at challenging the assumption that this is unchangeable)

- 'I worry about how the family would cope if I weren't here any more.'
  What could you do to ensure that you were here for them? (A type of circular question that elicits an action statement—a step toward making a plan and taking action)

As you can probably see, a patient's statements tell us what stops them adopting more healthy behaviour, and what might motivate them to change. In order to elicit these statements, we need to engage in active listening, questioning, and attending.

 See Chapters 8, 12, and 15 for more theory and practice in motivational communication.

Conclusion

In this chapter, we have looked at active listening and attending, and some of the techniques and applications for which they are useful. Active listening and attending underpin all communication as it helps the practitioner to understand the patient's perspective and therefore what their communication needs are, and how to respond. It is called *active* listening because it describes what the practitioner needs to do (act) in order to *listen*. This chapter has focused on the basic verbal and non-verbal skills that allow us to 'read' the other person and also to 'tell' the other person something about ourselves—by the way we act, move, and present ourselves. Basic active listening and attending skills are essential to developing the nurse–patient relationship, but also to delivering interventions such as assessment, information-giving, and motivating. Further chapters will build on these skills in specific healthcare practice areas and for specific needs.

 To find more resources to aid your learning, please now go online to
www.oxfordtextbooks.co.uk/orc/webb

Go to the Online Resource Centre for the video 'Active Listening 3,' to see active listening and attending demonstrated in practice.

Further reading

Burnard, P. (2006) *Counselling Skills for Health Professionals* (4th edn). Cheltenham: Nelson Thornes.

Dunne, K. (2005) 'Effective Communication in Palliative Care', *Nursing Standard*, 20(13): 57–64.

McCabe, C. (2004) 'Nurse–Patient Communication: An Exploration of Patients' Experiences', *Journal of Clinical Nursing*, 13(1): 41–9.

Peplau, H. (1988) *Interpersonal Relations in Nursing*. Basingstoke: Macmillan Education.

Rana, D. and Upton, D. (2009) *Psychology for Nurses*. Harlow: Pearson Education.

References

Adler, B. R. and Rodman, G. (2009) *Understanding Human Communication*. Oxford: Oxford University Press.

Asen, E. (2002) 'Outcome Research in Family Therapy', *Advances in Psychiatric Treatment*, 8: 230–8.

Barker, L. and Watson, K. (2000) *Listen Up: How to Improve Relationships, Reduce Stress, and Be More Productive by Using the Power of Listening*. New York: St Martin's Press.

Barrere, C. (2007) 'Discourse Analysis of Nurse–Patient Communication in a Hospital Setting: Implications for Staff Development', *Journal for Nurses in Staff Development*, 23(3): 114–22.

Burnard, P. (2005) *Counselling Skills for Health Professionals*. Cheltenham: Nelson Thornes.

Cox, M. (1978) *Structuring the Therapeutic Process*. London: Jessica Kingsley.

Davidhizar, R. (2004) 'Listening: A Nursing Strategy to Transcend Culture', *Journal of Practical Nursing*, 54(2): 22–4.

Engstrom, B. and Fridlund, B. (2000) 'Women's Views of Counselling Received in Connection with Breast-feeding after Reduction Mammoplasty', *Journal of Advanced Nursing*, 32(5): 1143–51.

Gilmartin, J. and Wright, K. (2008) 'Day Surgery: Patients Felt Abandoned During the Preoperative Wait', *Journal of Clinical Nursing*, 17(18): 2418–25.

Green, T., Haley, E., Eliasziw, M., and Hoyte, K. (2007) 'Education in Stroke Prevention: Efficacy of an Educational Counselling Intervention to Increase Knowledge in Stroke Survivors', *Canadian Journal of Neuroscience Nursing*, 29(2): 13–20.

Hall, E. T. (1966) *The Hidden Dimension*. New York: Doubleday.

Holloway, A., Watson, H., and Starr, G. (2006) 'How do we Increase Problem Drinkers' Self-efficacy? A Nurse-led Brief Intervention Putting Theory into Practice', *Journal of Substance Use*, 11(6): 375–86.

Jenkin, A., Abelson-Mitchell, N., and Cooper, S. (2007) 'Patient Handover: Time for a Change?' *Accident and Emergency Nursing*, 15(3): 141–7.

Kim, Y. and Kols, A. (2008) 'Factors that Enable Nurse–Patient Communication in a Family Planning Context: A Positive Deviance Study', *International Journal of Nursing Studies,* 45(10): 1411–21.

Morris, T. and White, G. (2007) 'Motivational Interviewing with Clients with Chronic Leg Ulceration', *British Journal of Community Nursing,* 12(3): 526–30.

Nelson-Jones, R. (2009) *Introduction to Counselling Skills* (3rd edn). London: Sage.

Peterson, W. (2006) 'Evaluation of a Multiple Component Intervention to Support the Implementation of a "Therapeutic Relationships" Best Practice Guideline on Nurses' Communication Skills', *Patient Education and Counseling,* 63(1/2): 3–11.

Selvini Palazzoli, M. P., Noscolo, L., Cecchin, G., and Prata, G. (1980) 'Hypothesizing—Circularity—Neutrality: Three Guidelines for the Conductor of the Session', *Family Process,* 19(1): 3–12.

Videbeck, S. L. (2009) *Mental Health Nursing* (1st edn, adapted for the UK by K. Ascott). London: Wolters Kluwer/Lippincott Williams and Wilkins.

5

Groups and teamwork

Lucy Webb

This chapter will help you to achieve competencies in:

- ⊙ acting appropriately in sharing information to enable and enhance care (with carers, members of the multidisciplinary team and across agency boundaries);

- ⊙ working within the context of a multi-professional team and working collaboratively with other agencies;

- ⊙ challenging practice of self and others across the multi-professional team;

- ⊙ taking effective role within the team, adopting the leadership role when appropriate;

- ⊙ working interprofessionally, and working confidently as part of the team.

Introduction

Understanding how groups work and being able to work with others are vital skills in nursing. You have perhaps already experienced working with fellow nursing and other healthcare students in university as part of inter-professional learning or within your own cohort to explore and share knowledge together in teams. It is important that nurses learn the skills of teamwork because it is a key feature of the nurse's clinical role.

The NMC Code stipulates that nurses must work effectively as part of a team and share information with colleagues in order to protect and promote health and well-being of those in our care (NMC, 2008). In practice, we are expected to work cooperatively, share our skills and experience, and at the same time respect the skill and experience of others and take advice when appropriate. We often share care management with other professionals from health and related care services and therefore need to use sophisticated communication and interpersonal skills to be effective team members. For many patient needs, the multidisciplinary team (MDT) is likely to include the medical team, ward or community-based nurses and key worker, a social worker, specialist members such as dietician, occupational therapist, and psychologist or physiothera-pist. Further-reaching collaboration may include inter-agency working with professionals from social services, education, probation, or specialist voluntary sector workers. The principle of holistic and person-centred care means that care is delivered as an inte-grated package, recognizing that aspects of health, social functioning, and environmen-tal factors all impact on the person's well-being. Therefore, MDT and inter-agency teamwork is vital in delivering holistic care.

Teamwork within and across healthcare disciplines is recognized as vital in order to protect vulnerable people. This importance is evident in the events of the Victoria Climbié case, in which a young child in the UK was abused and killed after 'falling through the net' of poor communication and coordination between health and social care serv-ices (Secretary of State for Health and Secretary of State for the Home Dept, 2003).

As a student, you will experience studying and learning in groups and be expected, as part of a team of students, to engage in self-directed study. This is often a challenge to students because the effect of being in a task-oriented group in itself is part of the learning journey: students will develop their self-awareness from the dynamics and feedback from the group members and will develop the communication and interper-sonal skills all group members that need to make a team function effectively.

This chapter will examine what teams are, what teamwork is, and how teams work. The chapter will also identify what the implications are for communication and interper-sonal skills development in both practice and academic roles for the student nurse.

Groups and group behaviour

There is a large body of evidence around teams and groups and how they operate. Many of the principles for groups apply to workplace teams, so we will look at the theo-ries that help explain groups and group factors. There are different kinds of group, but we will focus on two of the most relevant to nursing: work groups (teams) and families.

People in groups are shown to do things that they wouldn't necessarily do as individ-uals. Somehow, being with others and sharing a 'group identity' changes individuals' behaviour and even how they see themselves.

Conformity and identity

People in groups tend to form a **social identity**. Psychological studies, including famous experiments by Tajfel and Turner (1979) and Sherif et al. (1961), show how belonging to a group creates a common group identity and can create rivalry and divisions between groups (see Box 5.1).

Box 5.1 Sherif et al.'s (1961) group identity studies

In a US summer camp, researchers randomly assigned boys into two groups and encouraged them to socialize within their groups. After a week, they brought the two groups together for a series of inter-group competitions. In the first week, the groups developed leaders and group norms and gave their groups names (Eagles and Red Devils). During the competition week, hostility broke out between the groups, even when not actively competing in an activity, i.e. watching TV or eating meals.

This type of evidence suggests that we identify with the group to which we belong or are assigned and can conform to the values and norms of that group. This evidence, however, is based on artificial, experimental research with young people who, perhaps, do not have a well-developed sense of individual identity. However, it can show how a lack of self-awareness can lead people into conforming behaviour.

Another well-known study of conformity is by Asch (1955), as outlined in Box 5.2.

Box 5.2 **Asch's study of conformity**

A group of people were asked to match a line printed on a card with another line of equal length on another card. There was actually only one research subject in the group, while all of the others in the group were 'stooges' of the researchers. The lone subject did not know this. During the study procedure, the stooges constantly judged that the line matched another line of unequal length. This put pressure on the real subject to conform to the others' judgements, even though he or she may have thought their judgement wrong. Only around a quarter of the subjects actually disagreed with the other members of the group. Some even stated that they believed the answer the others gave, so demonstrating conformity not only of behaviour, but also of belief.

Evidence like this shows how the drive to conform to the group can be very strong, even to the point of changing the individual's own experience and creating doubt in their own perception. Such psychological theories of conformity and identity are often used to explain why people engage in destructive mob behaviour or join in with bullying. It is even thought to be fundamental to explaining the compliance with Nazi death camps and similar atrocities.

In a nursing context, a nurse may feel the pressure from the multidisciplinary or nursing team to adopt an attitude or behaviour with which he or she might not otherwise agree as an individual. This conformity is not just about knowingly going along with others, but also actually adopting the same values as the others in the group. See Practice example box 1 for a typical example.

Practice example box 1: Pressure to conform

An MDT meeting was discussing the care plan for an elderly lady who lived alone and presented a risk to herself due to increasing forgetfulness and disorientation. The key worker, an inexperienced staff nurse, came to the meeting intending to recommend that she have more support in her own home as a care home would increase the lady's disorientation and make her condition markedly worse. However, the other members of the team (consultant, social worker, and charge nurse) all agreed that a care home placement was best. The staff nurse realized no one was going to agree with her. When asked her opinion, she agreed with the idea of a care home. Although not comfortable with this idea, she thought that the others must know better and she was too inexperienced to recognize the dangers to this lady.

The staff nurse in Practice example box 1 appears to be socially inhibited by the pressure from the rest of the group, especially since they are more powerful and the nurse doesn't want to look silly in front of the consultant and the charge nurse. The nurse in this situation changes her perception of the risk this lady presents and believes that she should be moved to a care home.

....

➕ Learning point 1

What difference would there be if the nurse in Practice example box 1 were to have well developed self-awareness? What role would assertiveness play in this situation?

....

Nurses are often in multidisciplinary teams in which there are people in more authoritative or powerful positions (Ellis et al., 2005). And yet it is often the nurse who knows the patient best, knows what the patient and his or her family wants, and is in the best position to be an advocate for that patient (ibid.). A nurse in this situation would need to be aware of his or her own vulnerability to **conformity**, self-esteem needs (not to look naiive in front of other people), and feel confident enough to be assertive and dispute the group assumption that the lady should be in a care home.

Social roles

People in groups adopt different roles within the group, depending on what is needed and what suits the individual and other members of the group. This is often an unconscious process whereby people such as the leader will emerge. This can be despite

Table 5.1 Group roles

Common roles of work groups[a]	Description
The encourager	Sees positive angles and provides good morale
The observer/commentator	Provides reflection on the group process Can be quiet
The joker	Diffuses difficulty. Can be distracting
The recorder	Serves as the group's 'memory'
The agenda timekeeper	Helps the group to stay on track
The critic	Sees the negative or problematic side

Work 'types' and team participation[b]	
The 'plant'	Creative and good at solving problems
The coordinator	Confident, promotes joint decision-making
The team worker	Sociable, accommodating, listener
The completer-finisher	Conscientious, corrects errors
The specialist	Single-minded, dedicated

[a] Benne and Sheats (1948)
[b] Belbin (1981)

someone attempting to be the leader, but gradually deferring to someone else. A newly formed group will go through a process whereby these roles become clear. The roles adopted can be described as falling into two different categories: task roles and maintenance roles.

Task roles are those that focus on the task in hand—these are often the decision-maker, the problem-solver. The maintenance roles help the team to work towards the task and keep the group together—these roles may be encourager, observer, peace-maker, leader. See Table 5.1 for a description of some of the common group roles identified by Benne and Sheats (1948) and Belbin (1981).

⊕ **Learning point 2**

Consider a recent student group in which you have taken part. This may have been as a small study group during a taught lecture or a problem-based learning (PBL) group. What roles did people play? Was there a clear leader? Was there someone 'difficult' who caused problems? What was your role in the group?

In nurse education, PBL and small group work are commonly used to encourage self-directed study. They are very valuable for learning complex material in depth. However, people inexperienced in task-oriented work groups of this kind can find them challenging.

Often, there are perceived problems of unequal workload-sharing, poor leadership, disputes, and blame. These are usually normal group dynamics that expose student nurses to the learning process of working and communicating in groups and teams. Let's look at typical group dynamics and processes.

Group dynamics

Any group of people getting together to form a team will go through a process of group development toward some form of cohesion. Tuckman (1965) identified five developmental phases that can be seen in any type of group in which the group members adapt to roles, where group identity is formed and the task of the group understood. Table 5.2 outlines these phases.

These dynamics in group formation and working are often utilized by group facilitators when groups are important to achieving tasks. Institutions that train people use groups in order to help individuals to become socialized and to identify with their role in the institution. A classic example of this is the way in which the armed forces train recruits. Army personnel are put into small platoons and given tasks to perform together during training, such as raft-building and negotiating obstacle courses as a team. This **socialization** into group cohesion then translates into the individual's identification with the regiment and a compulsion to put comrades first in stressful situations such as battle. Soldiers will fight for their comrades because the bond between them is made up of their shared group identity. Nurse education and training often follows similar principles. A student cohort will be encouraged to work in small groups on tasks to develop teamwork skills and to develop a 'nurse' identity among the students.

Table 5.2 Tuckman's phases of group development

Phase	Characteristic	Effect on members	Outcome
Forming	Orientation, uncertainty, debate	Observing and testing out each other, looking for potential leaders and roles, becoming members or leaving group	Identification of common goals, early roles identified
Storming	Conflict, disputed control, anxiety, shifting identity	Disputes, challenges of roles, role change	Improved cohesion, trust, role definition and acceptance
Norming	Development of group identity and cohesion, practising and testing out group identity	Sense of belonging	Group rules established, focus on task of group
Performing	Goal-oriented activity, good morale	Individuals work for the group: committed to group rather than self	Able to work together to achieve goals
Adjourning	Closing down and reviewing of group identity and achievement	Reluctant to 'let go' of group identity, grieving processes	Group dispersed; individuals come to terms with loss of group role

When groups go wrong

Table 5.1 outlines a good working group. However, groups and teams can also be destructive and malfunctioning. What happens when individuals do not find a role or become the focus of blame for things going wrong? Or when role conflict and disputes remain unresolved? The 'storming' phase of a group can continue or be revisited in a group that does not gel well or is challenged by external forces. For example, when two people compete to be leader, this can cause a split in the group and may result in a subgroup being formed. When a group is challenged, stronger group members may find a weaker group member to blame and this individual becomes the **scapegoat**—the group adopts a belief that 'We'd be fine if it weren't for John'.

For student groups to work well, Price (2003) suggests that members recognize that everyone will have a different contribution to make, as inevitably some will be more knowledgeable and skilled than others. Roles will develop rather than be allocated, in recognition of members' diverse skills, but everyone has a role in collecting and disseminating learning. He suggests that a certain etiquette is helpful to the group process (see Box 5.3).

> ### Box 5.3 Study group etiquette (after Price, 2003)
>
> 1. Roles of leader (chair) and group secretary should be rotated and shared.
> 2. Meetings should be arranged in advance.
> 3. Investigative roles should be shared.
> 4. Members will listen to each other without interruption.
> 5. Discussion needs to be constructive.
> 6. The group facilitator will control and redirect the discussion.

Study groups need to be well led or organized and it is often the role of the tutor to guide students to operate a PBL working group according to a framework. However, more informal study groups are often rich material for learning about how we work in a group when we reflect on the dynamics of the group rather than merely look at the mechanics of why it is not working— that is, find someone or something to blame.

Another problem in real working groups can be when another member joins the group after the 'forming' phase has occurred. This means that the group must revisit the forming stage to accommodate the new member. A well-formed and functioning group may have difficulty finding a role for the new member. Does this sound familiar? It is a typical experience in nursing training in practice areas. Let's see Box 5.4.

> ### Box 5.4 **Student experience of a group role**
>
> On an extended community placement, a third-year student nurse felt that she had become a member of the team, with her own caseload and apparent acceptance as a valued contributor. The team decided to put staff photos on the wall to help patients to feel welcomed. The team eagerly arranged a photo shoot and included everyone in the team, including the cleaner and the community bus driver, but the student was not even considered for inclusion.
>
> This student's role in the group as an equal member could not be accommodated in the minds of the group as it would otherwise threaten the existing group roles of the team, even though the student felt that she was doing virtually the same job. The other team members saw the student role as temporary and not necessary for inclusion in the photo board of staff members that represented the stable and existing team.

Students often struggle to feel accepted and recognized for their contributions in the clinical area because the existing group has to maintain its own group identity when the student is not there. Also, the group has to accommodate the student in a role that necessitates protection, tolerance, and mentoring—something that doesn't apply to the rest of the team. The existing nursing team may have a 'reserved place' for someone in the role of 'pupil' that is filled whenever a student arrives, but cannot afford to constantly revisit the forming phase every time a new student arrives on the ward. After all, the existing nursing team is at the 'performing' stage and the student has to fit in with an existing dynamic.

> ### Box 5.5 **Survival tip: the student in a nursing team**
>
> It is useful to remember group dynamics when joining a new nursing team in order to reduce the defensive reaction of the group. Remember that everyone already has a role in this team and you will provoke hostility if you encroach on these. The team will accommodate a new person, but they will have preconceived expectations about what role you will take. The new group member will do well to have good self-awareness, understand how he or she comes across to others, and be aware that this team will only allow a temporary role for the student because it has to function effectively when the student is not there.

Group structures

Another way to look at groups and teams is to look at the structures they form: the leadership hierarchy and communication channels between members. Families provide good examples of group structures because they tend not to change quickly over time. So let's look at some family structures.

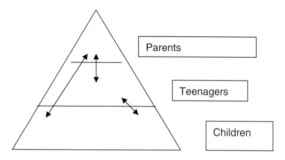

Figure 5.1 A healthy, democratic family structure

Families tend to have clear hierarchies because, usually, the parents are in charge and the children have power according to their ages and level of responsibility. Harry Wright, a nurse and family therapist, suggests three types of structure that affect the flow of communication between its members (Wright, 1990).

The healthy hierarchy of a group resembles a healthy family in which there is a clear delineation of responsibility, but good communication channels (see Figure 5.1).

This type of structure is often called a **democratic leadership** style in which roles are well defined, but all members have a say in the group functions.

A rigid hierarchy has overbearing authoritarian leadership and poor, or top–down, communication channels (see Figure 5.2). What the leadership say is what goes, no argument!

This is also known as an **authoritarian leadership** style in which the decision-makers are remote from the rest of the group and it can cause frustration, disinterest, and lack of motivation among group members.

The third type of hierarchy is a chaotic one (see Figure 5.3): no one seems to be in charge, group members are arguing and not working together; everyone has a say, but no one is listening!

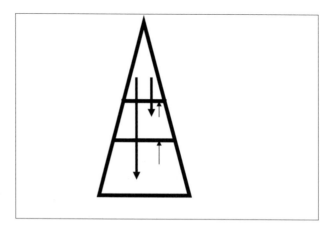

Figure 5.2 An authoritarian family structure

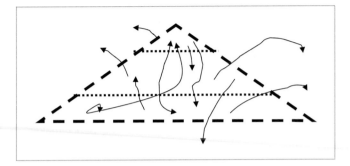

Figure 5.3 A chaotic, laissez-faire family structure

This is referred to as a **laissez-faire leadership** (anything goes) style and tends to be characterized by lots of arguing but nothing getting done.

Lewin et al. (1939) famously studied these leadership styles and found that the most effective group structure and leadership style was the democratic one that had a leader who listened and discussed ideas with the group, but who kept control.

....

⊕ **Learning point 3**

Have you ever experienced groups with these structures? How did you feel as a group member? Which one did you find most effective and enjoyable to be in and which one was frustrating?

....

Families and work groups both show these patterns of group structure. Children in rigid families often have little sense of having someone to talk to about their problems—often an older sibling or a grandparent acts as the parental guide instead. Families with chaotic structures often have chaotic dynamics; the parents lack authority, the children exhibit poor conduct and poor impulse control, and even the family dog misbehaves! Groups and families with problematic leadership often exhibit disruptive communication channels. Let's look at some common patterns found in both families and work groups.

Scapegoating

As mentioned earlier, a group member can carry the problems of the group by being blamed for all of its ills. An example could be when two people of equal status in a group can't agree, but also can't blame each other for the stalemate. So someone of a lesser status is blamed: two parents in marital difficulty may attribute their problems to a child's difficult behaviour or illness. The stress presented by the child acts as an excuse for the rift between the parents. Very often, however, it is the rift that has caused the misbehaviour or illness in the child and this continues while the two parents ignore their own problems.

Triangulation

Two group members need a third member to intervene and sort out their conflict—a common dynamic involving someone who becomes 'the peace-maker'. In families, a parent intervenes between two children or a child may be compelled to intervene between two arguing parents.

Overinvolvement

Overprotectiveness or interference from one member to another can often arise when a leader or peace-maker protects someone put into the role of being 'vulnerable'. In families, this is commonly a mother 'smothering' a child. In nurse training, this is seen commonly when a mentor is uncomfortable in allowing a student to take responsibility and is overcontrolling of what the student does.

Dyads

A **dyad** is the communication pattern formed by two (or more) people who have formed a small subgroup within a group, causing a bisection of the group. This is common in more rigid hierarchy groups in which communication is not encouraged. It will happen in teaching groups very commonly when two students explain to each other what the teacher has just said, instead of clarifying this with the teacher. We have all done this! In a family of authoritarian parents, two children will form a dyad, a subgroup apart from the parents, creating an 'us and them' dynamic. In a work group, subordinate members (students?) will ally themselves with each other when communication with the authority figures is difficult, perhaps because of lack of time, or remoteness of the leaders.

Triads

A **triad** is a communication link that brings more than one opposing perspective to the group, causing a three-way split. This could be perhaps a parent and an older child both opposed to the other parent, or two or more siblings of different ages individually opposing a parent. Divided work groups with remote and authoritarian leaders may create a triad where team members are divided about how to deal with the leader; they argue between themselves and cut out the leader from the group dynamics. The leader then becomes more remote and distanced from the group.

Look at the vignette in the Practice example box 2.

Practice example box 2: Student vignette

A mature second-year student joined a nursing team on a medical ward more
accustomed to inexperienced young first-year students. The mature student had worked
as a care assistant for many years, much longer than some of the qualified young
nurses had been in health care, and was highly competent with delivering hands-on care.
The student started showing the ward care assistants some of the 'tricks of the trade'
and frequently talked about her experiences as a care assistant. The young mentor for
this student found it difficult to teach the student anything because the student
frequently said 'I know that'. The mentor started to get frustrated, the care assistants
withdrew and only talked among themselves, and the other qualified nurses often gave
the mentor knowing looks and sniggered when the mentor and student attempted any
teaching interactions.

 Learning point 4

What group dynamics can you see occurring in the example in Practice example box 2?
Can you identify the possible patterns and roles? (See Tables 5.3 and 5.4.)

Groups and teams in practice

Professional groups

In the practice setting, a student is going to join several different social groups and work
teams. Socially, the student brings some group relationships to the practice area, such
as age group, sex, ethnicity, and cultural group identities. Also, the student will be placed

Table 5.3 Group and communication dynamics of Learning point 4

Question	Who	Why
Who forms dyads in this example?		
Who creates a triad?		
What is the result of this triad?		
Who is the leader?		
Who is likely to become isolated from the group?		

Table 5.4 Possible answers

Question	Who	Why
Who forms dyads?	Care assistants, the other qualified nurses	To separate themselves from conflict between the mentor and the student
Who creates a triad?	The student, mentor, care assistants and other nurses are all divided into subgroups	The care assistants feel threatened by the student, the other nurses are distancing themselves from the mentor, and the student is shut out of both groups
What is the result of this triad?		The working group is split into three subgroups and one individual
Who is the leader?	The mentor	The mentor is the one with the responsibility and power to change the situation
Who is likely to become isolated from the group?	The student	The established group normalize and the student will be scapegoated unless the mentor resolves this problem

in group roles by the practice setting, such as 'student nurse'. The student will also categorize colleagues into groups such as 'doctor', 'nurse', 'patient', as well as the social groups delineated by cultural perceptions of factors such as age, gender, ethnicity, level of authority. The student nurse, in joining professional groups, has to go through the process of forming, storming, and norming in order to find a comfortable match between what the student brings and what the student is allowed to offer by the group.

The nursing team is likely to offer more flexibility to the student's role because this is the team with which the student spends most time and in which he or she has more opportunity to assert his or her own needs and character. There is more opportunity for comfortable adjustment and the individual needs and contributions of the student. The MDT presents a more rigid group. There is less opportunity for the student to assert his or her own character and assets to this team, and there will be a more powerful set of dynamics and identity already existing in this team to keep the status quo. Channels of communication will be more democratic in nursing teams generally, except those that have authoritarian leadership and fixed hierarchical structures. In these, unfortunately, the student may be quite low in the pecking order!

Communication channels in MDTs are likely to vary depending on the structure of the group and leadership style. A strong and authoritarian medical consultant, for instance, will probably generate a top-down communication channel and only those close to the consultant in the hierarchy will have influence over group decisions. The student in these groups will need to communicate through the hierarchy chain of command—through the mentor or charge nurse—to get information across effectively. Multidisciplinary teams with democratic structures, however, will afford much more opportunity for the student to exercise assertiveness and contribute meaningfully to the group. The leader is likely to facilitate good communication channels while ensuring that members of the group have equal say and do not engage in destructive dynamics such as forming subgroups (see Practice example box 3).

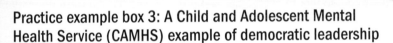

Practice example box 3: A Child and Adolescent Mental Health Service (CAMHS) example of democratic leadership

A MDT meeting among a CAMHS team was led by a strong consultant psychiatrist and consisted of nurses, social workers, psychologists, and occupational therapists. A new registrar had recently joined the team and was rather overenthusiastic about his own abilities. During a clinical meeting, he frequently interrupted the nurses who were giving their assessment and recommendations for a young patient. The consultant allowed some of these interruptions, but eventually reminded the registrar that all professional assessments would be heard, including his, and that the nurses' assessment was particularly important as they had spent a whole week with this patient, whereas others had only had an hour at a time to assess the different aspects of his needs.

The registrar kept quiet and others in the team looked at each other in relief that he'd finally been put in his place!

Patient groups

Families

Patients bring their group identities and roles with them into healthcare settings. They too are socio-culturally linked to gender, age, class, and ethnicity groups, and they also have occupational, social, and family group identities. Patients and their relatives often demonstrate powerful group dynamics when the patient is ill; the health problem is often a challenge to the equilibrium of their group as a family. The patient's role in the family is likely to change due to their illness and vulnerability. Other family members will take on roles of protectors, leaders, or decision-makers. Thus the patient's family as a group revisits the storming and norming phases of the group process. Television pro- grammes set in hospitals often relish portraying the storming aspects of families sud- denly in dispute because of an accident or illness of one of its members. There are usually dramatic bedside scenes involving family members arguing and then resolving their problems. Although fictional, these reflect in dramatic style the turbulence that families experience when the group is threatened by illness. As nurses, our role here is likely to be protection and care for the patien, but in recognizing the holistic needs of the patient, our attention should also be on the family and how they are coping with the challenges presented by both the illness and possibly the caring role that family members may have to take in the longer term.

Healthcare professionals are all charged with providing care for carers, therefore it is important that, as nurses, we take note of family dynamics and communication channels, role adoption, and group processes in order to understand how families interact and communicate. Perhaps then we can act to improve communication channels enough by encouraging members to talk to each other about the issues that concern the patient and the health challenge.

Case study 1: Family dynamics and communication

An elderly gentleman with Alzheimer's was admitted to hospital for assessment following concerns over his physical well-being. He lived alone with a daughter nearby and a son some distance away. It was found that this gentleman would need 24-hour care to maintain his safety. His daughter did not want to disrupt the family life at home for her children by having him living with her, but felt guilty about refusing to offer to be his carer. Her brother did not want to get involved as he lived on his own and had a career, but he too felt guilty about being unsupportive and insensitive. The nurse heard from both relatives independently how they were feeling, and that they did not want to share their anxieties with the other and be more of a burden to each other. The nurse facilitated a meeting between the brother and sister to talk about their feelings together, and they resolved to share the care. The brother had the money to fund a care home place near the sister, and the sister could visit regularly and ensure that the father was well cared for.

The case study outlines a very typical scenario involving a family adjusting to a relative in need. Dementia often challenges families to engage in role reversal within the family as the traditional head of the family becomes dependent and the 'children' become the decision-makers. Where several adult children are concerned, there is often a degree of storming as they adjust to new roles between themselves.

Clinical applications

Groups can be powerful tools for changing how people see themselves and with whom they identify. Becoming a nurse is a process of personal development because not only do student nurses acquire professional interpersonal skills, but they also come to identify with a professional body of people, which improves self-esteem and self-confidence. You may have already found that your personal self-confidence has changed if you have been nursing for some time. The power of groups is also effective in changing how patients see themselves, improving self-esteem and empowering patients to behave more assertively. Groups are used extensively by nurses in mental health practice, especially to improve self-esteem, change behaviour, and develop social skills (for example Thompson and Mathias, 2000; McLeod et al., 2007). Also, group work has effective application for health promotion and psychosocial skills in young people, people with learning difficulties, and parents of young patients (Gemmell et al., 2005; Popplestone-Helm and Helm, 2009).

The dynamics of groups—the challenges that occur during storming and norming—give group members feedback on how they are seen by others and help them to discover new things about themselves. Groups are also effective in delivering health promotion through education and rehabilitation programmes to patient groups for a range of chronic physical health needs (Ogden, 2004; Runciman et al., 2006).

....

⊕ Learning point 5

Remember the Johari window in Chapter 2? There are aspects of ourselves that we do not know about—the blind area and the unknown-to-self areas of the Johari window. A well-led group, with a trained and sensitive facilitator, will provide group members with challenges to their existing view of themselves, but the group will be encouraged to treat each member positively. In a therapeutic group, rejection or scapegoating is avoided and members are valued, and the group shares the burdens of each member, especially when one member feels challenged.

....

Other patient groups include educative and health promotion groups, perhaps run by community and outpatient nurses as a group clinic. Such groups may be convened to help patients with similar health problems to come to terms with managing their condition and learning from the facilitator and each other to cope with their health status and its implications. These groups might include a group for newly diagnosed patients with type II diabetes, where the group aims will be healthier eating, monitoring, and compliance with health regimes. Another common educative patient group may be an obesity clinic, for adults or children, or quitting smoking groups in GP surgeries, or supportive groups for informal carers of patients with dementia or learning difficulty. Each group will have its own aims, but these often include meeting motivational, educational, and self-esteem needs among members.

Conclusion

This chapter has provided only a brief overview of a large body of evidence around group dynamics, group communication, and the effect and application of group dynamics among professional and patient groups. For the student nurse, a major task is simply coping with the frequent changes in group membership that goes with changing clinical practice placements and coping with being a temporary member of existing teams. This task is difficult and should not be underestimated by students, mentors, or tutors. However, as training progresses and confidence, self-awareness, and assertiveness skills develop, the student nurse will soon be able to take these challenges in his or her stride and use these opportunities to develop teamwork skills that will be necessary in his or her future nursing practice.

 To find more resources to aid your learning, please now go online to **www.oxfordtextbooks.co.uk/orc/webb** See also the videos 'Specialist dementia nurse interview' and 'Nurse consultant in acute psychosis interview' for practitioner views on working with the MOT.

Further reading

McCray, J. (ed.) (2009) *Nursing and Multi-professional Practice*. London: Sage.

References

Asch, S. (1955) 'Opinions and Social Pressures', *Scientific American*, 193: 31–55.

Belbin, R. (1981) *Management Teams: Why They Succeed or Fail.* Oxford: Butterworth-Heinemann.

Benne, K. and Sheats, P. (1948) 'Functional Roles of Group Members', *Journal of Social Issues, 4*: 41–9.

Ellis, D., Jackson, S., and Stevenson, C. (2005) 'A Concept Analysis of Nursing Support', in J. R. Cutliff and H. P. McKenna (eds) *The Essential Concepts of Nursing*. Edinburgh: Churchill Livingstone.

Gemmell, S., Goodbrand, L., and Randall, F. (2005) 'Group Work', in M. Cooper, C. Hooper, and M. Thompson, *Child and Adolescent Mental Health: Theory and Practice*. London: Hodder Arnold.

Lewin, K., Lippitt, R., and White, R. (1939) 'Patterns of Aggressive Behaviour in Experimentally Created "Social Climates"', *Journal of Experimental Psychology*, 4(1): 19–31.

McLeod, T., Morris, M., Birchwood, M., and Dovey, A. (2007) 'Cognitive Behavioural Therapy Group Work with Voice Hearers: Part 2', *British Journal of Nursing.* 16(5) (8–21 March): 292–5.

Nursing and Midwifery Council (2008) *The Code, Standards of Conduct, Performance and Ethics for Nurses and Midwives*. London: NMC.

Nursing and Midwifery Council (2010) *Standards for Pre-registration Nursing Education: Draft for Consultation*. London: NMC.

Ogden, J. (2004) *Health Psychology: A Textbook*. Buckingham: Open University Press.

Popplestone-Helm, S. V. and Helm, D. P. (2009) 'Setting up a Support Group for Children and Their Well Carers Who Have a Significant Adult with a Life-threatening Illness', *International Journal of Palliative Nursing*, 5(5): 214–21.

Price, B. (2003). *Studying Nursing Using Problem-based and Enquiry-based Learning*. Basingstoke: Palgrave Macmillan.

Runciman, P., Watson, H., McIntosh, J., and Tolson, D. (2006) 'Community Nurses' Health Promotion Work with Older People', *Journal of Advanced Nursing,* 55(1): 46–57.

Secretary of State for Health and Secretary of State for the Home Department (2003) *The Victoria Climbié Inquiry.* CM 5730. London: HMSO.

Sherif, M., Harvey, O., White, B., Hood, W., and Sherif, C. (1961) *Intergroup Conflict and Cooperation: The Robber's Cave Experiment.* Norman, OK: University of Oklahoma.

Tajfel, H. and Turner, J. (1979) 'An Integrative Theory of Intergroup Conflict', in G. Austin and S. Worchel (eds) *The Social Psychology of Intergroup Relations.* Monterey, CA: Brooks/Cole, 94–109.

Thompson, T. and Mathias, P. (2000) *Lyttle's Mental Health and Disorder* (3rd edn). Edinburgh: Bailliere Tindall.

Tuckman, B. (1965) 'Development Sequence in Small Groups', *Psychological Bulletin,* 63: 384–99.

Wright, H. (1990) *Groupwork.* London: Scutari Press.

Application of communication skills in nursing

PART 2

Part 2 examines how the theory is applied in the practice setting. It begins by examining the application of the basic skills, demonstrating the theory–practice bridge in different but common fields of nursing care. In everyday life, there are challenges to successful communication and common scenarios from healthcare practice will be explored and solutions provided. Important aspects of nursing practice that have grown in importance recently and require each student nurse to develop a skills base are discussed in chapters on health promotion and information technology, as well as on writing and presenting.

Chapter 6 addresses interpersonal skills in a range of clinical areas. It examines the application of the basic skills. Chapter 7 extends this to typical practice applications that can present a communication challenge. It addresses the common scenarios that present barriers to communication, and outlines important strategies for overcoming these barriers. Chapter 8 examines the theory and application of communication in health promotion, an important part of the nurse's role. This focuses on how the nurse can use communication skills to enhance and change health behaviour. This chapter outlines the main theories and demonstrates common application scenarios. Chapter 9 also addresses a recent challenge to the nurse's role in communication: managing information technology. This chapter sets out find to explore and explain the challenges that information technology presents to nurses, and than addresses the skills needed to meet these demands for the future of health care. Chapter 10 addresses the expectations in writing and academic performance in nursing. It aims to help the student with academic writing and presenting, and acknowledges how these skills are part of continuing professional development for the modern professional nurse.

6

Theory to practice: communicating therapeutically

Eula Miller and Lucy Webb

This chapter will help you to achieve competencies in:

- ➔ acting as a role model in promoting a professional image and developing trusting relationships;
- ➔ being sensitive and empowering people to meet their own needs and make choices;
- ➔ acting professionally to ensure that personal judgements, prejudices, values, attitudes, and beliefs do not compromise care;
- ➔ using appropriate strategies to empower and support patient/carer choice;
- ➔ responding with kindness and empathy;
- ➔ using helpful and therapeutic strategies to enable people to understand treatments.

Introduction

We saw in earlier chapters that communication skills can be used in health care for a range of purposes, such as, patient assessment and evaluation, including a patient in planning care, and facilitating care through the nurse–patient relationship and use of self. In this chapter, the aim is to identify fundamental approaches in therapeutic communication in modern nursing practice and link them to practice-based care.

This chapter will focus on two specific paradigms of interaction between people pertinent to nursing care communication. These are the humanistic, or person-centred approach, and cognitive-behavioural, or behaviour change-centred approach. First, we will look at person-centred approaches.

Person-centred communication

Chapter 4 of this book looked at the nurse–patient relationship and emphasized the importance of developing a caring partnership between the nurse and the patient. Studies of modern nursing care and the nurse–patient relationship indicate that the essential components of the relationship are humanistic. That is, the relationship is one in which the patient is considered to be the person uniquely placed to experience their world, while the practitioner's role is to validate that experience and help the person to interpret it more effectively. Such studies include care delivery in wound pain and pain management (Kohr and Gibson, 2008), terminal cancer (Iranmanesh et al., 2009), mental health (Gaillard et al., 2009), surviving chronic illness (Fox and Chesla, 2008), rehabilitation (Sigurgeirsdottir and Halldorsdottir, 2008), and cardiovascular health promotion (Persson and Febe, 2009). The humanistic approach is often termed person-centred for the very reason that the person is seen as the 'expert' and has a unique perspective of their care needs and illness management. Many counselling styles are structured around this approach and one of its key theorists and exponents was Carl Rogers.

Rogerian counselling: the three core conditions of non-directive therapy

Carl Rogers (1961) was a psychotherapist who devised what is probably the most commonly used method of counselling and active listening in the health, social care, and education fields. It adopts the humanistic pre-concepts of adaptive development as encapsulated in **Maslow's hierarchy of needs** (Maslow, 1970), which holds that human development always strives towards becoming all that one can be. Rogers's **client-centred therapy** is based on the principle that the therapy is **non-directive**—that the relationship is one of equals, that the client (not 'patient') is able to grow and develop given suitable conditions, and that the practitioner's role needs to be **empowering** of the client's abilities to reach their human potential.

These three conditions are as follows.

- **Warmth and genuineness** on the part of the practitioner means that he or she is genuinely interested and personally engaged in the process. This means the practitioner cannot get away with a superficial pretence of caring. The practitioner needs to be genuinely concerned for the client.

- **Empathy** from the practitioner means that he or she is able to relate to the person's experience. This is empathy as opposed to sympathy. The practitioner needs to be able to understand the person's experience, but not necessarily agree with their interpretation of it.
- **Unconditional positive regard** from the practitioner will involve accepting the validity and value of the person's experiences. This also demands a division: accepting the person's views without necessarily agreeing with them. In fact, it is the difference between the practitioner's view and the client's view that often demonstrates the difference between coping and not coping. Therefore, the practitioner needs to have a more adaptive approach to the problem than the client.

In a nursing context, the humanistic approach complements holistic care in that it recognizes patient uniqueness and supports individualized care. It could be said that the nurse's role is to translate best practice evidence from what works for groups of patients to what will work for 'Mrs Smith' and 'Mr Jones'. To do this, the nurse is helped by models that structure the nurse–patient interaction.

Structuring the nurse–patient encounter

Boundaries of time, depth, and mutuality

A therapeutic process involving a practitioner and a patient is described by Murray Cox (1978) as being structured by time, depth, and mutuality. By this, he means that the structure of the interaction can be controlled by these three boundaries. 'Time' refers to the limit of the length of the encounter. 'Depth' refers to the degree of seriousness and involvement of the material being addressed, and 'mutuality' refers to the degree of shared personal psychological contact, or engagement, entered into by the practitioner and the patient. These boundaries define the nature and the quality of the relationship and indicate what is therapeutic and what is not. Let us deal with some key elements to these boundaries in a nursing context.

Time

When an interaction is short, it is difficult to convey the seriousness of the attention that we want to give our patients. With a seriously ill or upset person, we may feel the need to give them all of the time they may want. This is not always practical, nor indeed, necessary or therapeutic. It is therefore important to tell the person how much time we can give them, so that they know how to 'use' us.

Practice example box 1: The nervous patient

A gentleman due to have open-heart surgery is ready for his operation, but has not yet had his sedating medication. He is experiencing anxiety about the operation. He asks the nurse to repeat the explanation of what will happen during the operation. She doesn't have much time, but recognizes that he is anxious. She gives him a sympathetic look and tells him she can spare five minutes. She asks what it is that is really bothering him. He gives it some thought, looks embarrassed, and says: 'I think it's the procedure itself—what would happen if I woke up with my chest opened up?' She smiles and gives him an explanation of what the anaesthetist does to monitor the patient. She says he won't be aware of anything until he wakes up in the post-operative recovery room, where he will be monitored by a nurse. The gentleman appears reassured.

In Practice example box 1, the patient appears to be worried about the procedure. The nurse is busy, but recognizes that his need is important. The nurse structures this time for the patient by simply stating that she has five minutes. This may sound a bit abrupt, but the patient then knows that he needs to focus on what his real worries are. Have you ever noticed that people often blurt out something important at the last minute, just before you have to leave? By stating the time limit, the nurse flags up for the patient that they need to address the 'burning issue', whatever it is.

When time is abundant or the patient very needy, time structuring is also important. A needy patient can demand attention and use time ineffectively. The nurse can use time structure to effect better communication: for instance, by stating when and for how long the interaction will take place. The needy patient is then more likely to focus on the issues and use the time effectively.

⊕ Learning point 1

When you next go on placement (or thinking about your last placement), consider how the healthcare staff around you use time with patients effectively but therapeutically. Do effective staff members use certain phrases? Make a note of these and discuss with your mentor (or tutor) which would be appropriate, therapeutic, and effective for you to use.

Depth

This is the degree of disclosure and the amount of investment that the patient and the nurse are making. A therapeutic interaction, for Cox (1978), always moves towards disclosure of material. Cox divides disclosure of material in the therapeutic encounter as moving from:

Unconscious → Conscious-withheld → Conscious-disclosed

In Practice example box 1, the nurse aids the patient in exploring what is troubling him (what is in the unconscious), he is led to his own realization of what the problem is (conscious-withheld), and then reveals it to the nurse and so 'owns' it (conscious-disclosed). He perhaps didn't know at first what the problem was (unconscious), then realized he was scared of waking up, felt ashamed of admitting it (conscious-withheld), but, through the empathy of the nurse, 'owned up' to his fear and received reassurance.

Depth can also be divided into levels of disclosure. Cox (1978) identifies these as follows.

First-level (trivial)	'I see it is raining again.'
Second-level (neutral-personal)	'I don't like it raining all the time.'
Third-level (emotional-personal)	'The rain reminds me of my father's funeral.'

The first level of disclosure is just interpersonal chat, but it does set up a conversation and opens up opportunities for greater disclosure. The second is disclosure that is about the person, but has no emotional content. The person is disclosing a thought or opinion, but it is not personally important. The third, however, is both personal and emotional. There is emotional investment in the statement and often, for Cox, at a level that would not be revealed in a 'normal' conversation; it may be something revealed for the very first time. It could be regarded as a privilege to be given such trust by someone who makes a third-level disclosure to us.

Mutuality

The nurse–patient relationship is one made up of two people in alliance, with the aim of solving the patient's health-related problems. Cox (1978: 170) describes mutuality as referring to 'how much the [practitioner] discloses about himself in order to share with the patient the experience he is disclosing'. In other words, the nurse cannot hide entirely behind a professional facade and also be a 'person' to the patient. However, by 'disclosure', Cox is not referring to sharing stories of experiences. We cannot, as nurses, share the life experience directly with our patients. We probably do not know what it is like to be diagnosed with a serious illness, for instance. But we can put ourselves, personally, into the person's shoes and accept what they describe as their experience. Mutuality appears to be an applied form of empathy in that it is not enough to simply empathize. Mutuality is easier to apply when we like someone than when we cannot relate to the other person's experience or values. Cox gives an excellent example of this. In his work with psychopathic patients in Broadmoor Hospital, he was often challenged by a lack of ability to relate to the patients' direct experiences. He describes maintaining the therapeutic space of mutuality with one patient by adopting a framework for the interaction of 'One of us is a rapist' (Cox, 1978: 169).

We could translate this therapeutic space of mutuality in the nurse–patient relationship as follows.

> Nurse: *One of us has terminal cancer.*

Or as follows.

> Nurse: *One of us is going home at the end of the shift.*

This framework helps the nurse to identify his or her 'position' with the patient to enable the two people to discuss the issues. The nurse does not have to be able to say 'I know how you feel'. However, the nurse can say: 'I hear your experience and accept it without interpretation or judgement.' Mutuality is the genuine collaboration of two people who, while very different, can work together as human beings to address the patient's problems.

Time, depth, and mutuality work together to structure a therapeutic interaction or professional relationship. These three dimensions help us to map a relationship and evaluate its effectiveness. However, it is important that the practitioner has good self-awareness. For nurses, this may be a challenge unless personal and professional development are valued in the clinical setting and seen as equally important to care as more task-oriented skills. It may be that Cox's ideas of structure are easier to apply where interpersonal skills are a key part of the therapeutic care being delivered.

Egan's three-stage model

Cox's three dimensions form *structural boundaries* around the therapeutic interaction indicating what the practitioner uses to define the relationship. Egan's three-stage model could be considered as a model of the *process* of a therapeutic interaction, defining the stages of the relationship.

Egan (1986) suggests three stages to the process of counselling, which are also applicable to any practitioner–patient relationship (see Figure 6.1).

1. **Identification of the problem:** this may involve defining the problem or indeed exploring key aspects. This stage is often about facilitating the person to tell the story.

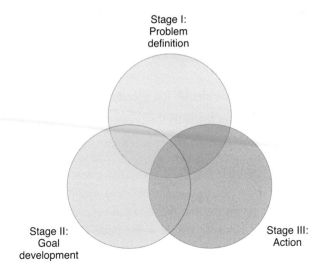

Figure 6.1 Egan's model of effective helping: an overview (Egan, 1986)

2. **Identifying goals that the patient may want to change:** this involves focusing on the problem and discovering the barriers to its solution.
3. **Making plans that aim at achieving the goals:** often, this involves finding new ways of looking at the problem.

This whole process sounds very much like the first half of the nursing process of assessment, planning, implementation, and evaluation. Indeed, it follows the same principles, but, critically, it is based on the patient's or client's values. Egan states that

Practice example box 2: Egan's stages of helping

Jane is a 16-year-old with Down's Syndrome. She is offered a place at residential college, but her parents are worried that she will not cope away from home. Jane feels uneasy because she wants to go, but doesn't want to leave her parents. Her key worker helps Jane discuss the issues involved around coping and identifying what she is afraid of specifically. They decide that Jane is afraid of upsetting her parents by saying she wants to go to college. Jane and the key worker identify that Jane needs to communicate her desire to go and that her parents need to come to terms with her leaving home. They decide to have a focused family get-together with the key worker and the education adviser to discuss how everyone is feeling and to allow everyone to air their concerns.

the model is developmental and cumulative in that the success of each stage depends on the effectiveness of the previous stage. Let's look at Practice example box 2.

In the example, we can see how Egan's model helps to map the three stages of the helping process:

Stage 1: The key worker and Jane identify the specific reason for Jane's anxieties.

Stage 2: Jane and the key worker focus on the problem and identify the goals.

Stage 3: They devise a plan to discuss the problem with the relevant people.

Egan's model is person-centred in that the problem identification and goals must be the patient's own ideas, and patient self-responsibility is key. The helper facilitates the person's problem-solving by guiding the problem-solving process, but not advising, or making suggestions or decisions on behalf of the patient. The model is also circular and overlapping as stages need to be revisited to tackle each problem that arises.

Summary of humanistic approaches

With both Cox's and Egan's approaches to therapeutic interactions, the humanistic principles as adopted by Carl Rogers can be seen to apply. Both regard the client as taking responsibility for problem-solving and being able to respond to empowerment by engaging in the problem-solving process. It is the patient who has the answers, but the nurse who facilitates their discovery.

It could be argued, however, that humanistic principles are impossible to achieve while there is a power difference between the nurse and the patient. Rogers (1961) was proposing a mutual relationship in a counselling setting in which the client seeks and uses the therapist in a form of self-healing. In healthcare professions concerned with public health in general, the agenda may be to change the unhealthy behaviour of populations and individuals and to deliver health promotion. Arguably, some aspects of health care go beyond the developmental needs of the individual patient toward population-based conformity with contemporary cultural health values, for instance, in forensic nursing in an environment such as a prison or mental hospital, which essentially challenges the notion of person-centred freedom of choice (Jacob et al., 2008). Furedi (2002) maintains that we currently live in a risk-averse society that sets an agenda of protection and prevention. A health example of this may be expectations of compliance with treatment, with health screening, and the promotion of healthy eating and smoking cessation.

Arguably, illness prevention and health promotion in nursing aim to change behaviour and make the assumption that they will be 'good' for the patient. The next section will look at a different approach to communication aimed at behaviour change.

Behaviour change and communication

Behavioural explanations of human existence maintain that people learn what is good and useful in the environment, and what is not good, not useful, or indeed harmful, by interacting with it. Socially, this means interacting with other people and striving to get on with others, and learning what to avoid. So, we learn as we develop socially and intellectually how to behave, think about, and understand our environment in ways that are 'adaptive'—that is, advantageous—and avoid doing things that we have learnt are maladaptive or disadvantageous.

As small children, we soon learn that hitting our younger sister is disadvantageous because we get told off. However, we also learn that picking on our younger sister is fun (advantageous) if we can get away with it. So we learn some very complex ways of behaving in our society as we grow up, and continue to learn how to adapt to new people, environments, and situations such as ill health through the principles of behavioural learning theory. The theory is often divided up into some key components, which we will examine.

Conditioning and reinforcement

When an animal, including a human, is exposed to an element in the environment for the first time, if something nice happens at the same time, the animal associates that element with something good.

You have probably learnt about Pavlov's experiment with dogs, in which the dogs heard a bell ringing every time they were fed. They soon anticipated food by salivating when they heard the bell, even when no food was present. A child will soon associate the chime of an ice cream van with a pleasant experience if they usually get an ice cream. Alternatively, a child may associate raised voices with fear of violence if they live in a violent household.

This process is called **classical conditioning** because it conditions someone biologically to expect a rewarding or punishing experience when an environmental trigger is present.

What humans and animals can also do is change their behaviour when faced with certain environmental factors. This could be to gain a rewarding experience or avoid a punishing one. This ability to learn to control events is called **operant conditioning** and was identified by a behaviourist called Skinner (1973), who trained rats to operate a lever in a cage to get a food pellet.

Suppose a child who lives in a violent household associates raised voices with being hit, or seeing someone they love being upset. By hiding or distracting themselves, the child does not get hit or see the violence. The next time the shouting starts, the child is likely to use that strategy again because it avoids the painful experience.

The child's avoidance behaviour is reinforced by a kind of reward—not having to experience as much of the trauma.

However, at school, this child may like the attention of a particular teacher, but the class is very big and the child doesn't stand out much. One day, the child is particularly frustrated and feeling bad and unloved, and hits another child. The child then gets lots of attention from the teacher. The next day, feeling bad, the child hits another classmate. This hitting behaviour has become a way of attracting attention and getting a positive stroke. Even being told off, for this child, is better than being ignored or being invisible.

This is called **reinforcement**, as the behaviour is 'reinforced' by the attention the child gets from the teacher. Reinforcement of behaviour requires a short-term association between the reinforcing stimuli and the 'pay-off' because it is learnt unconsciously. Humans can overcome this by learning consciously that longer-term consequences can be beneficial. For instance, most people would avoid the dentist, but we are aware that the pain is worth it in the long term. This is an important factor when it comes to overcoming unconscious learning. We will look at this in the next section, but, first, a quick reminder.

....

 Learning point 2: A reminder

Conditioning: Associating one trigger with a particular experience—positive or negative.
Reinforcement: A positive environmental effect that is a consequence of behaviour. It takes
the form either of a reward or of avoidance of something unpleasant.

....

Use of classical conditioning can be incorporated into specialist approaches to change serious maladaptive behaviour such as drug/alcohol addiction, and inappropriate sexual behaviour, but is probably most commonly used in nursing in child bedwetting, using an alarmed mattress that helps the child to associate the feelings of a full bladder with waking up.

Operant conditioning is often called behaviour modification and, apart from being used in specialist psychology, can be used effectively by nurses to target health behaviour change such as smoking cessation (Jansdottir and Jansdottir, 2001), wandering behaviour among people with dementia (Lai and Arthur, 2003), and obesity (Lindahl et al., 1999).

So, what has this to do with health communication? As health professionals, we are often faced with patients, relatives, and even colleagues who have learnt maladaptive ways of behaving and thinking that prevent them from adopting healthy lifestyles or having healthy relations with others. Let's look at some case study examples.

Case study 1: Maladaptive behaviour

1. A middle-aged divorced man with no current employment feels low, lonely, and worthless. He often drinks heavily to cheer himself up. This works in the short term, so every time he feels stressed, upset, or depressed, he drinks heavily. He has become alcohol-dependent, has liver damage, can't get a job because he is an alcoholic, and his teenage children don't visit him anymore.
2. A teenage girl used to be teased at school because she was fat. She went on a diet, and received lots of praise and attention for being slim. She now weighs 5½ stone, and is seriously underweight for her age and build.
3. An elderly gentleman with treatable bowel cancer refuses to go to hospital for an operation because he believes he will die on the operating table. Two years ago, his wife had a simple operation and died in hospital.
4. A boy with severe autism won't go to school without his Spiderman costume on as he associates it with being protected from other people. Without it, he has severe temper tantrums and anxieties, so his parents give in and let him wear his costume.

These examples are not uncommon patient problems. However, everyone we meet is subject to behavioural learning in some way, including ourselves. By understanding the principles of learning theory, we can incorporate them in our communication in professional relationships and aid people into more adaptive ways of engaging with health behaviour.

✚ Learning point 3

Before you read the answers below, take a minute to try to identify the likely conditioning triggers for the people in the case studies above, and what reinforcement they are getting for their unhelpful behaviour.

Possible answers to Learning point 3

1. This man is conditioned to associate alcohol with pleasure. His drinking behaviour is reinforced by avoiding negative feelings of stress and low mood by drinking. The more often he drinks, the more often he avoids feeling really bad, and therefore the more often he will use alcohol to avoid negative feelings.

2. This teenage girl is conditioned to associate being fat with being rejected by others. She has learnt that dieting/not eating avoids rejection and gains positive approval from others. Unfortunately, she has probably also associated not eating and feeling hungry with a sense of power over her body and other people and gets pleasure from resisting food.

3. This gentleman has probably learnt to associate the trauma of his wife's unexpected death with very powerful feelings of grief, shock, and possibly fear and mistrust. He is conditioned to link hospitals with fear of death and loss. By resisting invitations to go into hospital for treatment, he feels a sense of relief from his fear. He is using avoidance behaviour to reduce his grief and fear of death.

4. A severely autistic child usually finds other people and unfamiliar surroundings very threatening. This boy has associated Spiderman (and probably his identification with Spiderman) with safety and protection. The more he wears his Spiderman costume, the more he will associate safety with wearing the costume. He is also learning something else that is maladaptive: his parents give in when he has a temper tantrum, therefore this behaviour is being reinforced every time he gets his way.

The nurse–patient relationship has the potential to help service users to learn more positive ways of behaving and understanding situations through conditioning and reinforcement. The nurse can easily reward adaptive behaviour by communicating praise and positive attention, and help to reduce maladaptive behaviour with disapproval or lack of response (no reward). All of this is performed through communication. Let's look at some examples.

Example 1: avoiding reinforcing maladaptive behaviour

A depressed lady often makes herself feel worse by talking about how awful she feels. The nurse uses reinforcement to encourage the lady to talk positively and not dwell on her troubles.

Nurse: Hello, how are you feeling today?

Patient: Oh, nurse, I'm not good at all. I had those dreadful dreams in the night and woke up feeling worse than yesterday. I don't think I'll ever get better again.

Nurse (not responding to the negative comments): What are you planning today that will lift your mood?

Patient: I don't know. I can't think of anything.

Nurse: You liked the art group yesterday. What was it about that do you think that was good?

Patient: Well, it took my mind off things for a while.

Nurse: Good. That sounds like a great idea for today.

This nurse deliberately avoids rewarding the negative comments by ignoring them. Instead, the nurse encourages a positive comment and gives the patient a rewarding positive stroke when she says something less negative, and the nurse adds a suggestion that it was the patient's idea.

Incorrect use of power: teaching maladaptive behaviour

Conditioning can also be a very powerful factor in teaching maladaptive behaviour through inappropriate reinforcement. The power imbalance in the nurse–patient relationship can have a negative effect on people by reinforcing maladaptive behaviour. A good example of this is institutionalization, whereby long-term patients, such as those in elderly care, mental health rehabilitation, or learning disability homes, can become very dependent and compliant if overly controlled by the social environment (Goffman, 1961).

Example 2: punishing adaptive behaviour

A very reluctant child in hospital finally agrees to take his medication. The nurse has been getting frustrated by the child's previous refusals and replies as follows.

Nurse: So I should think, after all that fuss!

Here, the nurse has not rewarded the child for the adaptive behaviour, but made the child feel guilty (given punishment) for not complying in the first place. This child is unlikely to comply any more readily the next time.

Example 3: rewarding maladaptive behaviour

A patient in a psychiatric ward has deliberately cut her arm while feeling very upset and distressed. She shows the nurse the wound and the nurse says the following.

> Nurse: Oh your poor thing! You must have been feeling awful to do this. Let me stitch that up for you. What made you do this? I can't imagine what you must have been feeling to do this to yourself!

The patient needs attention, but not the sort that will encourage more self-harming behaviour. The nurse could attend to the wound, but talk about something else that is not rewarding. What she needs to avoid is both punishing the patient by telling her off and rewarding her by giving undue attention. The nurse could focus on what the patient could do instead of self-harming, such as talking to someone about how she feels, and encourage that behaviour instead with praise and positive attention.

 Learning point 4

Reflect on a situation you may have encountered in practice or in another aspect of your life in which you met someone who seemed to be seeking your attention and you couldn't get away. This may have been a patient who wanted to talk, or a child who wanted to keep showing you his or her toys. Considering the material above about rewarding through attention, what do you think were the factors that made this person persist in gaining your attention? What were you doing to reward this behaviour? What could you have done instead (politely!)? You might want to look forward to Chapter 7 and the section on assertiveness and saying 'no' for clues! You should also reflect on such incidents when they occur in practice and consider how you have used rewarding or non-rewarding communication to control the encounter.

Social learning theory

Modelling

We do not just need to experience the environment directly to learn what is rewarding or unpleasant. Another way in which we learn is through watching other people. The nurse can also become a role model of what is possible, or guide the person to other role models, reducing fear or anxiety and developing adaptive behaviour.

Have you ever watched a frightening film and been scared just because the characters in the film are scared? Why do you think you are scared? You are safe at home and there are no monsters or murderers lurking in the cupboards. What is happening is that you have 'identified' with the character in the film and are experiencing their environment vicariously (through their eyes). Alternatively, have you ever done something challenging because you have seen someone else do it successfully?

This is the principle of **vicarious learning** (Bandura, 1977): learning by observing others. People who have phobias about, for example, spiders will undergo exposure therapy. This may involve watching the therapist handle a spider before they handle the spider themselves.

The important element to this kind of learning is the relationship between the watcher and the person performing the behaviour. If the watcher cannot identify with the performer, they will not experience vicarious learning. You might watch a daredevil motorcyclist successfully leap a row of buses, but you probably would not identify with him or her and want have a go yourself.

The autistic boy in the last set of case studies associated safety with becoming Spiderman through watching a film. He learnt this vicariously, and this conditioning was reinforced by not coming to harm when he had his costume on.

Example 4: identification and role modelling

A 5-year-old child at the diabetes clinic is learning to have insulin injections. The nurse tells a story about how the teddy at the clinic has insulin injections, but he doesn't mind. The nurse shows the child how the teddy has his insulin and how teddy can then go and play. The nurse has communicated to the child that having an insulin injection is routine and allows people to lead a normal life. The nurse is using role modelling through the teddy and the child is learning vicariously by identifying with the teddy.

Example 5: role modelling unprofessional behaviour

An annoyed staff nurse walks into the office in which a student nurse and two healthcare assistants are sitting.

> Staff nurse: That doctor is so lazy! I've had to do all the bloods and observations for him while he just watched and ordered me about. He likes to show off in front of the patients! He doesn't know anything about teamwork!

This nurse, while obviously annoyed, has modelled unprofessional behaviour in front of junior staff by denigrating a member of the multidisciplinary team. The junior staff members are likely to copy this behaviour—even if it includes denigrating the staff nurse!

Self-efficacy

The last important element to learning theory that we will cover here is self-efficacy. Self-efficacy is the innate concept of ourselves that, whatever happens, we have the ability to do something positive, believe that we will survive, and have the confidence to rely on our own inner resources to get through. Albert Bandura described self-efficacy as the belief that one can perform effectively, and this is brought about best by actually overcoming feared or difficult situations (Bandura, 1977).

If you do something you never thought you'd be able to do, you are likely to experience a great sense of well-being, pride in yourself, and good self-esteem. If you perceive it as a major achievement, you are likely to go on to do other things that you previously thought were beyond your capabilities. Young people from deprived backgrounds who go on 'outward bound' courses and conquer mountains; a 'couch potato' who runs a marathon; learning disabled students who gain a degree: all of these are examples of people whose confidence is boosted by their achievements because their sense of self-efficacy has increased massively.

Nurses have the opportunity to develop another's self-efficacy by changing the way in which they see themselves and what they think they are capable of. For example, Lee et al. (2008) found improved and maintained exercise activity among older people when the theory of self-efficacy was incorporated into exercise programmes. These programmes included using verbal encouragement and helping people to feel good about their exercise (rewarding), vicarious learning (watching others achieve), and the experience of achievement (self-efficacy).

However, nurses are also in a position to reduce someone's self-efficacy by encouraging dependence.

Example 6: encouraging dependency—reducing self-efficacy

A nurse is with an anxious parent of a young boy with cerebral palsy. He has tantrums and becomes aggressive when he can't do things that his brothers can do. His mother is very stressed.

> Mother: I can't cope when he has a tantrum. He's too big for me to manage physically now. I don't know what's going to happen in the future. I won't be able to cope.
>
> Nurse: It is very hard. That's why you need lots of support. I and my colleagues will always be able to give advice and support when you need it.

Apart from promising support in the future that may not be there, the nurse is reinforcing the thought that the parent won't be able to cope on her own. This takes away the sense of self-efficacy that the mother needs to build up.

The nurse could have said the following.

> Nurse: You might not think so now, but you will discover ways of coping. What we could do now is explore those together and help you to find solutions.

This does not reinforce a sense of dependency. It encourages the person to be realistic but hopeful. It does promise collaboration, which is realistic, and coping better in the future.

Summary of behavioural approaches

Behavioural approaches to human relations could be seen as incompatible with the humanistic philosophy. They can be seen as empowering the practitioner to manipulate the patient into behaviour change. The result can often be that not only is the person behaving in a different way, but also they may not realize that they have been unconsciously guided into changing their behaviour. However, it may be as important to understand how nurses' power can affect patient's behaviour, and to avoid reinforcing and role modelling maladaptive behaviour and discouraging adaptive behaviour.

The cognitive behavioural approach

An approach that is expanding from its original mental health roots into other health settings is **cognitive behavioural therapy (CBT)**. It is described as a talking therapy by NICE (2006) and, over the last three decades, has been a therapeutic approach for depression and anxiety-related psychiatric problems (Hawton et al., 1989). However, it has expanded across a range of healthcare fields as a health promotion approach, especially where behaviour change and coping with chronic illness are key care needs, and has been shown to be delivered effectively by nurses (Brown and Marshall, 2006; Espie et al., 2008; Cort et al., 2009; Heslop et al., 2009; Moorey et al., 2009; Warrilow and Beech, 2009). Possibly an important element to the development of CBT is that it empowers the individual patient to make choices and change behaviour, and therefore may have a stronger claim to ethically based practice than perhaps does the purely behavioural approach.

Cognitive behavioural therapy is sometimes referred to as the 'three systems' approach (Richards and McDonald, 1990), or 'cognitive triad' (Beck, 1976), because it addresses behaviour, cognitions, and physical/emotional responses, and recognizes that these elements are dynamically linked. The principles of CBT are the same as behavioural and social learning theory, but, instead of focusing on what people do, it focuses on how people *think* about and *perceive* their situation. It recognizes that people are conditioned to associate one thing with another, but also that we often learn how to think about situations in ways that are maladaptive, just because they may have worked once or in the short term.

Figure 6.2 illustrates the sequence of events using the three systems of thoughts, feelings, and behaviour that link how we perceive a situation and consequently respond.

Box 6.1 illustrates a maladaptive sequence of events.

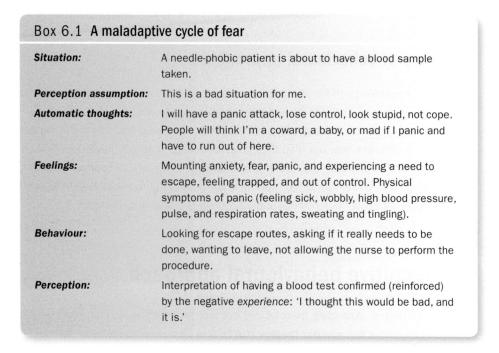

Box 6.1 A maladaptive cycle of fear

Situation:	A needle-phobic patient is about to have a blood sample taken.
Perception assumption:	This is a bad situation for me.
Automatic thoughts:	I will have a panic attack, lose control, look stupid, not cope. People will think I'm a coward, a baby, or mad if I panic and have to run out of here.
Feelings:	Mounting anxiety, fear, panic, and experiencing a need to escape, feeling trapped, and out of control. Physical symptoms of panic (feeling sick, wobbly, high blood pressure, pulse, and respiration rates, sweating and tingling).
Behaviour:	Looking for escape routes, asking if it really needs to be done, wanting to leave, not allowing the nurse to perform the procedure.
Perception:	Interpretation of having a blood test confirmed (reinforced) by the negative *experience*: 'I thought this would be bad, and it is.'

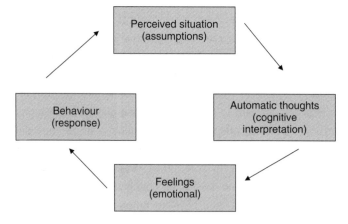

Figure 6.2 The three-systems cycle

We will add a good nursing intervention to this scenario. The nurse understands the cycle of panic that links thoughts to feelings and behaviour and notices that this patient looks worried. The nurse could use several different ways of interrupting this patient's cycle of maladaptive thinking, feeling, and behaving.

1. If the anxiety is mild: change the thoughts from negative to positive—remind the patient that it will help resolve their health problems when the results are back.
2. If more marked: distract the patient from thinking about what is happening— ask about their journey here, what they may be doing later, where they bought that lovely jacket from—anything that makes the patient focus on something rewarding about themselves rather than their fear.
3. If the anxiety is serious: put the patient in control—ask what would help the patient to have the procedure done less traumatically. Do they want to say when to do it? Do they want the door open/closed? Do they need privacy (to combat the 'everyone will think I'm stupid' thoughts)? Reassure the patient that other people hate needles and so it's not a stupid thing to worry about.

Many of us would perform these reassuring communications automatically to help a worried patient, but by understanding what may be happening for the patient, the nurse can easily assess the patient's perceptions and thoughts, and judge which communication intervention is most appropriate.

In the example in Box 6.1, certain automatic thoughts may seem absurd or irrational. However, we may have developed habitual use of certain ways of thinking. They epitomize how we see the world and interpret our role in it. In CBT, these 'unhelpful' or 'maladaptive' thoughts are regarded as dysfunctional because they stop us thinking about a situation realistically.

Dysfunctional thinking styles

Dysfunctional thinking has been defined as being 'beliefs which individuals hold about the world and themselves which . . . make them prone to interpret specific situations in an excessively negative and dysfunctional fashion' (Hawton et al., 1989: 55).

Certain words or phrases that people use indicate to the listener how they perceive themselves and the world. Nurses listening attentively can pick up on negative statements that are not realistic and challenge the patient to revise their way of thinking. See Table 6.1 for some examples of dysfunctional negative thinking and the kind of phrases that give clues to the patient's assumptions.

Table 6.1 Dysfunctional thinking beliefs

Common negative unrealistic thoughts (examples)	Realistic alternative (negative)	Realistic alternative (positive)
I can't . . .		
learn to inject myself	I might not be able to	I might be able to
It's not fair . . .		
I have this disease	My life will change for the worse	I don't know how my life will change
I will fail/die/look stupid . . .		
attending group therapy	I am afraid to try in case I don't fit in	I might fit in if I try. But it doesn't matter if I don't. (What's the worst that could happen?)
They won't like me . . .		
at the day centre	I am afraid to go in case I don't like it	It doesn't matter if I don't like it. I can go and see.

There's nothing wrong with recognizing the reality of a situation, but if the person is making an assumption, we can challenge their view of the world. The key to detecting unhelpful thinking is whether it is *realistic*. If the statement suggests that the person has a realistic understanding of the situation, this indicates helpful thinking. See Table 6.2 for some very common examples in health care.

Useful challenges to unrealistic thinking include: 'Why?' Who says? Where's your evidence? How do you know?

Table 6.2 Clues to unhelpful thinking

Unhelpful word	Example	Unhelpful because:
Can't	'I can't stop smoking.'	Restricts options and doesn't look at the evidence.
Should	'I should be able to remember . . .'	Why? Imposes too great an expectation on self and sets the person up to experience failure.
Shouldn't	'She shouldn't talk to me like that.'	But she does! That's the reality. Leads to unhelpful thoughts such as 'it's not fair'.
Must	'I must do better at . . .'	Who says? This makes an outcome dependent on certain behaviour. Sets the person up to fail.
Wouldn't	'I wouldn't have to do this if . . .' (Very common among nursing teams!)	How do you know? The reality is that the person *has chosen* to do this. There is always a choice.
Ought	'I ought to know better.'	Does not recognize the reality and sets unachievable standards. Expectations are too high.

Practice example box 3: Challenging negative thoughts

A patient insisted she couldn't go on a beach holiday because her burn scars looked so horrible. She said she would feel everyone was looking at her and thinking she should cover herself up in public. The nurse picked up on her assumptions about what people would think and identified that 'should' meant that people would judge her by her appearance. The nurse and patient examined the assumptions behind her thoughts and concluded that: 'People are unlikely to judge her negatively, think badly of her, and anyway what did it matter as it was their problem, not hers.' The lady went on the beach holiday.

Whenever you find yourself with a patient who appears 'stuck' in a form of unhealthy behaviour or not complying with treatment, listen to the reasons that the person gives for his or her behaviour. You may pick up on phrases or words used that suggest the person's unhelpful thinking style that may lie at the root of their problems in changing behaviour.

 You will find an example of humanistic and behavioural models working together in Chapter 15 on motivational interviewing.

Conclusion

This chapter links to previous chapters in Part 1 on the nurse/patient relationship and active listening, and further chapters in Part 3, particularly on promoting health. The earlier chapters outline the basic skills and theories of communication, and this chapter illustrates some of the models or approaches that provide a framework for those skills. Part 3 will address both the basic skills and the frameworks in application to specific health-related practice.

You will find an example of cognitive behavioural and motivational approach to interviewing on the Online Resource Centre. See also the video 'Active listening 3' for an example of eye contact for reading a level 3 disclosure.

 To find more resources to aid your learning, please now go online to **www.oxfordtextbooks.co.uk/orc/webb**

Further reading

Bennett-Levy, J., Richards, D., Farrand, P., Christensen, H., Griffiths, K., et al. (2010) *Oxford Guide to Low-intensity CBT Interventions*. Oxford: Oxford University Press.

Davies-Smith, L. (2006) 'An Introduction to Providing Cognitive Behavioural Therapy', *Nursing Times*, 102(26): 28–30.

References

Bandura, A. (1977) *Social Learning Theory*. Englewood Cliffs, NJ: Prentice Hall.

Beck, A. (1976). *Cognitive Therapy and the Emotional Disorders*. New York: International Universities Press.

Brown, M. and Marshall, K. (2006) 'Cognitive Behaviour Therapy and People with Learning Disabilities: Implications for Developing Nursing Practice', *Journal of Psychiatric and Mental Health Nursing*, 13(2): 234–41.

Cort, E., Moorey, S., Hotopf, M., Kapari, M., Monroe, B., and Hansford, P. (2009) 'Palliative Care Nurses' Experiences of Training in Cognitive Behaviour Therapy and Taking Part in a Randomized Controlled Trial', *International Journal of Palliative Nursing*, 15(6): 290–8.

Cox, M. (1978) *Structuring the Therapeutic Process: Compromise with Chaos*. London: Jessica Kingsley Press.

Egan, G. (1986) *The Skilled Helper: A Systematic Approach to Effective Helping*. Belmont, CA: Brooks/Cole.

Espie, C., Fleming, L., Cassidy, J., Samuel, L., Taylor, M., et al. (2008) 'Randomized Controlled Clinical Effectiveness Trial of Cognitive Behaviour Therapy Compared with Treatment as Usual for Persistent Insomnia in Patients with Cancer', *Journal of Clinical Oncology*, 26(28): 4651–8.

Fox, S. and Chesla, C. (2008) 'Living with Chronic Illness: A Phenomenological Study of the Health Effects of the Patient–Provider Relationship', *Journal of the American Academy of Nurse Practitioners*, 20(3): 109–17.

Furedi, F. (2002) *The Culture of Fear: Risk-taking and the Morality of Low-expectation Risk-taking*. London: Continuum.

Gaillard, L., Shattell, M., and Thomas, S. (2009) 'Mental Health Patients' Experiences of Being Misunderstood', *Journal of the American Psychiatric Nurses Association*, 15(3): 191–9.

Goffman, E. (1961) *Asylums*. Harmondsworth: Penguin Books.

Hawton, K., Salkovskis, P., Kirk, J., and Clark, D. (1989) *Cognitive Behaviour Therapy for Psychiatric Problems: A Practical Guide*. Oxford: Oxford Medical Publications.

Heslop, K., De Soya, A., Baker, C., Stenton, C., and Burns, G. (2009) 'Using Individualised Cognitive Behavioural Therapy as a Treatment for People with COPD', *Nursing Times*, 105(14): 14–17.

Iranmanesh, S., Axelsson, K., Savenstedt, S., and Haggstrom, T. (2009) 'A Caring Relationship with People Who Have Cancer', *Journal of Advanced Nursing*, 65(6): 1300–8.

Jacob, J., Holmes, D., and Buus, N. (2008) 'Humanism in Forensic Psychiatry: The Use of the Tidal Nursing Model', *Nursing Inquiry*, 15(3): 224–30.

Jansdottir, D. and Jansdottir, H. (2001) 'Does Physical Exercise in Addition to a Multicomponent Smoking Cessation Program Increase Abstinence Rate and Suppress Weight Gain? An Intervention Study', *Scandinavian Journal of Caring Sciences*, 15(4): 275–82.

Kohr, R. and Gibson, M. (2008) 'Doing the Right Thing: Using Hermeneutic Phenomenology to Understand Management of Wound Pain', *Ostomy Wound Management*, 54(4): 52–60.

Lai, C. and Arthur, D. (2003) 'Wandering Behaviour in People with Dementia', *Journal of Advanced Nursing*, 44(2): 173–82.

Lee, L.-L., Antony, A., and Avis, M. (2008) 'Using Self-efficacy Theory to Develop Interventions that Help Older People Overcome Psychological Barriers to Physical Activity', *International Journal of Nursing Studies*, 45(11): 1690–9.

Lindahl, B., Nilsson, T., Jansson, J., Asplund, K., and Hallmans, G. (1999) 'Improved Fibrinolysis by Intense Lifestyle Intervention: A Randomised Trial in Subjects with Impaired Glucose Tolerance', *Journal of Internal Medicine*, 246(1): 105–12.

Maslow, A. (1970) *Motivation and Personality*. New York: Harper and Row.

Moorey, S., Cort, E., Kapari, M., Monroe, B., Hansford, P., Mannix, K., et al. (2009) 'A Cluster Randomized Controlled Trial of Cognitive Behaviour Therapy for Common Mental Disorders in Patients with Advanced Cancer', *Psychological Medicine*, 39(5): 713–23.

National Institute for Health and Clinical Excellence (2006) *Psychological Therapies*. London: NICE.

Persson, M. and Febe, F. (2009) 'The Dramatic Encounter: Experiences of Taking Part in a Health Conversation', *Journal of Clinical Nursing*, 18(4): 520–8.

Richards, D. and McDonald, B. (1990) *Behavioural Psychotherapy: A Handbook for Nurses*. Oxford: Heinemann Nursing.

Rogers, C. (1961) *On Becoming a Person: A Therapist's View of Psychotherapy*. London: Constable.

Rotter, J. (1966) 'Generalized Expectancies for Internal Versus External Control of Reinforcement', *Psychological Monographs*, 30(1): 1–26.

Sigurgeirsdottir, J. and Halldorsdottir, S. (2008) 'Existential Struggle and Self-reported Needs of Patients in Rehabilitation', *Journal of Advanced Nursing*, 61(4): 384–92.

Skinner, B. (1973) *Beyond Freedom and Dignity*. Harmondsworth: Penguin.

Warrilow A. and Beech, B. (2009) 'Self-help CBT for Depression: Opportunities for Primary Care Mental Health Nurses?', *Journal of Psychiatric and Mental Health Nursing*, 16(9): 792–803.

Facing challenges in healthcare communication

Lucy Webb

This chapter will help you to achieve competencies in:

- ➲ recognizing and acting to overcome barriers in developing effective relationships with patients;
- ➲ being accepting of differing cultural traditions, beliefs, UK legal frameworks, and professional ethics;
- ➲ managing and diffusing challenging situations effectively;
- ➲ making appropriate use of the environment, self, and skills, and adopting an appropriate attitude;
- ➲ communicating effectively and sensitively in different settings, using a range of methods and skills;
- ➲ using appropriate and relevant communication skills to deal with difficult and challenging circumstances;
- ➲ selecting and applying appropriate strategies and techniques for conflict resolution and de-escalation in the management of potential violence and aggression.

Introduction

This chapter outlines some of the hazards and challenges often met when attempting communication in a range of health settings. We will give tips, advice, and guidance on common difficulties found in challenging circumstances such as in the patient's home, where there is cultural and communication difference, crossing professional boundaries, or where others are hostile or unwilling. This will also include skills development in helping the student to manage communication that they personally find difficult.

The domiciliary visit

The nurse in the community is required to deliver quality care outside the hospital environment and this often means in the patient's own home. This is the 'domiciliary visit' and can present several communication challenges from the outset, even before tackling the health need itself. As you have seen in Chapter 1, communication can be seen in light of power dynamics, where power is often enhanced for the nurse when the patient is out of his or her comfort zone, but the nurse is surrounded by supportive colleagues and the trappings of power, such as a uniform and institutionalized processes and customs.

Common problems

When we visit a patient in their own home, the balance of power shifts towards the patient. The nurse becomes subject to the rules and social customs of being a guest in someone else's house. We will need to be invited inside, may be required to take our shoes off when entering, will need to ask to use resources such as a basin, toilet, or rubbish bin, and may have to negotiate around offers of tea and coffee! As a health professional in the community, we may be on our own or as a student with a lone practitioner, while our patient may have family and friends present. Also, the environment itself can present factors we have little control over. Children love to be involved with whatever is going on and often seek attention. Pets can be similarly distracting. We rely on the patient or relative to control these distractions. People may have visitors when we call, or phone calls from chatty friends. It is remarkable how many people keep their televisions switched on when a visitor arrives. This is distracting for both the patient and the nurse and presents a communication barrier.

To get the best out of your patient–nurse interaction in the patient's home, you need to ensure that the environment is suitable for good communication. You may need to be assertive and take charge, whilst being sensitive to issues of consent.

Being assertive

Many people being visited at home by a health professional will view that person as an authority figure with skills they depend on. They will be quite happy for you to set the agenda for your visit, be business-like, and take charge. By being assertive from the outset, you are not likely to present the patient with anything unexpected. Assertiveness is a personal skill or quality that enables a person to give their opinions and manage their social boundaries without aggressiveness and without passive submission. An assertive person can give instructions to others and say 'no' to others in a way that demonstrates confidence and flexibility. So, how do we use assertiveness to control the environment in a patient's home?

Set the boundaries for the encounter at the outset

> Nurse: Hello. Are you Mrs Smith? I am [your full name], the student nurse from the surgery. I've come to check your dressings. It should only take about 10 minutes. Is now a good time?

This is a good opening. You have stated your intent, your time boundary, and your task boundary (what you are visiting for). You have also given the person an opportunity to give consent. After all, it might be a very difficult time for Mrs Smith—the boiler might have just exploded!

When inside, check the environment for anything that might present a communication barrier, especially if you are likely to have an exchange that requires privacy and sensitivity.

Which room is best to use? Mrs Smith is about to lead you to the kitchen, where you can see Mr Smith having his lunch. You can see that the living room is free.

> Nurse: Shall we go in here, Mrs Smith There's probably more room in here, and I don't want to disturb Mr Smith.

By simply directing Mrs Smith politely to what *you* want, you have asserted that your judgement is important. But you have given her the choice: after all, it is her home.

The television is on and quite loud, as Mrs Smith is a touch hard of hearing.

> Nurse: I'll just turn the television off, so that we can talk properly.

Get the television switched off rather than turning the sound down as pictures are distracting too.

Mr Smith wanders in when he's finished his lunch and takes an interest in what you are doing. You will have to judge if this is a problem for Mrs Smith, as it could constitute a breach of confidentiality or more simply interfere with any intimate issues that she might want to discuss with you. It may be up to you to protect the privacy and dignity of your patient. The nurse may be required to take charge of the situation and exclude Mr Smith, but asking someone to leave his or her own living room is ethically tricky. In this situation, it is appropriate to use the authority of the health professional, but you will still need to elicit cooperation and consent.

> Nurse: Mr Smith, I just need to see Mrs Smith alone for a few moments while I do my assessment. Would you mind waiting outside until I have finished?

Note the use of the word 'I': 'I', the nurse/health professional/expert, not 'we', Mrs Smith and I. This asserts that you, the professional, have a job to do and you are required to do this job in a certain way. It does not compromise the relationship between Mr and Mrs Smith.

Saying 'no' assertively

In many domiciliary situations, the health professional is more likely to be overwhelmed with kindness than need to direct others. This sort of scenario also requires assertiveness, because a community worker can only drink so many cups of tea a day and needs to get all of their appointments done before midnight! So, assertiveness is important in limiting the amount of time and attention that you can give. Start as you mean to go on by setting your boundaries.

> Nurse: This will only take 10 minutes.

This is a good start to flag up the time you have got.

> Nurse: No tea today, thank you. I've got quite a bit to do today. Now, let's have a look at that leg and you can tell me how you are getting on.

In other words: 'I can't stop for long, let's get down to business—but I still have time to hear your difficulties.'

There are loads of ways to say 'no', but not all of them are assertive. Look at the list in Box 7.1 and see which you think are assertive, and which are non-assertive (passive).

Box 7.1 Assertive and non-assertive statements

- No, thank you.
- I'd rather not.
- No, I'm fine, thanks.
- I don't think that's a good idea.
- No, not that way.
- That's not quite right.
- No.

Easy, isn't it? All of the assertive phrases have the word 'no' in them. We don't like to hurt people's feelings, but 'no' is the easiest way to say 'no'. Most phrases of refusal that do not contain the word 'no' are not as assertive as refusal phrases that contain the word 'no'.

And, when pressed, simply repeat the word—in another way if you like (see Box 7.2).

Box 7.2 Reinforcing assertiveness

- No, honestly, I can't.
- No, really.

⊕ Learning point 1

Next time you want to refuse something, note how you phrase it. Are you good at saying 'no'? When are you not good at saying 'no'? In what circumstances, with whom, and where?

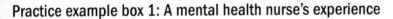

Practice example box 1: A mental health nurse's experience

'I was asked to see a teenager at home with his family because his key worker couldn't get to the root of his problem behaviour. On arrival, I found his architecturally designed house to be very open-plan, with no doors downstairs between rooms and an open space to the upstairs mezzanine floor. It was impossible to have a securely private conversation with him in the normal way.

'After assessing the risks, I interviewed him in his bedroom (it had a closable door). The disclosure that followed explained the root of his distress and also explained his reluctance to share this information with his family.

'His key worker was bound by risk protocol not to interview him alone, but as a registered nurse, I was able to make my own judgement and facilitate a therapeutic environment.'

(Mental health nurse)

Cultural difference and using interpreters

Whole books are written on culture and culture difference in health care, so this part of the chapter aims to focus specifically on problem-solving in order to reduce the communication barriers presented by culture and language difference. Further reading will be provided at the end of the chapter for those who would like to explore the subject in more detail for assignments.

Perhaps we can content ourselves with one definition of culture, from Mclaren (1998), who describes culture as including knowledge, belief, laws, and customs, and other attributes acquired by a person as a member of a society. We are all influenced by our culture, but often find it difficult to discern our own—which to us is 'normal', unless we are faced with 'difference'. Also we usually recognize the difference in communication 'rules' that suddenly present us with misunderstandings. Holland and Hogg (2010) warn that every nurse–patient relationship involves three cultures: of the nurse, the patient, and the organization. As we identified earlier in this chapter, the nurse is likely to be more comfortable with the organizational culture, putting the patient in a doubly uncomfortable position in this relationship.

The subtleties of meaning in interpersonal communication between two people of a similar culture or even subculture often come down to shared cultural phrases, facial expressions, gestures, and even inflections (DeVito, 1988). You only have to observe two young teenagers conversing to realize that their 'culture' of age and role in society confers shared language and communication norms all of their own. Verbal expressions can mean one thing to one social culture and quite the opposite in another. For example, it took a while for the older generation to realize that a young person may use the word 'bad' to mean 'good'! This could be very confusing unless the individuals on either side of the conversation make adjustments. The same could apply to gestures or inflections. If we extrapolate from the age difference culture to ethnicity differences, we can see that unless we all understand, recognize, and make adjustments to different cultural meanings, communication across cultural divides will be full of misunderstanding and miscommunication. This should be a concern for nurses who are committed to ensuring social inclusion and respecting diversity and the beliefs, rights, and wishes of individuals, groups, and communities, and are expected to challenge inequality, discrimination, or exclusion from access to care (NMC, 2010). It is recognized that certain cultural and ethnic groups have particular healthcare needs and face specific barriers to health care. Asylum seekers and refugees have specific health problems resulting from physical and mental trauma and often face social isolation, lack of understanding, and barriers of language and communication (Burnett and Peel, 2001). For instance, people from these communities may lack access to information on health and not understand how to access health care. Women are less likely to speak English or be the spokesperson for the family in traditionally male-led cultures, and unaccompanied children are likely to be particularly vulnerable and need social care and support (Burnett and Peel, 2001).

Let's have a look at some common problems.

Cultural difference

Clearly, the most obvious communication barriers are when two people do not understand each other's language. For some simple situations, and between people who at least share similar cultures, this may not be such a problem, as gestures at least are similar between the two. For example, take two Western Europeans who share a general ethnic culture, but not language. One could easily gesture a simple message, such as 'I'm in pain', which would be quite clear to the other, and indicate where the pain is and how bad it is.

Two people of markedly different cultures and language, however, may find this harder. For example, expressing pain may be socially unacceptable in the patient's culture, or pointing to signify 'you' or 'I' may simply confuse a patient who regards pointing as rude or aggressive. In Western medicine, health and illness are regarded as physical entities that are separate from spirituality or social well-being. In some health belief systems, however, there is no division between the body and the mind or spirit and illness may be explained in terms of the person's poor moral behaviour or being possessed by something evil. Understanding cultural expressions of health and illness requires us to take into account the values, norms, and ways of understanding with which the person has been brought up. The person's health beliefs may include the individual's cultural definition of health, their environment (including the physical, social, and symbolic environment they are and have been in), and cultural variations around their own health practices, beliefs, taboos, and rites of passage (Hogg, 2010). See Practice example box 2 for a real practice example of a clash of symbolisms that stem from different values and experiences.

Practice example box 2: Differences in cultural symbolism

A young black gay man brought up in apartheid South Africa was referred to a community mental health team in South Wales with worrying symptoms of paranoia. In discussing which nurse to refer him to, it was agreed that a particular male nurse would be suitable because of the match in age and sex. However, the nurse was a rugby-playing, white, and rather macho personality, and the patient had been brought up in a persecutory social environment in which white, male authority figures were often the persecutors and homosexuality was stigmatized. It appeared that the referral decision had not addressed the different values of masculinity (epitomized in rugby in both cultures), homosexuality, and social divisions between the patient and the nurse.

Expressions of culture in communication can also be different within areas of acceptable personal space, touch, and making direct eye contact. The health professional's awareness of non-verbal expression is important, as it can enhance the ability to deliver care. A case in point would be the experience of pain, which varies in communities due to the combination of language and cultural norms. People who are not used to the Western approach to medicine can be unused to the specific way in which pain is described or experienced. In a comparison between European mountain climbers and Nepalese porters, for example, the porters would not report the European's pain experience as 'painful', perhaps because they simply regard 'pain' as a normal experience (Halliday, 1992). Therefore, if a person with this belief system were asked 'where is the pain?', he or she may report that there is no pain.

In an important study of women with cervical cancer, Bond and Pearson (1969) found that expressed pain varied depending on the women's personality type: the higher the woman's emotionality, the more painkillers she requested. The essential skill of communication that a health professional should possess is to remember that cultural issues should not be reduced to obvious 'expressions' of culture (and religion) such as dress, food, or skin colour, but recognized as an aspect of care that is unique to each individual patient, whatever their background.

Burnett and Peel (2001) suggest six key points, summarized below, which may help to guide the health practitioner.

- People have differing experiences and expectations of health care. They are not a homogeneous group.

- Symptoms of psychological distress do not necessarily signify mental illness.
- Trained interpreters or advocates should be used.
- Community organizations can reduce isolation.
- Particular difficulties faced by women should no be overlooked.
- Support for children, especially unaccompanied, needs to be multifaceted and multi-agency.

Language difference and the use of interpreters

Nurses in many open societies are likely to encounter people with very little language and cultural understanding of the society: for example, migrant workers and their families, asylum-seekers, and refugees. In such cases, it may be seen that having an interpreter would be the ideal solution where language difference is a communication barrier, but this in itself can present problems of which it is helpful to be aware. Practice example box 3 illustrates a classic problem with using an interpreter.

Practice example box 3: The specialist sign language interpreter's perspective

'I try to remain simply an objective tool for interpretation, but this is often impossible. A deaf patient with a psychotic illness kept asking me to help him as he didn't trust the nurse conducting the interview. I tried to reassure him, but had to translate what I was saying for the nurse's benefit. If the nurse said anything to me, I needed to translate that as well to the deaf person. The patient wanted to see me as someone on his side and asked me not to translate everything he said. The nurse then got frustrated because he didn't know what we were saying. The nurse was unhelpful because he didn't recognize the difficulty I was having in remaining objective and kept including me in the conversation. In the end, I had to tell both of them how to use me in the role effectively.'

(Sign language interpreter)

It is difficult to have a third party present without that person becoming part of the triad rather than just facilitating a dyad.

 See Chapter 5 for an introduction to dyads and triads.

Nurses are now required to recognize the need for an interpreter (NMC, 2010) to support communication. To do that, we need to understand how interpreters can facilitate or present a barrier to communication. Research by Gerrish (2004) and Rhodes (2003) found that nurses had inadequate training, understanding, or support in using interpreters and usually relied on family members to facilitate communication with patients. Where professional interpreters were used, access to them was controlled by the nurse. This is seen as reducing the patient's access to health care through restricted communication and access to professional interpreters.

Professional interpreters are trained to keep their role as objective as possible but also to help the two interlocutors to understand each other's position. The professional interpreter 'interprets' meanings rather than just translates (Tribe, 2007). A sign-language interpreter, for instance, may advise the hearing person on their pace of speech or gestures. A language interpreter may also advise people of cultural misunderstandings associated with expressions or behaviour. For example, close proximity may be quite uncomfortable for one and normal for the other. A good interpreter will be aware of this and give advice.

Unfortunately, professional and specialist interpreters are rarely available for routine and daily communication, so healthcare workers often rely on health colleagues or family and friends of the patient (Rea, 2004). This presents many problems of which a practitioner needs to be aware.

1. **Using an adult relative:** this presents confidentiality problems and sometimes reluctance from the patient to divulge personal information. Also, a close relative often speaks *for* the patient rather than represents the patient's own communication accurately for example, 'my wife is fine, she doesn't want to make any fuss'.

2. **Using children:** often it is the case that children of first-generation immigrant families speak the host language better than the parents. This is a threat to confidentiality, but also risks parent inhibition, as parents may feel uncomfortable in discussing health and social issues with their children present. Importantly, using a child to interpret could be seen as exposing the child to harm. See Practice example box 4 for a real-case example.

3. **Using other non-professional interpreters:** again, there is a confidentiality issue if the interpreter is not a qualified health or social care professional. Also, non-professional interpreters have a tendency to get overinvolved with the issues being discussed. Additionally, where small minority populations are concerned, the informal interpreter may have knowledge of the patient. See Practice example box 5 for a real-case example.

....

➕ Learning point 2

When you start each placement, ask your mentor if there are trust or employer guidelines or policies on use of non-professional interpreters. Perhaps there is a local charity that provides interpreters in your area?

....

Practice example box 4: A child as an interpreter

A Tamil-speaking gentleman arrived in a London A&E with delirium tremens (DTs). He was hallucinating, distressed, and very frightened and suspicious. His wife and child (a boy aged 10) accompanied him.

A&E staff and the mother initially relied on the boy to translate information about what was wrong and pass on reassurance from the staff to the mother and the father. The boy was therefore present and witnessed his father behaving in a distressed manner, and had to translate details about his alcoholism, hallucinations, and anxieties. He also had to pass on reassurance to his parents in a form of parent–child role-reversal. Senior staff recognized that this situation was likely to put the child at emotional risk. The assessment was postponed until a Tamil-speaking doctor was found from another department to act as interpreter.

Practice example box 5: The informal interpreter

A Portuguese gentleman needed to give informed consent to a fairly routine, but personal, treatment procedure. A professional interpreter was not available for many hours, potentially delaying the procedure. However, a hospital-wide search found a member of the catering staff who was Portuguese and spoke good English. This lady was pleased to help and translated the information the gentleman needed, and he clearly consented to the procedure. On leaving the ward, the lady then said to the nurse as an aside that she knew his family, they were a bad sort, and she wasn't surprised he had become ill!

Guidance for working with interpreters

From the above examples and evidence, we can outline simple but worthwhile practices when dealing with language differences.

When using a professional interpreter

1. Be aware of the need to remain a dyad with a facilitator rather than allow the conversation to become a triad. Watch your boundaries.
2. Check with your interpreter beforehand for any cultural rules or guidelines that the interpreter needs you to follow.
3. Ensure that your interpreter remains professionally objective during the interview, but recognize that sometimes it is useful, and fairly likely, if the patient experiences relief and assurance at having someone to talk to in their own language.

When using a non-professional interpreter

1. Ensure confidentiality as much as possible—you can be guided by what is in the patient's best interests.
2. Check for any trust or employer guidelines or policies on use of non-professional interpreters.
3. *Do not* use children as interpreters for anything except simple and routine communication. Therapeutic, diagnostic, placatory, or other interventional communications are likely to place the child at risk of emotional harm.
4. Be guided by the potential harm and what is in the patient's best interests against loss of confidentiality, patient respect, dignity, and misinterpretation when using a non-professional interpreter.
5. Remember that the presence of a non-professional interpreter may mean that the patient has not disclosed relevant information.

You can find links to further advice and guidelines on:
www.mentalhealth.harpweb.org.uk

See the Online Resource Centre video 'Working with interpreters' for first-hand practitioner tips. Go to **www.oxfordtextbooks.co.uk/orc/webb**

Taking 'reasonable steps' to facilitate communication for informed consent

All healthcare practitioners need to be aware that communication difficulties can impair a patient's ability to give informed consent. Nurses in the UK are directed by the Mental Capacity Act 2005, the Disability Discrimination Act 2009, and the NMC (2008) to take 'reasonable steps' to facilitate information-giving, understanding, and expressing consent or withdrawal of consent as communicated by the patient. This includes using interpreters and other means of communication across cultural and language divides in order to demonstrate 'reasonable steps' under the law and in line with the NMC Code (NMC, 2008). Therefore, if we cannot understand our patients, or they cannot understand us, this does not mean that we can accept this as an inevitable barrier and continue to give treatment regardless, on the basis of it being in the patient's best interests. As nurses, we are expected to take reasonable steps to overcome cultural and language barriers in order to obtain informed consent before we deliver care.

Dealing with reluctance, resistance, and strong emotions

This leads us on to further barriers to delivering care that can come from reluctance, resistance, and strong emotions on the part of our patients. Many people may be unwilling to give consent to care and treatment because of fear, moral or personal objection, inability to accept the need (denial of a problem), or inability to understand what is being done to them (Miller, 1990). To overcome all of these barriers, the practitioner needs good communication skills.

Reluctance

This often comes about because the person lacks information about the situation and may be expecting worse outcomes than are realistic. A person may withdraw cooperation because they are in pain, disoriented, or even embarrassed (Miller, 1990). Let's look at one example case study.

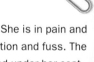

Case study 1: A reluctant patient

A 4-year-old girl has fallen at home and has probably broken her wrist. She is in pain and her mother is displaying a lot of anxiety by giving the child lots of attention and fuss. The nurse wants to examine the arm, but the child is keeping it firmly tucked under her coat against her chest.

This child is not cooperating because she is fearful of what may happen. Her mother is giving her mixed messages about the seriousness of the situation (by being overanxious) and this is reinforced by the pain the girl experiences every time she moves her arm. Duxbury (2000) suggests that communication strategies for fear and anxiety should be giving support and accurate, clear information, being empathetic, and cathartic. Following these guidelines we can suggest in our example that the nurse needs to:

- reduce the child's fear of pain and the mother's anxiety;
- reduce the child's expectations of harm;
- give realistic information about the situation.

The nurse can do this through communicating:

- the reality of the situation—that the pain is real, but won't do major harm;
- realistic expectations—that moving the arm will cause pain, but this needs to be done to solve the problem;
- that both the child and mother can trust the nurse.

First, the nurse is calm and matter of fact, while being empathetic of the pain experienced. Then, the nurse gives a simple explanation of the injury, why it hurts, and what can be done about it. This is followed by simple but direct and assertive instructions to the child (and the mother) about how and in what way it needs to be examined. The calmness and unflappable, authoritative demeanour of the nurse role-models the level of concern needed (not that much, but something needs to be done to the arm), delivered in a sympathetic but not overly concerned manner. It is important that the right phrase is used to communicate in a reassuring manner, as you can see below.

➕ Learning point 3

Look at the list below and see which phrase the competent nurse is likely to use in this situation.

1. Now then, there's no need for all this fuss. It doesn't hurt that much. Let me see it and we can have it fixed in no time.
2. I know it hurts, there is probably a small break in there. You need to show me so I can check. Just show me your arm. I won't touch it, but I know it might hurt a bit. The sooner I see it, the sooner we can get it mended.
3. Does it hurt a lot? I know, it's not nice is it. It's OK, though: it will mend. You need to show it to me so I can check it and we can stop it hurting.
4. Ooh, I bet that hurts! Never mind, it will be better soon. I need to see your arm to get it mended.

Suggested answer to Learning point 3

Hopefully, you preferred statements 2 and 3 rather than 1 and 4. Probably statement 3 is best, as it contains reassurance as well, although statement 2 also gives information.

Resistance

Resistance to care could be described as the intentional and deliberate choice of a patient or client to refuse care or engage in the care process. It can be passive or aggressive, manipulative or demanding (Miller, 1990), and can be for a range of reasons that stem from a different set of values around lifestyle choice or treatment approaches (Duxbury, 2000). For instance, people often refuse to take medication because of fear of side effects or lack of belief in their efficacy. People may refuse care because of fear of the intervention itself (some people don't like needles or blood) or they fear losing control of their own bodies or decision-making. Regardless of the direct reasons, a key problem is a lack of trust in the care practitioner and the treatment or care offered.

Responses to resistance are many and varied, depending on the reasons for resistance, but good communication skills are needed to get to the bottom of the resistance and to facilitate the cooperation of the person. Duxbury suggests communication strategies for a resistive patient need to include providing an appropriate environment and relationship (being catalytic), understanding the reasons for the resistance, ensuring privacy, being supportive, rewarding cooperative behaviour, and having firm boundaries.

Look at Practice example box 6. This is a real event in which the practitioner needed to address the environmental barriers, the nurse–patient relationship barriers, and overcome disclosure barriers to assess this care problem.

Practice example box 6: Overcoming resistance

A specialist drug and alcohol nurse was asked to see an elderly woman who was admitted in the night to casualty following a fall. The woman had old and fresh bruises to the outside of her arms suggestive of frequent falls and unsteadiness. Alcohol misuse was suspected, but no one tested blood-alcohol levels. On initial meeting, the nurse felt that this lady was reluctant to discuss the reasons for her accident as she repeatedly gave obscure and evasive answers. The environment was not at all private. The lady was dressed in only a backless nightgown and had been moved from a bed to a waiting area.

The nurse found the lady a blanket to cover herself with and moved the interview to the plaster room, which was the only unoccupied room that offered privacy. This action helped to establish a trusting and cooperative relationship between the nurse and the patient, and this environment provided uninterrupted privacy for the nurse to encourage the lady to make disclosures. It became apparent after careful and lengthy interviewing that her husband drank excessively while her own intake was moderate. However, the patient also disclosed that she obtained co-proxamol (an opiate-based analgesic) from her GP for a claimed back pain that she didn't have. She was using the analgesic for her husband who was otherwise aggressive and probably violent toward her. Her report of his behaviour suggested that he had become dependent on the opiate. She was also being visited by some youths in the neighbourhood who were buying the co-proxamol from her and would threaten her if she didn't give them any.

Table 7.1 Managing resistance

Incorrect information	Giving correct information
Lack of communication of fears	Encourage disclosure of fears
Lack of trust	Work on nurse–patient relationship
Realistic negative consequences of interventions	Empower the patient/client to problem-solve

This interview revealed three important factors about this lady. First, she was obtaining co-proxamol in order to supply drugs illegally (albeit under duress); second, she was experiencing domestic abuse and violence from her husband; and third, she was using the co-proxamol inappropriately on her husband. There were legal, social, and health management implications in the woman's life that needed rapid and careful management. If the nurse had not created an environment conducive to a private interview and taken time to establish and use a trusting relationship with the patient, none of this detail would have been disclosed.

Resistance can be caused by giving incorrect or no information, and can be solved, by giving correct information (see Table 7.1).

For more details on communication methods with resistance, see Chapters 12 and 15 regarding motivational interviewing.

Visit the Online Resource Centre (**www.oxfordtextbooks.co.uk/orc/webb**) and see the video 'Active Listening 2' for an example of intervening with a reluctant patient.

Dealing with aggression

Over the last few years, incidences of aggression in healthcare environments have escalated, and it is nurses who face the highest risk of assault in the healthcare workplace (NHS, 2006). This evidence helps to emphasize the importance of developing skills in recognizing and managing aggressive situations.

Aggression is inevitable and common in certain healthcare situations because it can be a symptom of illness. Therefore, its detection using good observation skills is part of the care assessment process. There are many organic causes of aggression. Common among these are hormonal disturbance, epilepsy, brain tumours, toxic states that cause hallucinations or psychosis (infections or exposure to chemicals), substance withdrawal, dementia, hyperthyroidism, functional psychosis (caused by mental illness), and hypoxia (lack of oxygen to the brain). However, there are also social and environmental causes that health professionals both contribute to and have the ability to manage.

Social and environmental influences of aggression

Certain care settings present greater trigger factors for aggression among patients and relatives than others because of the environment. Apart from care areas such as acute psychiatric and learning difficulty settings in which aggression is often part of the patient's condition, accident and emergency departments and GP surgeries present the highest risk for aggression from service users (NHS, 2006).

These settings present some of the typical factors that trigger aggression. In acute care settings, for example, Ferns (2007) identified several factors that contribute to aggression:

- poor communication;
- invasive and distressing procedures;
- noise;
- lack of sleep;
- perceived loss of control and powerlessness;
- pain;
- anxiety ;
- disorientation.

In certain care situations, anxious patients who are in pain, and relatives who feel helpless, encounter a care environment that involves waiting, lack of attention and poor information-giving, busyness, noise, and an alien and disempowering environment that they don't understand. Add to that staff who may be inappropriately chatting about what they did the night before or otherwise ignoring the waiting patients and this causes the potential for a build-up of frustration and anxiety that could turn into aggressive behaviour.

There are many longer-term management strategies that can reduce these triggers for aggression, but in the immediate or short term, we need to concern ourselves here with how good communication can prevent aggression arising or de-escalate aggression when it appears.

First, we need to use good observational skills to recognize when a patient is likely to engage in aggressive behaviour (Mason and Chandley, 1999). We need to recognize the **pro-dromal** (before onset of symptoms) signs of aggression, such as mounting anxiety, impatience, and irritability. Typically, as noted by Ferns (2007), these may be:

- commencement or worsening of stammering;
- pacing and staring;
- jaw and fist clenching;
- defensive posturing (such as covering head, standing square on, raising arms);
- exaggerated gestures and raised voice;
- tearfulness (as a result of frustration);
- self-hitting;
- withdrawal (becoming silent, uncommunicative or slow to respond).

De-escalation principles

Verbal de-escalation is a technique used to reduce potential aggression, which uses the nurse's personal social and communication skills, and should be preferred to any physical management (Herbel, 1990). At the pre-aggression stage, it is important that the nurse attempts to reduce the strong emotions that the person is experiencing, but also recognizes the threat involved. It is obviously important that the student nurse seeks supervision when facing possible aggression.

Evidence suggests that de-escalation responses should include a calm, non-confrontational approach, being listened to, personal space, and diversion (Farrell and Gray, 1992; Mason and Chandley, 1999; Duxbury, 2000). To summarize, a person who is at risk of engaging in violent behaviour needs:

- a sense of being in control of the environment or situation;
- time to think;
- space around them in order to feel in control;
- information to allow them to make sensible decisions;
- empathetic support from someone 'on their side';
- ability to move around and expend energy and adrenalin.

When faced with possible aggression, there are things that a nurse can do to disarm the situation:

- adopt a comfortable and relaxed demeanour (avoid 'mirroring' the person's aggressive body language);
- continuously assess the risks to safety;
- be genuine and warm;
- take time—do not rush the person;
- be respectful of the person's views and feelings;
- listen actively;
- speak clearly, slowly, and in short sentences;
- maintain a large personal space (for the nurse and the person concerned!).

In doing the above, the nurse is then in a position to engage the person in conversation about their feelings, without them feeling threatened. There are some sensible communications that the nurse can adopt to reduce the person's strong emotions:

- encourage the person to talk and identify the problem;
- avoid disagreeing or saying that you know how they feel (you don't);
- describe what has been happening (give the person the information they need);
- identify and suggest possible coping strategies if possible (such as getting some fresh air outside, phoning a friend, getting a cup of tea from the canteen);
- provide ways of resolving the situation if possible.

Common communication mistakes that nurses can make in such a situation include:

- arguing or raising your voice (unless you need to be heard);
- displaying your own strong emotions—getting angry, upset, or frightened;
- approaching the person without back-up (continuous risk assessment is required);
- using sarcasm and humour (this is neither the time nor place);
- touching the person (this is guaranteed to inflame a volatile situation).

In the event of actual aggression or violence, the student nurse is not expected to manage the situation. Specific training in dealing with aggression is only given to qualified staff. In the case of actual aggression, the only course of action for the student is to get out of the situation and call for help. If a student nurse finds him or herself in a situation that threatens to become violent, the student must remove him or herself from the situation and facilitate staff to intervene.

Conclusion

This chapter has attempted to address some of the challenges to communication that are not dealt with specifically in other chapters in this book, but are likely to present themselves in all branches of nursing. The domiciliary visit deprives the nurse of the power of the institution and demands skills in assertiveness and management of the environment. The use of interpreters is becoming more common in a world in which borders have become flexible to workers, visitors, and refugees, and in which immigration represents a major social change to the society. The ability to work effectively with interpreters is likely to become increasingly important to nurses in a future in which global mobility is increasing.

This chapter has also addressed the basic knowledge and skills for dealing with aggression, which, like language barriers, is increasingly demanding effective communication skills from nursing staff. This can be a specialized area of nursing, particularly in mental health and learning difficulties, but applies to all nurses and in many areas and environments of health care.

One of the factors that defines communication challenge is often its unusualness. No two situations are exactly the same, but, by applying the basic skills, we can negotiate our way through most of the common challenges.

> See the Online Resource Centre video 'De-escalation of aggression' for an example of aggression symptoms and de-escalation as well as the videos 'working with interpreters' and 'Active listening 2'.

 To find more resources to aid your learning please now go online to **www.oxfordtextbooks.co.uk/orc/webb**

Further reading

Mental Capacity Act 2005.

Disability Discrimination Act 2009 Both available from: Office of Public Sector Information (OPSI) at: www.opsi.gov.uk

Burnard, P., and Gill, P. (2008) *Culture, Communication and Nursing*. London: Pearson Education.

Holland, K. and Hogg, C. (2010) *Cultural Awareness in Nursing and Health Care*. London: Hodder Education.

References

Bond, M. and Pearson, K. (1969) 'Psychological Aspects of Pain in Women with Advanced Carcinoma of the Cervix', *Journal of Psychosomatic Research*, 13: 13–19.

Burnett, A. and Peel, M. (2001) 'Health Needs of Asylum Seekers and Refugees', *BMJ* 322: 544–77.

DeVito, J. (1988) *Human Communication: The Basic Course* (4th edn). New York: Harper & Row.

Duxbury, J. (2000) *Difficult Patients*. Oxford: Butterworth Heinemann.

Farrell, G. and Gray, C. (1992) *Aggression: A Nurses' Guide to Therapeutic Management*. London: Scutari Press.

Ferns, T. (2007) 'Factors that Influence Aggressive Behaviour in Acute Care Settings', *Nursing Standard*, 21(33): 41–5.

Gerrish, K. (2004) 'Bridging the Language Barrier: The Use of Interpreters in Primary Care Nursing', *Health and Social Care in the Community*, 12(5): 407–13.

Halliday, T. (1992) 'Touch and Pain', in T. Halliday (ed.) *The Senses and Communication*. Buckingham: Open University Press.

Herbel, K. (1990) 'Management of Agitated Head injured Patients: A Survey of Current Techniques', *Rehabilitation Nursing*, 15(2): 66–9.

Hogg, C. (2010) 'Understanding the Theory of Health and illness Beliefs', in K. Holland and C. Hogg (eds) *Cultural Awareness in Nursing and Health Care*. London: Hodder Education.

Holland, K. and Hogg, C. (2010) *Cultural Awareness in Nursing and Health Care*. London: Hodder Education.

Mason, T. and Chandley, M. (1999) *Managing Violence and Aggression*. Edinburgh: Churchill Livingstone.

Miller, R. (1990) *Managing Difficult Patients*. London: Faber & Faber.

National Health Science (2006) *Violence Against NHS Staff Survey: 2006 Report*. London: Information Centre for Health and Social Care, NHS Security Management Service.

Nursing Midwifery Council (2008) *The Code: Standards of Conduct, Performance and Ethics for Nurses and Midwives*. London: NMC.

— (2010) *Standards for Pre-registration Nursing Education: Draft for Consultation.*
     London: NMC.
Rea, A. (2004) 'Now You're Talking My Language', *The Psychologist*, 17(10): 580–2.
Rhodes, P. (2003) 'A Problem of Communication? Diabetes Care among Bangladeshi
     People in Bradford', *Health and Social Care in the Community*, 11(1): 45–54.
Tribe, R. (2007) 'Working with Interpreters', *The Psychologist*, 20(3): 159–61.

8

Health promotion and communication techniques

Maxine Holt

This chapter will help you to achieve competencies in:

- ➔ actively helping people to identify and use their strengths to achieve their goals and aspirations;
- ➔ promoting health and well-being, self-care, and independence through teaching and empowering people;
- ➔ discussing sensitive issues in relation to public health and providing appropriate advice and guidance to individuals, communities, and populations;
- ➔ working within a public health framework to assess needs and plan care for individuals, communities, and populations;
- ➔ supporting people to make appropriate choices and changes to eating patterns;
- ➔ discussing in a non-judgemental way how diet can improve health and the risks associated with not eating appropriately.

Introduction

In 1891, Florence Nightingale stated: 'I look forward to the day when there will be no nurses of the sick, only nurses of the well.' Of course, we can interpret her meaning of this in the context of that particular era, but if we were to consider it from a health promotion and prevention perspective, despite twenty-first-century technological advances in health care and nursing, Nightingale might be disappointed to discover that nurses still face huge challenges in improving the health and well-being of the patients and families with whom they work. The reason for this is multifaceted and often complex, however, good communication in health promotion is crucial if we are to fulfil the modern nurse's role.

This chapter will explore the different levels and types of method that we use to communicate health messages to the different groups with which we will work in our nursing role. It will examine the different settings within which we work as nurses and how these may be used to communicate health promotion across a diverse range of patients.

Defining health promotion

To enable us to appreciate the importance of communication in health promotion, first and very briefly, we need to consider what we mean by 'health promotion'. The World Health Organization (1986) has played a key role in refining its modern definition. Health promotion is concerned with enabling positive health and well-being by adopting a holistic concept of health. It recognizes factors that influence health and well-being and is a process that endeavours to strengthen both individual and community skills to tackle the factors that affect health. Health promotion practice addresses individual risk factors in order to improve outcomes: for example, physical inactivity, poor diet, and nutrition. This is undertaken alongside addressing socio-economic and environmental factors that determine health and well-being: for example, poverty.

The promotion of health and well-being is an integral feature of the assessment of health needs and the planning of care delivery, and, as such, is a crucial part of the nurse's role. It requires that nurses are competent in a number of skills and effective communication is one important skill that nurses need to develop. If we just take a few moments to consider the vast range of health promotion campaigns that occur both in the UK and globally and the huge number of different topics that such campaigns address, we can perhaps understand why nurses need to be able to communicate health promotion in a clear and concise way, drawing upon a range of methods available to them. As a nurse, you will meet a lot of patients who have diverse health promotion needs, which are influenced by many factors. These may include factors related to culture, sex, or age, those related to educational attainment, or perhaps a physical or mental illness. Effective communication in promoting health and well-being ensures that health promotion interventions are tailored to meet the different needs of our patients.

Individual and population levels of communication in promoting health

First, we need to think about the different levels we use to communicate health promotion as nurses. Think back to the point above regarding the range of health promotion campaigns and the topics and how they are communicated. We can begin to see that these can occur on a large scale, targeting the population in general, or, alternatively, some health promotion campaigns may be aimed at specific organizations, groups, or individuals. Consider the National Health Service flu vaccine campaign poster (see Figure 8.1): do you consider this to be a means of communicating a health promotion message to individuals or groups?

It is a very familiar campaign that we see occurring each year around October and through the winter months to protect people against current strains of flu. It is communicated to the general public by the Department of Health and aims to reach particular 'at risk' groups in society. Nurses are very much involved in communicating the campaign to patients on an individual basis and do this in a variety of ways: for example, a practice nurse may discuss the need for a patient to consider the vaccine during a routine clinic visit to the asthma clinic.

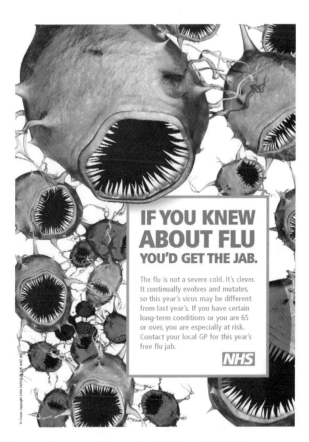

Figure 8.1 NHS flu vaccine campaign poster © Crown Copyright

> Nurse: Well, John, your asthma symptoms are really well under control at the moment, but winter is a tricky time for anyone who has asthma, with all the colds and flu viruses that are around, so you might want to consider having a flu jab to protect you. Here: have a look at this leaflet, which explains a little more about it, and if you have any questions, ask me. If you decide that you want to have the vaccine, we can do it today so that you don't need to make another appointment.

 Learning point 1

Can you think of other ways in which nurses can communicate the vaccine message to patients?

Nurses working in other areas, such as outpatients and medical wards, can provide at-risk patients with the necessary information and direct the patient to the appropriate means of receiving the vaccine. Community nurses may provide information to groups within residential or nursing care homes. The point here is that, as nurses, we are in a position to communicate health promotion from the community level through to individual levels. This will be dependent upon our nursing role or area of work, but it is important to consider that, as nurses, we are able to communicate health promotion in a variety of ways and this may be by working with patients or by designing, planning, and influencing health promotion campaigns or policies.

Nurses as role models in communicating health

Another level of promoting health to patients that needs consideration is that nurses and other health professionals act as role models for the patients and communities that they serve, and there are a number of studies that reveal that nurses are aware of this (Clark et al., 2003; McCann et al., 2005). However, the idea of nurses acting as role models does appear to cause some dissonance amongst some nurses. Some of my own research (see Box 8.1) has revealed that nurses would not embark on a dialogue with patients around topics that might cause emotional discomfort or challenges for both the patient and the nurse: for example, topics such as smoking—particularly if the nurse is a smoker.

Box 8.1 Practitioner comments

'I wouldn't suggest to patients that they need to give up smoking because I'm a smoker and I'd feel that I was being a hypocrite. (Nurse's quote)

'How can I really discuss or ask a patent about their alcohol intake when we go out at weekend and probably drink more than the recommended amount?

(Nurse's quote) (Holt, 2008)

Clark et al. (2003) and McCann et al. (2005) suggest that a significant number of nurses do not appreciate that role modelling involves not smoking or promoting a non-smoking lifestyle. Others, such as Rush and Cook (2006), suggest that, as nurses, we do not always act as credible health promoters. They use a comment from the husband of a patient to illustrate: 'My wife was dying of cancer and if you went out in the corridors you could see the nurses sat outside smoking their heads off—people dying of cancer, it doesn't make sense you know' (cited by Rush and Cook, 2006: 384). Patients do watch, observe, and listen to us, and it is important that we understand that our own health behaviours can be another means of communicating health messages to patients.

True commitment to health promotion may only be achieved when nurses and their colleagues not only understand the meaning of good health as the influential factor but internalise this to such an extent that this directs their personal and professional behaviour.

(Dines and Cribb, 1997: 197)

Where is health promotion communicated?

We have begun to appreciate the scope of communicating health promotion as nurses and we now need to consider the range of settings in which we can communicate health. The idea of promoting health within different settings originates from the concept of the settings approach to health promotion. The Ottawa Charter (WHO, 1986) appreciated the links between communicating health promotion in environments in which we work, learn, play, and love. As nurses, we both live and work in such settings. People may obtain information about their health from a variety of sources both inside and outside of the hospital and doctors' surgeries. This was clearly demonstrated in the document *Choosing Health*, which suggests that health professionals 'make the most of the millions of encounters that the NHS has with people every week' (DoH, 2004) and within more recent government papers such as *Our Health, Our Care, Our Say* (DoH, 2006b) and *Healthy Live, Healthy People* (DoH, 2010).

Learning point 2

Make a list of as many settings as you can in which health promotion can be communicated.

Suggested answers to Learning point 2

Health promotion can be communicated both inside and outside the NHS and below are some settings that you might have included in your list.

- **Educational:** schools, colleges, universities, pre-school nurseries, afterschool clubs
- **Health care and social care:** hospitals, dentists, GP surgeries, police stations, NHS walk-in centres, elderly care homes, pharmacists, polyclinics, prisons
- **Social/environmental:** pubs, night clubs, supermarkets, workplaces, neighbourhoods, churches, gyms, over-60s clubs, red-light districts, homeless shelters.

The above are just a few examples; the list of settings in which to communicate health is continually growing and has become a global initiative. One of the advantages of using different settings is that it enables the whole problem to be tackled by taking a holistic approach. Another advantage is that it enables us to communicate with those who are often difficult to reach, such as the young, elderly, disadvantaged, or marginalized in some way. There are some disadvantages to the idea of identifying settings for the communication of health promotion, one being that health promoters working with other agencies may fail to grasp their organizational agendas and structures, resulting in victim blaming (Corcoran and Bone, 2007). For example, promoting safe injecting practices among heroin users may seem to some to be encouraging drug-taking. If you consider the above list, there are many venues that offer the nurse an opportunity to be involved in communicating health.

 Learning point 3

Think about your own area of nursing work or a recent practice placement you have experienced and identify the opportunities that you have/had for communicating health promotion.

Suggested answers to Learning point 3

You might have initially considered your first contact with the patient or family and how you both began the process of assessment of their needs and subsequent planning of care to meet those needs. It may be that, when you prepared a patient due for discharge, they needed advice on how to take their medication or how to access other services for the continuation of their care. Another example is during a procedure such as a dressing or assisting with personal hygiene or when teaching a patient a skill: for example, administration of insulin to a newly diagnosed diabetic. A school nurse will be involved in screening programmes and providing health education sessions within school to children, teachers, and parents. Occupational health nurses are involved in providing advice and communicating with the workforce and the managers on health issues.

As you can begin to see, the opportunities across different settings are vast and it is important to remember that communication in health promotion may not always be directly with patients. Health promotion involves communicating and working with other partners and stakeholders to develop health promotion initiatives, developing or directing policy, providing written papers and other documents. As nurses, we are very much involved in such areas and need to acquire good communication skills for a diverse range of situations.

How is health promotion communicated?

In this chapter so far, we have explored the different levels and settings available for the communication of health and well-being. We now need to consider the different methods used and how, as nurses, we can utilize and develop these methods. The use of the mass media is perhaps the most popular and frequently used method to provide information about health issues and promote behaviour change. The media is a powerful means of communication and just to give you an example of how powerful it can be, listen to this broadcast at your earliest convenience (you can stream it from this website: **www.archive.org/details/OrsonWellesMrBruns**).

You will realize that this is not a health promotion campaign as such, although it did, in fact, have a significant effect on the health and well-being of a million people for a short time on 10 October 1938. It is, in fact, a radio broadcast clip from the H. G. Wells sci-fi story *The War of The Worlds*. Such was the power of the story and the way in which it was communicated that it is estimated that a million people fled their homes in terror as they believed that the world was being invaded by aliens. A headline in the *New York Times* on 31 October 1938 read 'Many Flee Homes to Escape "Gas Raid from Mars"—Phone Calls Swamp Police at Broadcast of Wells Fantasy'.

....

 Learning point 4

Can you think of some examples from health promotion that may be said to have had similar effects?

....

Suggested answers to Learning point 4

Modern-day examples of this form of health promotion can be identified as those relating to early campaigns on HIV and AIDS, or the spread of SARS and the recent MMR debate. Many of the patients whom we nurse and their families will access their health information via the mass media and, as nurses, we need to be able to recognize the influence that this may have on their beliefs about, and ability to act upon, such information. Let us consider first what we mean by the term 'mass media'. Naidoo and Wills (2004) suggest that it is a form of communication to the public that does not require person–person contact. Corcoran and Bone (2007: 74) propose four categories of mass media and how these may be applied to health promotion (see Table 8.1).

⊕ Learning point 5

The far right-hand column of Table 8.1 has been left blank for you to consider how you might use the types of media example suggested by Corcoran (2007) in your nursing role. Complete the column, giving examples of how, as a nurse, you may apply this form of communication in your health promotion work. See Table 8.2 afterwards for suggestions.

Table 8.1 The approach of the media to health promotion

Type of media	Example	Ways to use media	Ways nurses may use media for health promotion
Audiovisual broadcast	Television, radio	News, documentaries, soap operas, advertisements, public announcements	
Audiovisual non-broadcast	Videos, DVD, CDs, cassette tapes,	Self-help packages, teaching packages	
Printed material	Newspapers,magazines, leaflets,booklets, billboard posters, journals, games	Advertisements, news items, stories, magazine features	
Electronic material	Internet, CD ROM, mobile phone, computer packages, touch screen	Websites, text messaging	

Source: Adapted from Corcoran (2007).

One of the important features of the mass media is that it has many purposes in our society such as educating people through information-giving or entertainment, providing or clarifying meanings for people about health topics, and influencing behaviour and lifestyle. As nurses, the use of the mass media to communicate health is one that underpins the goals of health promotion. These are to provide objective and accurate information on health and risks to health to the patients and families we work with and to contribute to policy development. Let us now consider some of the examples that you may have given in the previous exercise.

The opportunities for nurses to use the mass media to communicate health are very broad indeed and the below are just a few examples. We have, of course, to recognize that there are some problems with using the mass media as a means of communicating health promotion. It can be very expensive—a fact that nurses would need to consider if planning any campaigns. The media can also promote health-damaging behaviours rather than health-promoting behaviours: for example, the current debate around the 'size zero' models and the influence that these may have on young girls' body image and eating disorders. We will, as nurses, experience instances in which patients may turn to us for advice about something they have seen in one of their favourite soap operas, or read in the newspaper, believing it to be a miracle cure. As nurses, we need to be able to support patients whose health and well-being is influenced by what they

Table 8.2 Suggested uses of the mass media

Type of media	Example	Ways nurses may use the media to communicate health promotion
Audiovisual broadcast	Television, radio	Public announcements, i.e. the flu vaccine campaign on local radio. Local initiatives identified as part of local delivery plans: screening services or well persons clinics. School plays that represent a particular theme e.g. drug misuse.
Audiovisual non-broadcast	Videos, DVD, CDs, cassette tapes	Self-help packages for newly diagnosed diabetics, asthmatics. Educational cassettes on living with specific conditions such as cancer. Relaxation therapies and techniques for stress management.
Printed material	Newspapers, magazines, leaflets, booklets, billboard posters, journals	Leaflets on healthy eating or other lifestyle and health behaviours. Patient newsletters, i.e. the stroke club or the local 'breathe easy' group. Posters on current health topics or services available.
Electronic material	Internet, CD ROM, mobile phone, computer packages, touch screen	Practice or ward website for patients to access information possibly about a forthcoming hospital stay or GP practice/clinic appointment. Touch-screen information on travel immunization requirements. Computer games in schools.

Source: Adapted from Corcoran (2007).

read or hear in the media by giving accurate and objective information. In addition, we must appreciate that while media materials that communicate the promotion of health are available to us, as nurses, to utilize, such materials should be, wherever possible, used to reinforce verbal information.

Example 1

> Nurse: Ok, Joan, we have discussed how you might want to stop smoking and how nicotine therapy may help you with this. Just so that you can recap on our discussion about the different types available to you, take this leaflet away and read it a little further in your own time, and then we can discuss this again in a couple of days. Is that ok?

So the key is to use the different resources such as leaflets or booklets to support our health promotion communication and this has been found to be effective in improving knowledge and reducing anxiety about certain health issues (Dyer et al., 2004). There are some other important factors that we need to consider when using information materials to communicate health promotion and these are in relation to the appropriateness of the materials that we are using. Some information can be confusing for patients simply because it can change so often.

Example 2

> Patient: I am really confused, nurse, about whether to take HRT because of the risks of breast cancer. The newspapers now say it reduces your risk. I just don't know what to do.

It is important that the information we communicate to patients and their families is current and underpinned by sound evidence. As nurses, we need to be able to direct patients to sources of good-quality health information, including health-related websites. Some examples that you might want to use are:

www.patient.co.uk/

www.nhsdirect.nhs.uk/

Learning point 6

In advance of your next placement, look at these sites to see what information is available on the health conditions or issues you are likely to encounter on that placement, as well as information for any health promotion opportunities that may arise. When you arrive on placement, ask your mentor and colleagues to direct you to other resources that they have.

We also need to ensure that the materials we use are suitable for our patients; Ewles and Simnett (2003) suggest a checklist for nurses to consider when using or designing resources to communicate health messages.

- Is the resource appropriate for achieving the intended aims?
- Would another type of medium be better?
- Is the information clear and to the point?
- Are the key themes emphasized?
- Does the resource communicate the message in a language that is easily understood by the patient or their family?
- Does the resource look appealing (colour, use of pictures, size, etc.)?

 ## Learning point 7

Look again at the NHS flu vaccine campaign poster (Figure 8.1). How do you think it addresses the above checklist?

Suggested answers to Learning point 7

We can see that the use of the poster for this topic area is appropriate for meeting the overall aims, which are to target the 'at risk' population. For this particular campaign, there are other resources available, such as leaflets for patients to take away and read or pass onto others and also an MP3 audio file format for those with a visual impairment. The information is brief and to the point, emphasizing key points. The poster is certainly eye-catching, using the theme of nasty bugs with sharp teeth to emphasize the seriousness of the message. The leaflets are also available in eleven languages.

You will find further examples on the following webpage: **www.dh.gov.uk/en/ Publicationsandstatistics/Publications/PublicationsPolicyAndGuidance/ DH_087455**

Learning point 8

We have discussed above how, as a nurse, you might use different resources with patients to communicate health promotion. Consider now another aspect of health promotion: that of communicating to the general public to address or raise local health agendas. How might you do this?

Suggested answers to Learning point 8

It is suggested that nurses are not really proactive in using the mass media as a means of reaching audiences to communicate health (Whitehead, 2003). One of the ways in which nurses can use the local press is through the use of stories on health topics that depict, for example, a positive message, such as success stories addressing a local issue (remembering confidentiality and data protection issues). Other ways are through letters or articles in the local GP practice or primary care trust newsletter. Communicating health promotion is also about working across disciplines to develop policy or interventions and relies on good communication skills in working with other partners.

Factors that may influence health communication

We have so far considered the different methods that nurses can draw upon to communicate health promotion. We now need to consider some of the factors that may influence our communication with the diverse patients with whom we will work and their ability act upon health promotion. As mentioned previously in this chapter, health promotion is influenced by a multitude of sometimes complex factors, which include policy, political, and societal agendas. It is important, then, that we are aware of such factors and are able to take these into consideration when communicating health promotion, both with patients and other related parties or stakeholders. It is also worth noting that, in the broader sense of health promotion work, we are more likely to gain resources and financial support if our interventions are in line with current policy and health promotion agendas at both a national and local level. Barton and Grant (2006) offer a diagrammatic picture of factors that influence health and well-being (see Figure 8.2).

The individual is placed at the centre, together with the factors of age, sex, and genes that shape their health potential. Surrounding them are layers of environmental factors. The closest layer is personal behaviour and ways of living that can promote or damage health. Next, we have social and community influences, which may have a

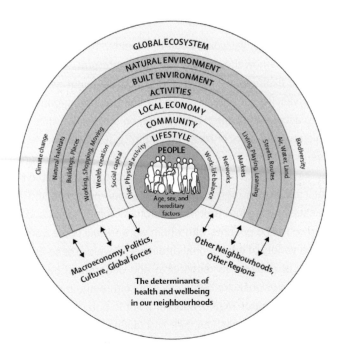

Figure 8.2 Influences on health and well-being (from H. Barton and M. Grant, 'A Health Map for the Local Human Habitat', *Journal of the Royal Society for the Promotion of Health*, 126 (2006), 252–3 repr. by permission of Sage.)

positive or negative effect on the individual. They suggest that the links between the community and sustainability of healthy communities are fundamental in promoting our health and well-being. In order to consider how we may communicate health promotion, let us begin by considering social factors that may influence our patients.

⊕ **Learning point 9**

Let us consider the example of the NHS flu vaccine campaign. Look at the Department of Health website:

www.dh.gov.uk/en/Publicationsandstatistics/Publications/PublicationsPolicyAnd Guidance/DH_087455

What social factors would you need to consider when using the leaflet to communicate the message to the following:

● a 70-year-old with coronary heart disease?
● an 8-year-old child with asthma?

Suggested answer to Learning point 9

There are several things that we would need to consider. For example, the age range of our patents will influence how they are able to apply, interpret, and react to language. If we look at the above example, we can see that how we might describe the problems with not having the vaccine will vary between the different age groups. Older adults are likely to be able to access the written information on the poster, while children will love the graphics, which tell the story of nasty bugs that cause disease.

One word of caution is not to assume that all patients in each age range will respond in the same way. We need to remember that respones may be affected by other factors such as physical, cognitive, or mental disability or impairment. Age and gender are also factors that influence how we interpret health promotion messages and how we want to be communicated with. The patients with whom we work will come from different social classes and have a variety of educational attainment levels. These are factors that will influence the ability of patients to respond to and understand health messages. We have also highlighted previously that ethnicity and culture are important factors in com-munication in health promotion. Again, another point to note here is not to assume that all patients who do not have English as their first language automatically read their own language. Many may speak their mother tongue, but not read it, dependent upon their age and length of time in the country. Other factors, such as the attitudes and beliefs of our patients, are also influential in the communication of health promotion and there are a number of theoretical models that seek to predict responses to these in an effort to change behaviour.

 These are discussed in more detail in Chapter 15 of this book.

Using the nursing assessment to communicate health promotion

We have considered the use of different resources that nurses can use to communi-cate health promotion, and now need to consider how we can use our own nursing assessment tools for the same means. Nightingale's contemporary understanding of the theories of health and sickness suggest that, as nurses, one of our most important jobs is to ensure that the patient is placed in the correct circumstances to ensure their optimal health and well-being. In order to do this, we are required to develop a sound knowledge base and skills in observation and communication to assess, inform, and educate patients and their families (Holt, 2008).

Many nurses have the skills that enable them to incorporate health promotion principles into their existing work, and without doubt this is the suggestion within cur-rent government and nursing policy (DoH, 2006a; 2004; RCN, 2007). The theoretical principle that underpins the nursing assessment is that of a gateway for the building of the nurse–patient relationship to enable the assessment of the patient's needs and goal-setting. Within this ideology, the opportunity to assess health and well-being and to initiate health promotion interventions is perhaps inevitable as part of the process, yet the literature and feedback from student nurses would suggest that, in reality, this is often not the case (Holt and Warne, 2007; McCarthy and Holt, 2007; Holt, 2008).

The theory that underpins the patient assessment is that of being an opportunity for the nurse to develop a relationship with the patient in order to assess their needs, set goals, and plan interventions to meet those goals. It is a significant opportunity for the nurse to engage in communicating with the patient about their health and well-being, and offer advice and support where and if necessary. It is suggested, however, that such opportunities are often missed and that, in reality, the nursing assessment is 'perfunctory in nature' (Porter and Ryan, 1996), and that it is more an exercise in completing charts and tick boxes (Foner, 1994; Johnson and Webb, 1995; Costello, 2001). Let us now consider, then, how we may use the nursing assessment to communicate health promotion.

There are many theoretical nursing models that we can use to guide our nursing practice and which we use will depend upon the particular area of nursing we work within. The Roper, Logan, and Tierney model of nursing (1983) is based on activities that, as humans, we need to be able to perform in order to carry out activities of living (ALs). These are as follows.

1. Maintaining a safe environment
2. Communicating
3. Breathing
4. Eating and drinking
5. Eliminating
6. Personal cleansing and dressing
7. Controlling body temperature
8. Mobilizing
9. Working and playing
10. Expressing sexuality
11. Sleeping
12. Dying

Many of the nursing assessment documents that you will see and use in practice are designed to reflect these ALs. The model enables the nurse not only to assess the actual problems, that the patient may have, but also to place as much emphasis on prevention and health promotion. As a nurse, you will, at some stage, spend time with the patient discussing their problems, from which you will jointly develop a plan of care. It is during this process that you may be able to use the opportunity to begin a dialogue with the patient about a health issue. See the case study for an example.

Case study1: Assessment opportunities for health promotion

Mr D, who is 60 and of Pakistani origin, arrives on the ward from A&E after having a dizzy spell following a fall at home whilst getting up to go to toilet during the night—something that he says he often has to do. He has just retired from being a taxi driver, early, due to ill health. He has type 2 diabetes, is hypertensive and obese. He takes diuretics and anti-hypertensive therapy, although occasionally forgets, and has a regular blood pressure of 150/100. He and his wife are due to go on their Haj pilgrimage to Mecca within the next week.

 Learning point 10

Can you identify any opportunities for using the nursing assessment to communicate health promotion for Mr D?

Suggested answer to Learning point 10

The following is not a complete assessment of Mr D's needs, but suggests examples of how nurses can use the opportunity of the nursing assessment to communicate health promotion. It must be stressed here that this is an integrative process and that health needs also reflect those that aim to promote and protect health and well-being, in addition to those that may present as immediate or existing problems (see Table 8.3).

As nurses, we can use the assessment process as a means of getting to know and understand the patients with whom we work. It facilitates a discussion with the patients on the factors that influence their health and well-being and opens up opportunities for us to use this information to communicate health promotion.

Conclusion

This chapter has enabled you, as a nurse, to consider the different levels in which health promotion is communicated and the different settings in which you may communicate health promotion. It has helped you to recognize that communicating health promotion occurs both in primary and secondary care, and at community and individual levels. The key to successful communication in health promotion is to take the core principles of communication and apply them to health promotion, whilst appreciating the diversity of the patients and people with whom we work in promoting health.

Table 8.3 Mr D's likely needs

ALs	Health promotion opportunity
Maintaining a safe environment, personal cleansing and dressing	Medication advice: Mr D fell whilst getting up to use the toilet during the night. He takes diuretics and quite often patients do not follow the directions on medication bottles. He may therefore be taking his diuretic in the evening rather than the morning, resulting in him having to get up during the night. Foot care advice: Both he and his wife are going to Mecca in the near future. This can involve walking in bare feet. The feet of a diabetic patient are very prone to injury, which can have devastating effects.
Communicating, eating and drinking, mobilizing	Consider the need for an interpreter if necessary: patients who do not have English as their first language may often not comply with instructions and may not understand colloquial terms for health that we may use. Discuss the need to maintain healthy body weight and relationship to high blood pressure. Promote healthy eating and perhaps involve Mrs D in discussion. Refer to dietician. Teach how to take, record, and interpret own blood pressure. Involving Mr D in his own management of his blood pressure and how to keep a record of it, and when to consult for further advice. Provide leaflet and audiotape in Urdu on foot care and diet for diabetics. Mr D may or may not read Urdu, so check this first. He may find an audiotape useful. Give him these whilst he is on the ward so that he can read or listen to them and then ask further questions if necessary.

 To find more resources to aid your learning, please now go online to
www.oxfordtextbooks.co.uk/orc/webb You will find exercises and advice
relating to the chapter, and a video entitled 'The health promotion practitioner.

Web links

www.patient.co.uk/
www.nhsdirect.nhs.uk/

References

Barton, H. and Grant, M. (2006) 'A Health Map for the Local Human Habitat', *Journal of the Royal Society for the Promotion of Health*, 126: 252–3.

Clark, E., McCann, T. V., Rowe, K., and Lazenbatt, A. (2003) 'Cognitive Dissonance and Undergraduate Nursing Students' Knowledge of, and Attitudes about, Smoking', in H. Nicholl and A. Higgins, *Issues and Innovations in Nursing Education*. Oxford: Blackwell Publishing.

Corcoran, N. and Bone, A. (2007) 'Using Settings to Communicate Health Promotion', in N Corcoran and A. Bone (eds) *Communicating Health: Strategies for Health Promotion*. London: Sage.

Costello, J. (2001) 'Nursing Older Dying Patients: Findings from an Ethnographic Study of Death and Dying in Elderly Care Wards', *Journal of Advanced Nursing*, 35: 59–68.

Department of Health (2002) *Health Promoting Prisons: A Shared Approach*. London: HMSO.

—— (2004) *Choosing Health White Paper: Partial Public Sector Impact Assessment— Supporting NHS Frontline Staff in Health Improvement*. London: DoH.

—— (2006a) *Essence of Care on Promoting Health Benchmarks*. London: HMSO.

—— (2006b) *Our Health, Our Care, Our Say: A New Direction for Community Services*. London: HMSO.

—— (2010) *Healthy Lives, Healthy People: Ours Strategy for Public Health in England*. London: HMSO.

Dines, A., and Cribb, A. (1997) *Health Promotion: Concepts and Practice*. Oxford: Blackwell Science.

Dyer, K., Fearon, K., Buckner, K., and Richardson, R. A. (2004) 'Diet and Colorectal Cancer Risk: Impact of a Nutrition Education Leaflet', *Journal of Human Nutrition and Dietetics*, 17(6): 576.

Ewles, L. and Simnett, I. (2003). *Promoting Health: A Practical Guide* (5th edn). London: Balliere Tindall.

Foner, N. (1994) *The Caregiving Dilemma: Work in an American Nursing Home*. Los Angeles, CA: University of California Press.

Holt, M. (2008) 'The Educational Preparation of Student Nurses as Communicators of Health and Well-being', *Journal of the Royal Society for the Promotion of Health*, 128(4): 159–60.

—— and Warne, T. (2007) 'The Educational and Practice Tensions in Preparing Pre-registration Nurses to Become Future Health Promoters: A Small-scale Explorative Study', *Nurse Education in Practice*, 7(6): 373–80.

Johnson, M. and Webb, C. (1995) 'Rediscovering Unpopular Patients: The Concept of Social Judgements', *Journal of Advanced Nursing*, 21: 466–7.

McCann, T. V., Clark, E., and Rowe, K. (2005) 'Undergraduate Nursing Students' Attitudes Towards Smoking Health Promotion', *Nursing and Health Sciences*, 7: 164–74.

McCarthy, J. and Holt, M. (2007) 'The Complexities of a Policy-driven Pre-registration Nursing Curricula: Rhetoric Versus Reality', *Nursing Standard*, 35(4): 35–8.

Naidoo, J., and Wills, J. (2004) *Public Health and Health Promotion: Developing Practice*. London: Balliere Tindall.

Nightingale, F. (1891) *Notes on Nursing: What It Is and What It Is Not*. London: Harrison.

Porter, S. and Ryan, S. (1996) 'Breaking the Boundaries between Nursing and Sociology: Critical Realist Ethnography of the Theory–Practice Gap', *Journal of Advanced Nursing*, 24: 413–20.

Roper, N., Logan, W., and Tierney, A. (1983) *Using a Model for Nursing*. Edinburgh: Churchill Livingstone.

Royal College of Nursing (2007) *Nurses as Partners in Delivering Public Health: A Paper to Support the Nursing Contribution to Public Health, Developed by an Alliance of Organisations.* London: RCN.

Rush, B. and Cook, J. (2006) 'What Makes a Good Nurse? Views of Patients and Carers', *British Journal of Nursing*, 15(7): 382–5.

Whitehead, D. (2003) 'Using Mass Media within Health-promoting Practice: A Nursing Perspective', *Journal of Advanced Nursing*, 32(4): 807–16.

World Health Organization (1986) *Ottawa Charter for Health Promotion.* Ottawa, ON: Canadian Public Health Association.

9

Using health information (informatics)

Jacqui Gladwin

This chapter will help you to achieve competencies in:

➲ providing accurate and comprehensive written and verbal reports based on best available evidence;

➲ acting appropriately in sharing information to enable and enhance care (carers, MDT, and across agency boundaries);

➲ working within legal frameworks for data protection including access to and storage of records;

➲ acting within the law when confidential information has to be shared with others;

➲ sharing information safely with colleagues across agency boundaries for the protection of individuals and the public.

Introduction

Health informatics as a subject deals primarily with the equipment, resources, and methods used in the acquisition and management of information within healthcare organizations. This does not merely relate to the use of computers or electronic equipment, but includes other methods such as clinical information systems and clinical guidelines.

Coiera (2003: xxii) defines health informatics as 'the study of information and communication systems in health care'. This primarily focuses on the following areas:

● understanding concepts of information and communication systems in use within healthcare settings;

● developing systems to improve the quality of data collection and storage;

- evaluating the impact of these systems on the way in which organizations or individuals work or the outcomes of specific interventions, such as patient care.

The Royal College of Nursing (2006) suggests that information communication technology is primarily about managing information, which is absolutely fundamental to effective nursing practice.

This chapter will explore the concept of health informatics and how it relates to communication within patient care. It will address the main issues involved with collecting, storing, and sharing information, and the possible benefits that this may bring to health organizations and patients. There are a variety of activities and reflection points within the chapter designed to develop your knowledge and understanding of the concepts discussed and how they may apply to your practice.

It is important that nurses understand that the use of information in health care includes a range of issues for both patients and staff. Patients are increasingly aware of the types of information available and, as nurses, we need to ensure that we can manage information appropriately in order to meet the needs of our patients. This means understanding policies and legislation related to information-handling and storage in order to protect patient information and ensure patients access information appropriately.

Terms in informatics

In health care, we use different terms for different types of information.

- **Data:** this relates to facts such as clinical observations—for example, a temperature recording or a pulse rate for a specific patient.
- **Knowledge:** this relates to understanding the relationships between data— for example, a temperature recording of 38.5 degrees celsius and a heart rate of 130 beats per minute, in conjunction with the patient history, may lead us to suspect the patient has an infection. This knowledge will only be effective, though, if we understand the relationships between the data.
- **Information:** this generally relates to a situation in which we apply interpretive knowledge to data and identify something new or monitor change. In the above patient scenario, this may relate to the administration of antibiotics, the treatment effectiveness of which would be indicated by a reduction in temperature and heart rate. These data would provide us with information about the patient's condition and support the decision-making processes by confirming the diagnosis and indicating the effectiveness of infection treatment. This can also be defined as evidence.
- **Evidence:** this can be used to develop information in the format of clinical guidelines such as those issued by organizations designed to support or

direct our practice,such as the National Institute for Health and Clinical Excellence (NICE). These guidelines can then be used to justify our practice and guide our management of specific situations.

The requirement for evidence-based medicine and nursing practice (NMC, 2010) means that we must engage with collating, interpreting, and validating the information about patients and their treatment in order to determine its reliability as evidence (Cullum, 2002).

....

⊕ Learning point 1

Using the above definitions of information (terms of informatics), consider your experience in practice and identify the sources of information that you use on a daily basis to help you in your work.

....

Table 9.1 Sources of information in health care

Source of information	Information and examples of its use
Nursing kardex/patient notes	Information relating to individual patients and their care, previous medical history, etc. Used to assess, plan, treat, and evaluate care.
Patient prescription sheet	Identifies specific drugs prescribed for an individual (incl. allergies etc). Record of when and by whom drugs were dispensed.
Staff intranet	Information regarding organizational policies and procedures, guidelines, training opportunities, etc. Can be used by staff to keep up to date with organizational issues, policies, and to report incidents, identify risks.
Internet	Online sources, clinical databases, evidence-based websites, professional databases, i.e. Nursing & Midwifery Council, Royal College of Nursing
Policy manuals	Hard-copy sources of individual policies and procedures available in the place of work
Patient observation charts	Physiological/behavioural data from individual patients used to determine state of health and severity of illness
Laboratory results	Results of investigations that influence treatment for patients, i.e. blood tests, urinalysis
People	Largest source of information, handover between staff, histories from patients and families, conversational information, teaching, and mentoring

Sources of information in health

Nurses rely on information in order to make everyday decisions on a number of issues including patient care. There are different types of information that nurses can use to support their decision-making to ensure that effective care is delivered to patients.

When you consider the numbers of people and services who have input into a single episode of care, you can quickly appreciate the vast amount of personal information generated in a single episode. For example, Mr Jones, a 74-year-old man, is referred by his GP to accident & emergency with a chest infection.

Figure 9.1 demonstrates the amount of information recorded and shared in one episode of care for Mr Jones.

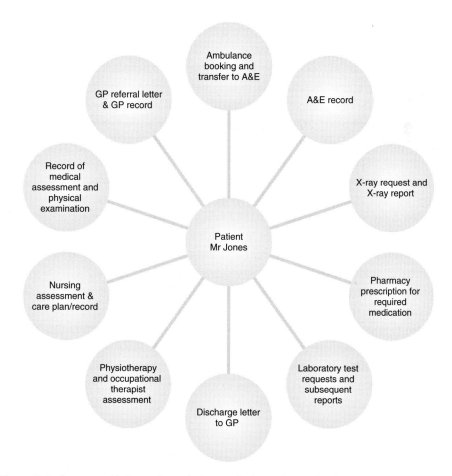

Figure 9.1 Sources of information relating to single patient episode

Learning point 2

Consider how many people will be involved in the process and how many times personal information relating to Mr Jones will be shared. Effective communication is essential to ensure that the information is accurate and shared appropriately.

When a lot of information is collected, patients can feel they have to give the same information to a variety of people repeatedly. Work has been carried out to reduce the amount of assessments and repetition of information through more effective information-sharing between the care team (Dickinson, 2006; Roberts et al., 2006).

Use of electronic formatted information allows documentation and information to be shared across a large organization more readily than handwritten notes. A single assessment process can be commenced by one member of the healthcare team—for example a nurse—and other healthcare professionals can add to the information without repeatedly documenting similar information collected from the patient again.

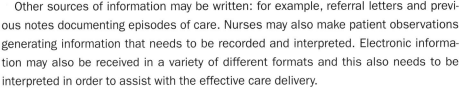

Patient information may come from a verbal interaction between the patient and the clinician and the role of the nurse is to interpret the information in order to identify patient needs. The use of model-based electronic care plans is now common in many settings. Mills and Rajwer (2005) suggest that electronic patient care plans provide an opportunity to link patient problems, goals, and interventions to related policies, procedures, and guidelines. This further supports the principle of evidence-based care and also facilitates links to specific patient-focused health promotion information.

Other sources of information may be written: for example, referral letters and previous notes documenting episodes of care. Nurses may also make patient observations generating information that needs to be recorded and interpreted. Electronic information may also be received in a variety of different formats and this also needs to be interpreted in order to assist with the effective care delivery.

Finally, there are the policies, protocols, and guidelines that underpin the organizational processes, the professional role of the nurse, or the care of the patient. It is important to ensure that nurses understand how to access and interpret this information in order to provide safe and effective care for patients. Many healthcare trusts now provide **clinical intranet systems** that store all of their organizational documentation and provide care professionals with links to relevant national organizations and agencies the policies and protocols of which impact on care delivery.

 Learning point 3

Student nurses in any field of care may be able to access their trust's clinical intranet system. If you have not already come across the one used by your trust, ask your mentor to show you the intranet system for the trust in which you are training. There may also be hard copies available for you to see.

Organizational communication systems

Each commercial and public organization has a set of systems designed to facilitate and support communication across and within it. Examples of this may include people, policies, and equipment such a paging systems, email, telephone and answering systems, diaries, handover books, and whiteboards. Employees within the organization need to be able to select the appropriate communication system for the message that they wish to convey. Understanding the appropriate format for communicating information is an integral part of a nurse's role.

Format of information

Information can be presented in a number of formats, including written, electronic, visual, or verbal. Different formats work for different types of information. The selection of the format will often depend on the intended purpose and audience involved. The following section will discuss the collection and use of different types and formats of information in more depth.

Written

It is common for nursing notes and patient records to be handwritten or typed. The use of a model or framework for assessment can reduce the amount of time required to undertake the process and can ensure consistency of assessment and standardized documentation for every patient. In most instances, handwritten information is completed on standardized pro formas that the organization applies to all patients.

Nursing records of daily care are often written in free text and may be very subjective. The use of free text can often lead to the use of jargon and abbreviations that only the nurse making the entry may understand. This may lead to misunderstandings between staff regarding recording of events or the care delivered. NMC (2009) outlines the principles that should be adhered to when recording and using patient information and gives specific reference to the legibility and accuracy of written information.

....

➕ Learning point 4

Consider some of the abbreviations you have come across in practice. Do you know what they all mean and what impact do you think the use of abbreviations in a patient's notes may have?

....

Nurses use a lot of abbreviations when handing over and discussing care and in their documentation, but it is important that records are clear and transparent both in their legibility and translation. There are hundreds of abbreviations used within health care.

Acceptable ones may include C&R (control and restraint), A&E (accident and emergency), COPD (chronic obstructive pulmonary disease) CVA (cardiovascular accident), DDA (Disability Discrimination Act 1995). Many organizations produce a glossary of acceptable abbreviations for that specific workplace. It is vital that health professionals do not invent their own abbreviations that may cause confusion in patient records or prescriptions, for instance. Any doubt in the interpretation of the abbreviation should be checked to maintain safe and effective care.

Handwriting is often very difficult to read, and if the information is unclear, then it is easy to see how errors may occur. Inferences are drawn by the reader about what the writer meant. The person who has written the information may have a different understanding of the information from the person reading it.

Misinterpretations of information account for many clinical errors. According to the National Patient Safety Agency (2009), there were 85,085 medication errors reported in 2007. Of these, 32 per cent were attributable to prescribing errors and many were due to the prescription being unclear.

 Some examples of good and poor practice in relation to record-keeping are available on the Online Resource **www.oxfordtextbooks.co.uk/orc/webb**

Electronic

The use of information technology in health care means that many forms of communication are now completed electronically. The use of email is commonplace in many organizations and, within the NHS, there are many examples of electronic systems for data collection and information storage.

Electronic information may be sent in written format or by pro forma completed online using a set of pre-existing criteria. An example of this is an electronic incident reporting system. The incident report number is generated by the system automatically and a series of pre-set criteria are utilized by the person reporting the incident to outline the type of incident, date, time, and details. Comparisons could be drawn here with using an online booking system for an airline. The system is set up to offer choices of pre-set information; the user clicks on the appropriate choice and the system then records that choice.

Electronic systems may allow a combination of pre-set information and free text. The example of the incident reporting system may combine both options.

Care planning systems are also available in practice that use set frameworks to allow the nurse to assess a patient, plan, and record care. Some systems have pre-set criteria that assist the nurse in defining the process required for assessing a specific patient, but the disadvantage may be that they do not always meet the needs of individual patients. Other systems may be more flexible and allow free text input, which ensures that the nurse can meet the needs of the individual patient (see example in Figure 9.2).

 This picture is available at: **www.cncplan.com/**

The use of electronic forms of communication is growing rapidly and many people have personal computers and electronic devices such as Internet-enabled phones. Electronic communication is commonplace and social networking sites such as MySpace and Facebook have revolutionized the way in which the world communicates. In 2009, there were thought to be over 200 million users registered on MySpace (Marketing Genius, 2009). This has led to many healthcare organizations developing policies regulating their use, but also exploring the possibilities of using them to engage with the public to communicate health information and to provide discussion forums and patient feedback.

Electronic formatting of information facilitates easy storage and extraction of data. This supports the audit process, which can assist with identifying errors and therefore improving the overall quality of patient records (Audit Commission, 2009), and enables information to be gathered from a range of sources to aid the planning and design of services for specific groups of patients. Electronic clinical information is usually coded to assist with the extraction process and this enables clinicians to measure uptake of specific services—for example, smoking cessation—or to identify patients with specific conditions or risk factors for targeted interventions. One such example would

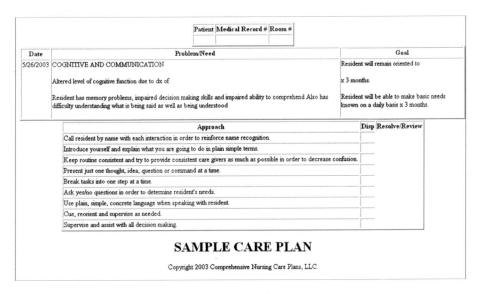

Figure 9.2 Example of electronic care plan © Comprehensive Nursing Care Plans

be inviting vulnerable patients for a flu vaccination. Electronic information can be identified much more quickly than if one had to go through the handwritten notes of thousands of patients. The impact of coding information for patients may be that they won't necessarily understand the nature of the coding or its relevance to them.

However, the accessibility of electronic information allows nurses to access a huge range of clinical information at the point of care. Clinical guidelines and protocols that underpin nursing practice are available for us to view both within staff intranet systems and the wider Internet. The Map of Medicine is one such evidence-based practice site, which brings together a range of conditions and treatments linked to specific evidence bases, providing a framework for treatment for approximately 400 conditions. The use of such systems can enhance the care given to patients, but they can also limit it if not specific to every group of patients. A study by Leach and Segal (2010) found that clinical guidelines used in clinical practice did not always cover specific minority groups of patients and, as such, could impact on the standard of care offered. Another example would be NHS Evidence, which is a comprehensive collection of accredited evidence supplied within the National Institute for Health and Clinical Excellence (see web links at end of chapter). The use of clinical evidence databases such as NHS Evidence, Best Bets, and the Cochrane Database allows practitioners to identify the specific guidelines or treatments that are recommended for patients and promotes safe and effective care across the NHS (see Figure 9.3). It is vital however, as Verhoeven et al. (2010) identify, that nurses understand how to retrieve and critique this information to ensure that the care they deliver is effective and safe for the patient.

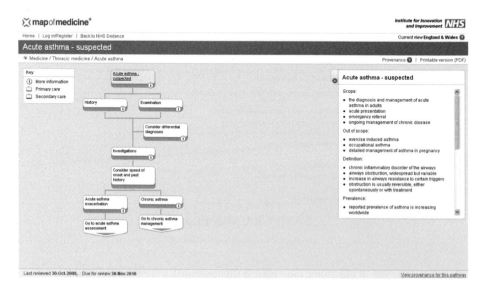

Figure 9.3 NHS evidence page © Map of Medicine

This picture, and more from this site, are available at: **www.mapofmedicine.com/ accessthemap/directaccess/**

Visual images

Visual images are often useful in documenting specific care of patients. Pictures can represent the stages of wound healing that provide more accurate information than the written word. This would be particularly useful if the patient's care were being delivered by a range of people and over a prolonged period of time, as it would allow them to see the difference between the stages of wound healing without having seen the actual wound.

Images can also be stored to represent cases or specific diseases that help us to develop our knowledge and understanding in relation to a specific subject. The use of visual images often helps to illustrate a subject or a point of view in a way that words simply could not. Examples include the use of diagrams to represent family trees in a patient's record or diagrams of the body to document the distribution of a patient's injuries.

Verbal

As we have seen throughout this book, verbal communication undoubtedly remains the most important skill that a nurse has to offer. The ability to modify language and apply different types of verbal communication to different situations is one of the guiding principles of nursing. All aspects of patient care require verbal engagement between the patient, the nurse, and often the family and the wider members of the healthcare team. Therefore, in terms of health informatics, it is important that nurses capture the information that is gained through verbal communication, record it, and interpret it accurately in order to maintain safe and effective care delivery (National Patient Safety Agency, 2007). According to Nadzam (2009), this can be challenging, as she suggests that nurses are trained to be narrative and therefore descriptive rather than analytical. This can lead to misinterpretation of information between health professionals and this, in turn, may compromise the safety of patient care.

There are different formats of information and different ways in which to communicate it. In order to select the appropriate format, nurses need to consider the purpose of their message. If a nurse needs to convey information urgently—for example, if a patient's condition deteriorates—it would not be appropriate to use email or a written format. It would instead be appropriate to use verbal communication via a phone or paging system or direct to the person who needs to be informed.

However, if a ward manager were to need to communicate to staff that a meeting was to take place, it would be appropriate to inform people in writing, either using electronic or handwritten formats. Diaries and whiteboards are often used in clinical environments to communicate important dates or tasks.

Whichever form of communication is used, it is important that all staff know which formats are used for which purpose and what communication processes exist within that clinical area.

 Learning point 5

When you are next on placement, ask your mentor which format of communication it would be appropriate for you to use and for which purpose. Ask for feedback on examples of your work.

Collecting and using patient information

As nurses, we have access to vast amounts of information and have a responsibility to ensure that the information is collected, stored, and utilized appropriately. The Data Protection Act 1998 provides specific legislation regulating the collection, storage, and accessibility of information, and outlines the following principles in relation to the protection of information:

- Data should only be used for the purpose for which they were intended.
- Data should not be disclosed to other individuals/organizations without the consent of the individual to whom they pertain unless there is legislation or an overriding reason permitting such a breach.
- Individuals have a right to know what information is available pertaining to them.
- Personal information must be kept up to date and should be kept no longer than is necessary or than statute permits.
- All organizations holding personal information relating to individuals must have adequate security measures in place to protect the information stored.
- An individual has a right to have any information that is proven to be factually incorrect, corrected.

The Code: Standards of Conduct, Performance and Ethics (NMC 2008) identifies the following principles to which any registered nurse should adhere within their practice.
As a nurse, you must:

- respect people's right to confidentiality;
- ensure that people are informed about how and why information is shared by those who will be providing their care;

- disclose information only if you believe that someone may be at risk of harm (in line with the law);
- keep clear and accurate records of the discussions you have, the assessments you make, the treatment and medicines you give, and how effective these have been;
- ensure that all records are kept securely.

These principles uphold the main regulations outlined within the law for collecting, using, storing, and sharing information, the basic premise being that we must maintain patient confidentiality and ensure that all patient records are secure.

The NHS also has a specific Code of Practice relating to *Information Security Management* (DoH, 2007). This covers the collection, use, and storage of any digital, electronic, or hard-copy information that exists within the context of the NHS as an organization.

The NHS Code of Practice outlines the following requirements for utilizing information within the NHS.

- Support patient care and any underlying associated business processes.
- Support evidence-based clinical practice.
- Support health promotion and guidance for the public.
- Support administrative and managerial decision-making.
- Meet legal requirements ensuring adherence to legislation—that is, the Data Protection Act 1998.
- Support audit.
- Support research, clinical effectiveness, and required improvement programmes.
- Archive information.
- Support patient choice and design of services to meet patient need.

In addition to the NHS Code of Practice, each NHS organization has a 'Caldicott guardian' who is responsible for overseeing the arrangements for using and sharing person-based clinical information (Griffith and Tengnah, 2008). He or she ensures that patient information is only shared for justifiable purposes and that the legal requirements of the Data Protection Act 1998 are adhered to.

....

⊕ Learning point 6: Ethical and legal issues—using, storing, and sharing information

Consider the following questions below, and write down your answers and justification for them. Use the information you have gained from reading the first part of this section to support your answers.

1. A text message reminding a 15-year-old about her appointment with the practice nurse is sent to her phone; her mother reads it and questions her daughter why she has made an appointment. Does this breach confidentiality?

2. A patient with learning disabilities has given permission for his brother to have access to his full medical records online. A community nurse dressing a wound on his foot requests to see them. Do you think that there are any ethical issues here and should she have access to the full record?

3. A patient's notes are left in the patient's room following a ward round. Her son reads them whilst she is in the toilet and discovers his mum has cancer. He demands to know why he hasn't been informed. Should he have been informed?

4. A student nurse downloads a patient's record onto a USB stick to use for her assignment. The USB stick subsequently gets lost with the information on it. What are the legal issues here?

5. A patient discovers that information about him has been posted in a discussion between two people on a social networking site. They are subsequently identified as being qualified nurses at the trust where he was treated. What are the legal and ethical issues here, and what areas of the NMC Code have been breached?

6. A nurse forgets to log off from the PC in the ward office and another member of staff accesses the PC on their user name. A routine IT audit identifies inappropriate use and access to Internet gaming sites. This access is traced back to the nurse who was deemed to be logged on at the time of the usage. What are the issues here?

See Table 9.2.

....

Sharing information about patients in any format must adhere to the legislation as outlined above. Information gained from patients must be stored safely and with the full knowledge of the patient. The individual must consent to their information being used for any other purpose other than that for which it was supplied. This means that information gained from patients that is to be used for the purpose of supporting their care should not be used for the purposes of research or academic purposes without gaining their consent first.

Furthermore, nurses must respect confidentiality at all times and take account of the environment in which their conversations may take place both electronically and face to face. Discussion of intimate patient details between two people on a public social networking site may be thought to be a private conversation between two people. However, it has the potential to have the same effect as a nurse sitting in a crowded room shouting out the same details to another nurse. The conversation is visible and audible to others.

The impact of electronic information being stolen or lost is often more serious than handwritten notes, as vast amounts of data can be stored on a disk or electronic device in comparison to the same amount of data in handwritten format.

Table 9.2 Suggested answers to Learning point 6

Question	Discussion
1	It could be argued that the patient has the responsibility to maintain the security of her own phone if she does not want her mother to read her messages. The girl would have had to sign up and consent to the information being sent to her in text format. The practice has not sent any confidential information via the message, so it would not be deemed a breach of confidentiality.
2	There are ethical issues here. Did the patient have the capacity to consent to allow his brother access to his medical records? These issues would be dealt with before he was given access to the records. Once the patient has given his brother access, he still has the right to limit who else views them. The nurse can request to see them and the patient or his brother can decide whether or not they wish her to see them. The patient or next of kin are not likely to object to her seeing the record, but a nurse has a responsibility only to access information that is required for the direct benefit of the patient in their care and would not necessarily require access to the full record in this instance. In this case, the nurse should explain why she requires access and what information she is looking for.
3	Any patient information is confidential and nurses must protect that information unless the patient has asked for it to be shared. In this case, confidential notes have been left in a place that is accessible to others and therefore this would constitute a breach of confidentiality. The patient may have decided she did not wish her son to know and would have every right to have that information kept confidential. It can be very difficult to deal with these situations, as relatives are often very anxious and want to know how their relative is. The nurse's role would be to talk to the patient and her son and explain that the information has been accessed and try to support both of them in discussing the implications of the diagnosis. This would have to be recorded as a clinical incident and an investigation would be conducted to establish the circumstances surrounding the breach.
4	Under the Data Protection Act 1998, data should only be used for the purpose intended and if the patient had not consented to this information being used for this purpose, then a breach would have occurred. The organization could be held accountable for the fact that the information was able to be downloaded onto a non-secure storage device. All personal data should be encrypted if it is stored on any portable device. It is unlikely the student would be prosecuted, but he or she could be subject to professional suitability or disciplinary proceedings by the university for not protecting the confidentiality of the patient.
5	The use of social networking sites is commonplace and the chat between users of them is often visible to many other people. In this case, a patient has seen information relating to him. Professionally, the qualified nurses have breached his confidentiality and, dependent on the nature of the information divulged, they could be subject to both disciplinary proceedings from their employer and the NMC. The NMC Code identifies the following areas in relation to this incident that have not been upheld: 'Respect the people's right to confidentiality'; 'Ensure people are informed about how and why information is shared by those who will be providing their care'; 'Disclose information only if you believe someone may be at risk of harm. In line with the law'.
6	Anyone issued with a user name and password to access a database of information is responsible for maintaining the security of it. Every login on a system can be traced back to the username, so it is vital that your user name and password are kept secure and that you log on and off using your own username. Leaving a computer workstation logged on has the potential to allow someone who shouldn't have access to see confidential information. In this case, the person used the workstation to access inappropriate material on the Internet. If the person who has logged on cannot prove that they were not the person accessing the material, then potentially they could be subject to disciplinary procedures within the employing organization and also the NMC.

In the same way that a nurse would not seek to leave confidential notes lying around in a corridor or on a table accessible to the public, we must not leave confidential material accessible to people on a PC, laptop, or other electronic device.

The use of passwords and user names ensures data security and enables the tracing of users via their login details. It is vital that any password or user name issued to an individual is kept securely and that, once the individual has finished accessing information, they log out to maintain the security of the system.

No system of storing information will ever be completely secure. However, it is an important part of the role of the nurse to maintain the confidentiality of information relating to an individual, regardless of what format it takes. This means ensuring the safety of any passwords that enable access to electronic systems and ensuring that documentation relating to patients is not left unsecured.

Accessing and sharing information with patients

Patients have been able to apply for access to health records formulated after 1991 following the introduction of the Access to Health Records Act 1990. However, in practice, this has often proved difficult for patients or their relatives as the application process was often confusing and, if the patient did gain access, they could not take the record away and scrutinize it. In addition, handwritten records were often found to be incomplete or difficult for patients to read.

The Data Protection Act 1998 provided further regulation governing the storage, use of, and access to specific personal data in written or electronic formats. This was followed by the Freedom of Information Act 2000, which confirmed the right of an individual to have access to information that is held by a public authority in relation to themselves.

The introduction of electronic patient records has led to an increase in the number of patients being able to apply for and access their own health records. There are currently several systems in operation in the UK that allow patients to access their records electronically. One example of this is the PAERS/EMIS system **www.patient. co.uk/emisaccess.asp**, which allows patients to access their whole GP-held record via a secure password that they can access via the Internet. The patient has to consent to the access and will receive information to assist them to understand some of the information they may access. Patients can also book non-urgent appointments and order repeat prescriptions online.

 This picture is available at: **www.ardleighsurgery.nhs.uk/Emis-Access%20 Medication.htm**

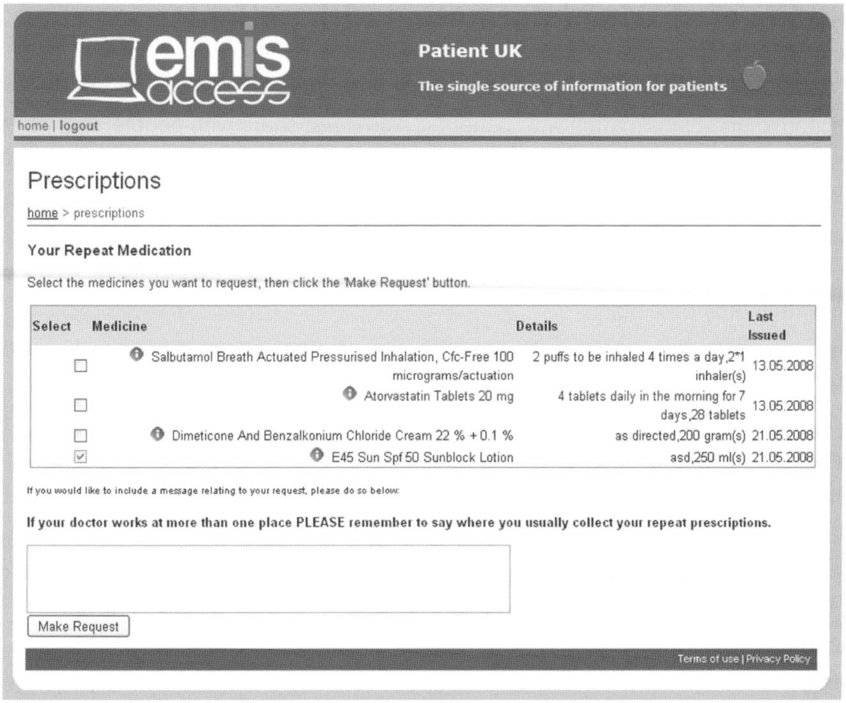

Figure 9.4 Example of Emis online booking system

Another example is available via **www.healthspace.nhs.uk**. The NHS plans to enable every patient in England to have access to a summary care record, which will be stored electronically. Around 486,000 patients have already registered access to a summary of their healthcare record online (DoH, 2008a). This record will only contain certain details relating to an individual's health and will be accessible to the patient and health professionals involved in their care. A log of who accesses the information will be maintained centrally by the NHS and the patient will be told who has access to their record.

The benefits of this system are obvious in that the patient has complete ownership of their record and can choose with whom they share it. Its accessibility means that patients can access it any time and anywhere via the Internet. This is valued by patients, as they feel they have ownership of their record and can choose where, when, and with whom they share it (Gladwin, 2007).

Check out this video of a patient describing benefits of accessing their electronic patient record: **http://wiki.patientsknowbest.com/PAERS**

Benefits of sharing information with patients

The Code: Standards of Conduct, Performance and Ethics makes the role of the nurse explicit in sharing information with patients: 'You must share with people, in a way they can understand, the information they want or need to know about their health' (NMC, 2008). Decisions about patient care should always involve the patient and, if appropriate, the family. Effective decisions about care require effective communication, and the nurse's role should include informing the patient about care decisions or associated goals within their care plan.

How we share information with patients and whether or not there are benefits to doing so is an issue worth discussion. Sharing information with the patient helps to establish trust, and we need trust to underpin the professional relationship that we have with a patient.

There are many examples in which the professional relationship between healthcare professional and patient has been damaged by the negligent or criminal actions of a specific registrant. Cases such as Beverley Allitt (DoH, 1994) and Harold Shipman (DoH, 2005) have highlighted to the public that those in the medical and nursing professions cannot automatically be deemed trustworthy. High-profile cases such as these in which health professionals, either doctors or nurses, abuse their privileged relationship with patients by causing them harm has demonstrated the need to ensure our practice is transparent and that we establish a partnership of trust with our patients.

Although there is little evidence to support the fact that sharing records with patients reduces the likelihood of errors occurring, common sense dictates that it is a possibility. If patients are able to access and understand their records, they will be best placed to identify any inaccuracies or omissions in the data. How we subsequently deal with the information that the patient provides us regarding any errors will either strengthen or weaken that partnership of trust.

Knowledge can be viewed as power, and if a patient is given all of the relevant information needed to make decisions about their health, they are more likely to feel an equal part in the relationship. Many aspects of a nurse's role should involve working in partnership with patients.

....

 Learning point 7

Think about the experience you have had in practice in which you have either observed or participated in partnership working with a patient or family. How did you feel about it? Do you think the patient benefited from this approach?

....

Suggested answer to Learning point 7

Partnership working could include: setting goals for achievement in managing long-term conditions or supporting patients and their families to deliver treatments or care; teaching practical skills such as tube feeding; or enabling them to give injections to themselves or others.

There is evidence to support the belief that patients feel empowered by being able to access their records and that sharing information makes patients feel involved in their care (Pagliari et al., 2007). Empowering patients is a key function of a nurse and requires effective communication between the nurse and the patient.

The nurse's role is pivotal in ensuring that the patient has the information in order to understand their records, and that support mechanisms are in place should the patient have difficulty understanding the terminology, abbreviations, and coded entries. Of course, there will be challenges in ensuring that everyone has equitable access to records and not everyone will be an appropriate candidate to have access to their full records.

There may be occasions on which it is deemed inappropriate for a specific patient to view their whole record, for example, a mentally ill patient may be deemed to be a risk to themselves or others if given access to information within their file. There are procedures in place to ensure that decisions that have to be made about access are considered in a fair and equitable way. The Social Care Record Guarantee (NIGB, 2009) identifies best practice as sharing information between patients and healthcare professionals; it provides a framework for local authorities to manage patient information and addresses issues in relation to this.

The exciting thing for patients and health professionals is that electronic records have the capacity to be linked to information points, allowing the patient to learn more and in their own time. This will allow the nurse, particularly in the community, to ensure that patients understand their conditions and the treatment options available to them.

One example of this may be a patient who has been newly diagnosed with depression and commenced on a specific drug. The patient would be able to access their record and click on the drug that they have been prescribed; information relating to that drug, including side effects, would then appear on the screen. The patient would also be able to click on the screen to find out information, including support networks or services relating to depression, and then read about it in their own time. This could help the patient to identify any areas of concern or questions for the next time they see the nurse or their GP. This could help to make the time within the consultation more effective for both the patient and the clinician.

Of course, not all patients will choose to engage at this level or have the capacity to make decisions about their care. Nurses will need to recognize those patients who want to engage at this level and ensure that all patients are given the same opportunities.

Case study 1: Challenges in granting access to online records

Mrs Begum, a 58-year-old lady who has ischaemic heart disease, is clinically obese and at risk from further health problems such as stroke and diabetes. She is on regular medication to reduce her cholesterol and her GP has advised her to lose weight as she is awaiting a coronary artery bypass graft. She has regular checks with her practice nurse to monitor her weight and cholesterol. English is not her first language as she speaks Urdu and communication can often be difficult for her. At one of her appointments, the nurse suggests that she sign up to access her records online so that she can keep track of her appointments and the advice she has been given.

 Learning point 8

Consider the challenges this may present to the nurse and Mrs Begum in the case study. How may this approach benefit both the patient and the nurse?

Suggested answer to Learning point 8

The challenges for the nurse are likely to be ensuring that Mrs Begum understands the process of signing up for access to her records and that she is able to read the notes once she has accessed them. It may be that Mrs Begum decides to allow a relative to access them for her. If this were the case, the benefits of Mrs Begum managing her records would be lost. If Mrs Begum were able to understand her records and could use the information points to understand her condition, she could become more informed and would possibly be more likely to engage with health promotion advice.

It would be vital that the nurse ensured that any information that was given to Mrs Begum to help support her in her weight loss and maintaining a healthy lifestyle was accessible to her and in her own language.

Another significant challenge may be ensuring that Mrs Begum has the necessary skills to enable her to access her records electronically. If she hasn't the skills, then how will the nurse support her to develop these? There are numerous organizations that exist to assist people from all backgrounds to develop their reading, writing, and IT skills.

The main challenge will be for the nurse to understand what level of engagement Mrs Begum wishes to have in this case. The nurse will need to ensure that Mrs Begum understands the choices and options she has and support her to develop them if she wishes. If she does not wish to engage, then the nurse needs to respect this and continue to support her in a more traditional nurse–patient relationship.

The challenge for nurses will be ensuring that they have confidence in their own knowledge and skills and do not feel threatened by patients who embrace information and seek it out for themselves. The increase in information available at our fingertips means that patients are often well informed and attend appointments armed with the latest downloads relating to specific treatments and conditions for which they have spent hours trawling the Internet.

Much of this information may be of poor quality and lack credibility, and nurses need to be able to explain to patients confidently why the information that they have found may not be applicable to them. This can be extremely challenging and nurses may feel threatened by an informed, or misinformed, patient.

However, empowered and informed patients are more likely to work in partnership with us to manage their own health and are therefore more likely to comply with treatment options. This will, in turn, lead to less need for acute intervention and patients will be able to recognize and be proactive in managing any future health crisis.

According to the Department of Health (2009a), there are 15.4 million people in the UK with long-term conditions, and with an ever-increasing ageing population, this figure is likely to continue to rise. The development of 'Expert Patient' programmes (DoH, 2009a) has seen a significant increase in those people who are becoming empowered and informed about their condition in order to remain healthier for longer.

There is likely to be an increase in the emphasis on enabling and supporting self-care within communities and empowering patients with information will become a requirement that will underpin the nurse–patient interaction of the future.

The five pillars of self-care identified by the Department of Health (2009a) comprise the following.

1. Information
2. Skills, knowledge, and training
3. Tools and self-monitoring devices
4. Healthy lifestyle choices
5. Support networks

The process of sharing information with patients, particularly electronically, can help to facilitate self-care. Patients provided with information can decide for themselves what lifestyle choices they wish to make. There is a vast array of support networks available for patients to help them make informed choices and to provide them with access to information from experts and others experiencing similar problems.

Evans et al. (2009) indicate that the earlier in the diagnosis a patient becomes informed and empowered, the more likely they are to engage within their own care and follow a self-care pathway. This highlights the need for nurses to ensure that patients are given relevant and appropriate information about their condition as early as possible. They will also need time to discuss their care and have access to support when they require it.

Learning point 9

Consider the skills, knowledge, and tools a patient may need to enable them to access their records, identify support networks, and enhance their understanding relating to their condition and their treatment. How do you view your role in developing these for the patient?

Suggested answer to Learning point 9

Nurses in the future will play a key role in supporting patients to manage their own conditions. To empower patients, the nurse must be able to help them to gain knowledge and to signpost where they can get the information. Patients may require very practical information relating to how to use the information available to them and how to access it. Nurses need to be able to identify what information is useful to patients and to help them to understand it. Patients may require very practical skills-based assistance to enable them to access their records and nurses can help them to understand the importance of checking the accuracy of their records and make suggestions as to how they may use them effectively to manage their health.

The future of health information and communication

As discussed within this chapter, the future of health care in the UK will involve technological advancement and changes to the way in which we communicate with patients and record, access, or store information. The review conducted by Lord Darzi (DoH, 2008b) puts quality right at the heart of the future direction of the NHS. Many of the improvements and standards that he suggests involve ensuring the information available to both patients and clinicians is of good quality, is managed appropriately, and that technology is utilized to enhance both communication and the care of patients.

Examples of future technologies that are either already being used in practice or will become more common are as follows.

- Hand-held electronic assessment systems are designed to be used at the bedside to assess and plan care. Information can then be downloaded at a docking station centrally to be stored as part of the patient's main record.
- Electronic prescription services mean that patients will no longer have to travel to their surgeries to pick up paper prescriptions.

- Electronic systems for recording drug administration are designed to highlight errors and omissions and will help to reduce the amount of clinical drug errors.

- Online booking systems for clinics and GP practices allow patients to book appointments ahead of time and to see the GP of their choice.

- Mobile phones can be used to monitor health information from patients and to provide health promotion advice either on an individual or population basis.

- Remote technology can be used to monitor patients with long-term conditions and to support them in managing their own health needs.

- Nurses using video links or digital imaging can provide support for patients or other healthcare professionals.

- Coded information can be extracted from patient data to predict trends in health, design, and audit services, and to identify potential target groups requiring health intervention and specialist services.

- Social networking sites may be used to engage with diverse groups of patients or to gain feedback about services.

The potential for working differently and being able to provide services or support remotely will continue to increase as technologies develop. This will increase the flexibility of our healthcare delivery systems and allow us to reach more people. The continuous advances in communication technologies mean that the possibilities for the future are virtually endless.

Developing skills to meet the future challenges

Managing information and communication is an integral part of a nurse's role. The future of healthcare delivery will undoubtedly involve an increase in technologies designed to support and enhance communication across professional groups and to ensure safe and effective care for patients. However, as Moore (2009) highlights, the use of technology within nursing should not detract from human interaction, which should continue to underpin our practice.

It will be essential that nurses in the future are able to meet the ever-increasing needs of their patients and are equipped with the skills to manage the information technology that will exist in health care and which will become an integral part of nursing care.

A report conducted for the Royal College of Nursing (RCN) (Baker et al., 2009) identified that many nursing students felt unprepared for working in an e-health environment. It will be beneficial for student nurses to identify early on in their education any skills gaps or learning needs they have in relation to utilizing information technology and managing health information. This may include being able to conduct a comprehensive search for, and critical appraisal of, evidence to support practice and patients.

Most students are fully conversant with using word processing and the Internet, but may not be able to manage or store information appropriately, nor fully understand the issues relating to data protection and confidentiality. *Connecting for Health and Learning to Manage Health Information Programmes* (DoH, 2009*b*) has designed specific courses to prepare nurses and other health professionals for the challenges of managing and using electronic resources within their practice.

 Learning point 10: Planning for professional development

Return to the NMC principles relating to confidentiality and data protection outlined on pp. 166–7 and identify what knowledge you already have following completion of this chapter. Identify what knowledge or skills you still require in order to meet them. How might you address any identified learning needs and what resources could you utilize? This will be individual to you, and should include an action plan for how you intend to develop your knowledge and understanding in relation to the learning outcomes.

 You can read more about professional development in Chapter 16.

Conclusion

There is no doubt that the future of communication in health care and particularly nursing will involve technology to aid our practice. The basic premise of communication being at the heart of what nurses do will never change, but technology will give us opportunities to enhance our practice and develop more of a partnership with our patients. Patients will have access to an increasing range of information about their own health and the technologies available to manage and treat them. The nurse's role will need to develop in order to understand these technologies and to be able to help patients to make the right choices for their own health.

The public demand for instant access to information and services is increasing, and technology exists and is accessible to facilitate this. Nurses have an important role to play in facilitating the use of technology to deliver services that our patients want and need. In the same way that conversations are held in real time in a virtual environment, and goods and services can be purchased online and delivered the next day, health care must keep up with the pace of change in order to meet the expectations of our patients.

 To find more resources to aid your learning, please now go online to
www.oxfordtextbooks.co.uk/orc/webb

Web links

www.connectingforhealth.nhs.uk/

www.evidence.nhs.uk/default.aspx

www.mapofmedicine.com/

www.nhs.uk/

www.nmc-uk.org

Further reading

Nursing and Midwifery Council (2009) *Record Keeping: Guidance for Nurses and Midwives*. London: NMC.

References

Access to Health Records Act 1990. Available at Office of Public Sector Information: www.opsi.gov.uk/acts/acts1990/ukpga_19900023_en_1 (accessed October 2009).

Audit Commission (2009) *PbR Data Assurance Framework 2008/09: Key Messages from Year 2 of the National Clinical Coding Audit Programme*. London: Audit Commission.

Baker, D., Clark, J., and Bullock, I. (2009) *How Well Prepared are Nursing Students for Working in an eHealth Environment? Phase One: Report of an Online Survey*. London: RCN.

Coiera, E. (2003) *Guide to Health Informatics* (2nd edn). London: Arnold.

Cullum, N. (2002) *IMP 2-11 Nurses' Use of Research Information in Clinical Decision Making: A Descriptive and Analytical Study*. London: DoH.

Data Protection Act 1998. Available at Office of Public Sector Information: www.opsi.gov.uk/acts/acts1998/ukpga_19980029_en_1 (accessed October 2009).

Department of Health (1994) *The Allitt Inquiry: Independent Inquiry Relating to Deaths and Injuries on the Children's Ward at Grantham and Kesteven General Hospital during the Period February to April 1991*. London: HMSO.

—— (2005) *Shipman: The Final Report*. London: HMSO.

—— (2007) *Information Security Management: NHS Code of Practice*. London: DoH.

—— (2008a) *Health Informatics Review: Report*. London: DoH.

—— (2008b) *High Quality for All: The Next Stage Review Final Report*. London: DoH.

—— (2009a) *Your Health, Your Say: A Guide to Long-term Conditions and Self-care*. London: DoH.

—— (2009b) *Learning to Manage Health Information: A Theme for Clinical Education, Making a Difference*. London: DoH.

Dickinson, A. (2006) 'Implementing the Single Assessment Process: Opportunities and Challenges', *Journal of Interprofessional Care*, 20(4) (August): 365–79(15).

Freedom of Information Act 2000. Available at Office of Public Sector Information: www.opsi.gov.uk/Acts/acts2000/ukpga_20000036_en_1 (accessed October 2009).

Gladwin, J. (2007) 'Giving Patients Open Access to Medical Records Would Help Nurses Improve Care', *Nursing Times*, 103(25): 14.

Griffiths, R. and Tengnah, C. (2008) *Law and Professional Issues in Nursing*. Exeter: Learning Matters.

Leach, L. and Segal, M. (2010) 'Are Clinical Practical Guidelines (CPGs) Useful for Health Services and Health Workforce Planning? A Critique of Diabetes CPGs', *Diabetic Medicine*, 27(5): 570–7.

Mills, C. and Rajwer, M. (2005) 'Care Planning with the Electronic Patient Record', *Nursing Times*, 101(37): 26.

Moore, R. (2009) 'How Technology Can Help Nurses Improve Patient Care', *Nursing Times*, 105(19): 29.

Nadzam, D. M. (2009) 'Nurses' Role in Communication and Patient Safety', *Journal of Nursing Care Quality*, 24(3): 184–8.

National Information Governance Board for Health and Social Care (2009) *Social Care Record Guarantee for England*. Available at: www.nigb.nhs.uk/bookletlr.pdf (accessed October 2009).

National Patient Safety Agency (2007) *Recognising and Responding Appropriately to Early Signs of Deterioration in Hospitalised Patients*. London: NPSA.

—— National Reporting and Learning Service (2009) *Safety in Doses: Improving the Use of Medicines in the NHS*. London: NPSA. Available at: www.nrls.npsa.nhs.uk/resources/?entryid45=61625 (accessed October 2009).

Nursing and Midwifery Council (2008) *The Code: Standards of Conduct, Performance and Ethics for Nurses and Midwives*. London: NMC.

—— (2009) *Record Keeping: Guidance for Nurses and Midwives*. London: NMC.

—— (2010) *Standards of Education for Pre-registration Nursing Programmes*. London: NMC.

Pagliari, C., Detmer, D., and Singleton, P. (2007) 'Potential of Electronic Personal Health Records', *British Medical Journal*, 335: 330–3. Available at: www.bmj.com/cgi/content/full/335/7615/330 (accessed June 2009).

Roberts, H., Hesley, Z. M., Thomas, G., Meakins, P., Powell, J., Robison, J., Gove, I., Turner, G., and Sayer, A. A. (2006) 'Nurse-led Implementation of the Single Assessment Process in Primary Care: A Descriptive Feasibility Study', *Age and Ageing*, 35: 394–8. Available at: http://ageing.oxfordjournals.org/cgi/reprint/35/4/394 (accessed October 2009).

Royal College of Nursing (2006) *Putting Information at the Heart of Nursing Care: How IT is Set to Revolutionise Health Care and the NHS*. London; RCN.

Verhoeven, F., Steehouder, M. F., Hendrix, R. M. G., and van Gemert-Pijnen, J. E. W. (2010) 'How Nurses Seek and Evaluate Clinical Guidelines on the Internet', *Journal of Advanced Nursing*, 66(1): 114–27.

White, L. and Clegg, A. (2009) 'Encouraging and Supporting Patients Living with Long-term Conditions to Self-care', *Nursing Times*, 105(32): 14–16.

10

Professional communication skills for student survival: self-management, writing, and presenting

Lucy Webb

This chapter will help you to achieve competencies in:

- ➔ communicating effectively both orally and in writing so that your meaning is always clear;

- ➔ recording information accurately and clearly on the basis of observation and communication;

- ➔ effectively communicating people's stated needs and wishes to other professionals;

- ➔ providing accurate and comprehensive written and verbal reports based on best available evidence.

Introduction

This chapter is about helping students with skills and techniques in presenting written and verbal information in the practice setting. It acknowledges the difficulties that students often face in adapting to the dual role of being a university student and a learner healthcare professional. The kinds of skills needed range from how to communicate as a member of a team, how to represent your patients to fellow professionals, and how to share your learning with others. In essence, this chapter aims to help the student to manage the journey from novice student to professional nurse in the way in which he or she communicates with colleagues and interprets how they communicate with them.

At the same time, the student nurse has to cope with being a student, accommodating the life and expectations of university, and acquiring academic skills to support their studies. Therefore, this chapter will look at challenges in practice, including socialization, roles, stress, learning, as well as writing skills in clinical documents, academic writing, and making presentations.

The challenges facing the student

A lot of communication advice for the student nurse aims to develop professional skills with patients and relatives, and covers those skills that could be described as therapeutic, such as developing the nurse–patient relationship and applying active listening skills. This is incredibly important, but this chapter seeks to target the broader communication skills that help the student to develop as a person in a professional setting— the kinds of skills that are needed to work in an often stressful environment and within a team that needs a certain standard of interpersonal skills in order to function effectively. It also recognizes the typical workload of a student nurse in having to balance placements and academic work, including assignments, at the same time.

Health care is a stressful profession to enter, in any role or at any level, because it involves dealing with people who are stressed, distressed, and demanding. To become effective in such an environment demands personal skills, as well as professional ones, to meet the demands of the job. All health students go through a process of 'professional **socialization**' into the role of the professional (Mackintosh, 2006). This is stressful in itself as old aspects of oneself are discarded and new characteristics are adopted. Any nurse can tell you that training to be a nurse changes people. A person finishing a nurse education programme will be a very different person from the one who started. Along the way, many new personal skills have to be acquired and practised. Let's consider some of them that you will encounter.

The nurse role

On the first placement as a student, you may have already experienced being called 'nurse'. When you adopt the nurse role, put on the uniform, or simply start your shift, you, the person, have become you, the nurse. People have greater expectations of nurses, they expect a particular type of behaviour that would be extraordinary in any other context. First-year students often find that their lack of skills and knowledge, and their lack of self-awareness or identification as a nurse, undermines their confidence and creates anxiety (Chesser-Smyth, 2005). However, we are all 'nurses'. In one sense, this is a realistic expectation, as the *Guidance on Professional Conduct for Nursing and Midwifery Students* expects similar personal and professional conduct from the student as the qualified nurse (NMC, 2009a).

To adapt to that level of expectation, the student has to 'become' that person while in the nurse role. This can be very uncomfortable if that role is not like our real selves at all. For example, you may be expected to be dynamic and active and lead a social sing-song for elderly residential patients, even though you are really a quiet, thoughtful person, or to hold a stranger's hand while they cry, despite such intimacy being quite alien to you.

At these times, we discover the difference between the nurse 'role' and our personal identity—when we are out of our 'comfort zone'. Students do develop these skills, or develop coping strategies for those 'out of the comfort zone' moments (Brennan and McSherry, 2007). But it takes training and self-development to learn how to do this, and can be very stressful along the way.

The student role

Many students commencing nursing training have left their school/college days behind them and had some experience of the working world. Indeed, many nursing students come into nursing in later life, having years of experience of adult roles such as being a parent, partner, or employee. In other words, many student nurses have an adult sense of responsibility and autonomy and find university life a little bit overprotective and even infantilizing. Universities are often regarded as delivering adult-style learning in which the student takes responsibility for their own motivation and is self-directed. However, Bedford and Wilson (2006) warn that it can be easy for the child–parent form of relating to inhibit adult learning if the university culture reinforces this student role by having strict parental-style rules and structures. Arguably, nurse education and training can impose institutional parenting through attendance requirements, assignment deadlines, and the provision of personal tutors, student counselling, and learning support. For Bedford and Wilson (2006), it is therefore important that student nurses be aware of the need to maintain motivation and self-direction in their learning and maintain that 'adult' ego state we addressed in Chapter 3.

 Refer back to Chapter 3, which outlines transactional analysis, demonstrating how, when one person adopts the role of a parent, the other is forced into the role of a child.

Nurse training can be particularly confusing for students, whether they are school-leavers or mature students, as they are subject to conflicting roles (Brennan and McSherry, 2007). The nurse student has to be a 'nurse' in practice, but has other identities as a student, parent, or a professional role from their past. It is fortunate that most nurse trainers understand this conflict of roles and strive to emphasize and support the need for the maturing of personal qualities among nurse students and the development of professional responsibility, confidence, and skills. Evidence suggests that the more skills and knowledge are acquired in practice, the more confident the student becomes and the easier it is to identify with the role of the nurse (Brennan and McSherry, 2007).

Working with others

Most healthcare professionals work as a team. That means working with people we sometimes don't like, don't gel with, or even can't stand. Nevertheless, the professional needs to separate their personal values from their professional values and judge the situation in terms of effectiveness for the patient, rather than what should or shouldn't happen according to a personal viewpoint.

Conflict with other people in our team is inevitable. It might be a clash of personalities or a professional difference in opinion or approach. Either way, it is very difficult to 'get on with the job' unless we develop some personal strategies in the way in which we communicate with our colleagues that separate the 'professional' persona from our own identities.

The challenge of learning and practising

It is very anxiety-provoking to attempt new skills, especially with real patients who depend on you. Being on a practice placement is about learning and practising new skills all of the time, not just about being one of the members of staff on that shift. Therefore, for the student, the practice episode can be more stressful than for the other members of staff who work there all of the time (Chesser-Smyth, 2005). On a new placement, the student has to meet all of the new people and establish a working relationship with each person, learn new routines and practices, seek out learning opportunities to meet learning objectives, and integrate themselves into an established team in order to be accepted and welcomed. It is quite a tall order when you think about it. A successful placement relies on communication skills and relationship-building on both sides, but the student needs to work on those relationships. All students will be assigned a mentor and the quality of the student–mentor relationship can be the main factor in making the placement a successful one (Roberts, 2010), so it is important that the student uses his or her communication skills to develop a working relationship with that mentor.

Becoming a confident practitioner

Many students say that their biggest challenge is becoming confident in practice. Studies have shown, however, that this is natural and does not mean that they are not competent (Lauder et al., 2008). There are many situations that can deflate a student's confidence in the practice setting, just as there are situations that can boost confidence. However, a student is putting themselves in the way of new challenges all of the time, so it is inevitable that many situations and events will be new, unexpected, and difficult, and often lead to unsatisfactory outcomes. That is the learning process.

This process is about communication because it is about personal development and maturity. How we communicate with others is influenced by our self-confidence and assuredness in what we are doing. Therefore, the student's confidence needs to grow in order to communicate professionally and effectively at each stage of the learning process. An essential skill to learn for any health professional is how to manage stress effectively. Here, we will focus on those techniques and skills that involve communication specifically.

Managing stress: using communication skills

The obvious technique in managing your own stress is to communicate with other people. A problem shared, as the proverb goes, is a problem halved. Well, up to a point: it depends with whom you share it and how. Let's look at this.

There are some simple 'rules' that can guide us to effective stress management by communicating our problems with others.

Share your problems with friends or other non-work colleagues

Yallom (1970), an influential psychoanalyst, identified that sharing problems with others, even if they don't help us to solve any problems, helps us to feel like we're not alone. We can realize that others have faced similar problems, other people can empathize with us, take our side, and, in effect, validate our stressful experience. Sometimes, people might use phrases like 'I know what you mean', 'that happened to me', or 'that must have upset you'. Yallom calls this effect '**universality**' because we realize we share similar feelings with others: it's not just us! This is a good approach when you are stressed by things that you can't easily change, such as your assignment deadlines or practice setting.

Explain your problems to colleagues

This is a different approach from sharing because, by explaining the cause of your stress to colleagues, you are seeking to solve a problem or looking for help in managing the problem better. There is a goal involved here: you are not just 'offloading' on to others as in the above example.

Learning point 1

Why do you think it is better to explain a problem to colleagues rather than to 'offload' your feelings?

Suggested answer to Learning point 1

We can see that simply 'offloading' onto colleagues would be sharing a problem that they also experience and possibly already have an opinion about. Yes, they may agree with us, but work colleagues are in the same situation as us and we will not get that sense of 'universalism' from people 'in the same boat'. However, if we are seeking to solve a problem, work colleagues are often in the best position to help as they know the situation and the options available. Problem-solving is even more effective if we can include a line manager, clinical supervisor, or personal tutor who is in a position to make any necessary changes. We can also make ourselves more stressed by thinking stressfully.

Have a look at Tables 6.1 and 6.2 on dysfunctional thinking in Chapter 6. Do you recognize any of these unhelpful thinking styles? Beware the student's favourite unhelpful thought: 'It's not fair!'

You can find more advice on managing stress in ch. 16 of Sue Hart's *Nursing: Study and Placement Learning Skills* (2010).

Writing in clinical practice

Nurses are required to keep written records in relation to care in their workplace (NMC, 2008) and students need to develop these skills to a professional standard in order to qualify for registration. Student nurses are often all too aware that academic writing is part of the assessment process in training, and qualified practitioners will also have to write academic essays in order to acquire post-registration qualification and demonstrate continuing professional development. We will look first at writing in the practice setting.

Documenting practice: enhancing care and safeguarding patients

See Box 10.1, which lists the standards for record-keeping according to the NMC standards of conduct (NMC, 2008).

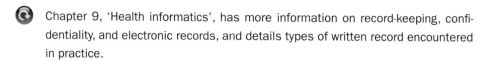 Chapter 9, 'Health informatics', has more information on record-keeping, confidentiality, and electronic records, and details types of written record encountered in practice.

Care plans and patient records are regarded as legal documents that can be used as evidence in a court of law; therefore it is vital that nurses record data accurately, realistically, and without prejudice and bias. It is important that entries on patient records are worded in such a way as to convey objective and observable facts, and that these facts are true, supportable, and include all important details and do not exclude important and relevant details. The wording and style of writing is important to reflect the elements of record-keeping listed below.

Objectivity

Data that are objective are free from bias and assumptions. The only element of subjectivity may be the professional opinion of the practitioner who is, by virtue of his or her skills and knowledge, able to make a degree of professional judgement equal to his or her training and experience. Data also should be free from moral judgement based on values and norms of the practitioner and free from stigma or prejudice.

Observable and supportable

Data entered into patient records or care plans need to describe measurable and observable behaviour and facts. The nurse has to be able to account objectively for the data on what they have observed. Data should only be based on evidence for which the nurse can be accountable. This therefore rules out the nurse's opinion (outside professional judgement) or assumptions. A nurse can describe that a patient 'appeared upset', but should not simply say 'the patient was upset'. If a patient says that they are upset, the appropriate objective recording of this would be 'the patient reported being upset'.

Relevant

Recorded data should be demonstrated to relate to aspects of the patient's care. If a specific nursing model or approach is used, nursing observations may be structured according to the elements of the model. For instance, in Roper's model using activities of daily living (ADL) (Holland and Rees, 2008) observations will reflect an ADL. Sometimes, entries are made that relate to ADLs, but are not relevant to care. For instance, the often overused 'slept well' may not have anything to do with a person's reasons for needing care. Nurses still record this, however, and it is not usually supportable information anyway, unless the nurse sat by the bedside and observed the patient snoring happily all night!

Entries for patient records should aim to aid the evaluation aspect of the nursing process and record whether interventions were carried out and how they were carried out. Care plan entries should clearly state specific care instructions, which include the rationale for interventions and the aims or goals. Look at Boxes 10.2 and 10.3 below for examples of good practice and poor practice in record-keeping.

....

 Learning point 2

Looking at the care plan examples in Boxes 10.2 and 10.3, can you identify:

1. words that describe observable data?
2. words or phrases that describe value judgements or assumptions?
3. words that give specific and relevant instructions?
4. words or phrases that give vague instructions?
5. words or phrases that are not relevant or inaccurate?

....

Suggested answers to Learning point 2

* **Words that describe observable data:** 'restfulness', 'three times', 'active', 'lay on bed', 'appeared to sleep'—all specific timed events.
* **Words or phrases that describe value judgements or assumptions:** 'normal sleep pattern'—need to establish what is 'normal' for this patient when well; 'pt. suffers from bipolar disorder, in manic phase'—assumes overactivity is due to diagnosis, also assumes patient 'suffers' because of the diagnosis; 's'lept well—assumes that the patient actually slept and this was good-quality sleep, which is not observable.
* **Words that give specific and relevant instructions or information:** all data in Box 10.2; time of sleep plan as an action and 'review diary in one week', in Box 10.3.

Box 10.2 Care plan and notes for patient X

Rationale (assessed need)	Patient demonstrates 24-hour over-activity, has difficulty getting to sleep and maintaining sleep for more than two hours during the night.
Aim (plan)	For the patient to establish a stable sleep pattern.
Action (intervention)	(1) To encourage patient to adhere to planned sleep/wake regime, 11 pm–6 am rest period. (2)–(10) [*] (11) To monitor patient's periods of restfulness in bed.
Evaluation	(1) Record observed sleep pattern in sleep diary.
	(2) Obtain patient's report of sleep pattern.
	(3) Review sleep plan weekly.
Notes	Day one: (1) Patient reminded of sleep plan three times between 11 and 11.30 pm. (2)–(10) [*] (11) Patient lay on bed in day clothes by 12 pm. Remained till 2.30 am. Active in ward till 4 am, then returned to bed and appeared to sleep until 5.30 am. Active on ward to present (7 am). Patient reported having slept 'most of the night'.

* Details omitted in this example for brevity

Box 10.3 Care plan and notes for patient Y

Rationale (assessed need)	Patient suffers from bipolar disorder, in manic phase.
Aim (plan)	Patient to establish normal sleep pattern.
Action (intervention)	(1) Encourage patient to get to bed at 11 pm and stay in bed till 6 am. (2)–(10) [*] (11) Observe sleep pattern.
Evaluation	(1) Complete sleep diary. (2) Review diary in one week.
Notes	Day one: Patient went to bed late evening. Got up once during night, otherwise slept well.

* Details omitted in this example for brevity

* ***Words or phrases that give vague instructions:*** most in Box 10,3, except as above; Box 10.2 contains some necessarily vague instructions that are open to nursing judgement, such as *'stable', 'restfulness', 'encourage', 'monitor', 'reminded', 'active'.*

* ***Words or phrases that are not relevant or inaccurate:*** *'pt. suffers from bipolar disorder'*—the patient's diagnosis is irrelevant; his behaviour (overactivity) is relevant to the care need (sleep); *'observe sleep pattern'*—how will this be observed and how recorded?; *'review diary'* (Box 10.3)—this is not supported by a clear aim except a

normal sleep pattern; Box 10.2 at least relies on something measurable—a *stable* sleep pattern (that is, regular, consistent).

  You will find further guidance on record-keeping in NMC (2009*b*).

Academic writing: how to get your message across

Writing an essay, and other kinds of academic assignment, is an essential skill for nursing students, as this element constitutes a high proportion of the material by which you will be assessed. The main reason for examining nurses by written work is to have evidence of the student's ability to understand the theory behind practice, to demonstrate their depth of understanding by evaluating and critically analysing theoretical evidence, and a practical ability to make links between theory and practice. Hence many marked assignments actually ask students to evaluate or critically analyse some aspect of theory and apply it to a practice situation. Most written assignments in nursing are likely to take this form in one way or another. So, while whole books and courses can be dedicated to improving student writing skills, this section will focus specifically on aiding you to identify what exactly is being asked of you in an assignment, and how to answer that question so that you are communicating to your lecturers that you have attained the right level of understanding and knowledge.

Identifying what is being asked of you

Assignment writers need to set a task that gives a fair opportunity for the student to demonstrate key learning outcomes on specified theory/practice themes. These key learning outcomes guide the marking process and are easy to spot in the marking criteria and assignment brief. They are specific words called **descriptors** in educational language, and they are always verbs or adverbs (words that describe actions or words that describe *how* an action is performed) in the assignment and criteria sentences (see below).

Descriptors tell you what to do, and how to do it.

Describe a nursing model and *critically discuss* its use in a practice setting.

The two descriptors above are 'describe' and 'discuss'. The sentence also tells you *how* to perform one of those tasks: 'critically discuss'.

Next, the assignment will tell you what the topic is. This is what you are expected to talk about. In the above example, the topic is 'a nursing model'.

The final element of an assignment like this is the context, and in nursing this is invariably some form of nursing practice context—clinical, managerial, or research-based.

In our example here, the context is 'a practice setting', so we can take it that this means clinical, although there is no reason in this case why we couldn't also look at the impact of a model on the care management element of practice.

➕ Learning point 3

Look at the assignment examples below and identify:

(a) what the student is being asked to do (the verb descriptors);
(b) how the student is to do it (the adverb descriptors);
(c) the topic the student should address;
(d) the context in which the student should address the topic.

Examples

1. Choose a chronic illness and describe and discuss three health promotion strategies that enable patients to adopt self-care to better manage their condition.
2. Critically evaluate any nursing intervention of your choice in relation to improving patient safety in the hospital setting.
3. Identify a specific health need commonly encountered in community nursing, and describe and critically evaluate the key service provision resources provided to meet that need.
4. Identify and describe a reflective model and critically analyse its effectiveness in aiding an aspect of professional development.

Suggested answers to Learning point 3

1. (a) Descriptors: describe, discuss. (b) Adverb descriptors: no adverb descriptors given. (c) The topic: three health promotion strategies (of your choice). (d) The context: patient self-care.
2. (a) Descriptors: evaluate. (b) Adverb descriptors: critically. (c) The topic: improving patient safety. (d) The context: a hospital setting and care need (of your choice).
3. (a) Descriptors: identify, describe, evaluate. (b) Adverb descriptors: critically. (c) The topic: service provision resources. (d) The context: a common community health need (of your choice).
4. (a) Descriptors: identify, describe, analyse. (b) Adverb descriptors: critically. (c) The topic: a reflective model (of your choice). (d) The context: one aspect of professional development (of your choice).

Sometimes descriptors, topics, and contexts can be obscured in the sentence construction. It can help in those circumstances to rewrite the sentence yourself to make it clearer. The example in Box 10.4 identifies the key elements of a complex question that aid the simplification.

Box 10.4 Assignment task

Using a patient or client for whom you have cared in practice, *choose* one aspect of care and discuss and critically *analyse* the evidence underpinning the nursing care given. *Discuss* how well the care given complied with the need to apply evidence-based practice in nursing care.

This can be reworded for clarity, as Box 10.5.

Box 10.5 Rewritten version

Using a case study and one aspect of care, *discuss* and critically *analyse* evidence that supports the care given. *Discuss* how well it complied with evidence-based nursing practice.

Notice that the descriptors (in italic) and the topics to be covered are still there.

The descriptors, topic, and context also tell us what not to do. If the words 'describe', 'list', 'identify' are not there, it can be assumed that lengthy descriptions of, say, Roper's model or diabetes are not necessary. We can save words and get straight on with 'discussing' or 'critically analysing' because that is where the marks will be offered.

  You can find advice on using evidence for student assignments in another book in this series: Holland and Rees (2010).

Structuring your answer: how to write an essay

An essay is a story, but in a different form. It has a beginning, a middle, and an end. The example below will help you to 'tell your story' for most essays in nursing.

Beginning: the introduction

Say what you are going to talk about and say why this topic is important (to health care). That's it! There is no need to go on at this point. Most students waste word space here. It is unnecessary.

Middle: your discussion/critique/evaluation

You don't need to repeat what you have already said. Get on with addressing the descriptors in the assignment guidelines or question. See examples below.

1. Describe: your topic and the context in which it takes place.
   Roper's model (Roper et al., 1981) is . . .
   Patient X was a 43-year-old man with type II diabetes and needed . . .

2. Discuss: the relevance/importance of the patient's needs to the topic.

   Patient X's main need appeared to be best met by Y aspect of the model because . . .

3. Evaluate: the effectiveness of the topic in the context of care.

   Roper's model helped nurses to identify and meet the patient's needs, however, Orem's self-care model may have been more useful in identifying the patient's self-care abilities such as . . .

4. Critically analyse: use the material that you have described, discussed, and evaluated to then explain why you think the situation was as it was. You can also suggest what could improve the situation.

   Roper's model was probably used in this case because the nurses were familiar with . . . Lack of skills development may have limited staff members' flexibility of model use and so . . .

This section of the essay should contain all of the key evidence that demonstrates your knowledge, understanding, and ability to discuss, evaluate, and critically analyse the topic in the specific context.

The end: your conclusion or summary

The golden rule is not to introduce new material in this section. However, the section is often the students' saviour because, if there hasn't been much critical analysis or evaluation before, here is the last chance to demonstrate these skills. This section should aim to remind the reader what the 'argument' has been, and a simple sentence within the conclusion can do this. For example,

> Therefore, it could be argued that adoption of one model on a ward can limit flexibility in meeting the wider holistic needs of some patients.

A good summary shows the reader that you understand the implications of what you have detailed previously. So, *don't* repeat yourself, but *do* sum up your 'take-home message' in one or two sentences in this section.

You can find more advice on writing assignments in ch. 6 of Hart (2010).

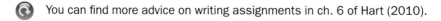

⊕ Learning point 4

Look up some examples of past exam papers or assignments in your academic institution.

1. Identify the descriptors, topic(s), and contexts that are required.
2. Rewrite long or complex assignment briefs into your own questions. Try to be as succinct and clear as possible without changing the task.

3. Write a very brief outline of headings you might use for such an assignment within the introduction, discussion, and conclusion.

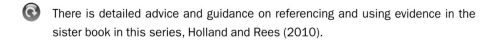

There is detailed advice and guidance on referencing and using evidence in the sister book in this series, Holland and Rees (2010).

Surviving making presentations

Making a presentation to colleagues, fellow students, or for a formal assignment is usually seen by students as very stressful and challenging. Few of us feel comfortable speaking formally to an audience, even if they are friends. Student nurses have to demonstrate their ability to disseminate knowledge and provide learning to others, so it is an important communication skill that needs to be developed. The good thing is, once you have done a few presentations on the course, you will feel much more confident when doing them professionally. We all need to be able to develop skills in disseminating good practice to our colleagues as a requirement of the NMC Code (2008); we may also be required to deliver educational or health promotional material to students, patients, or patient carers: for example, on sexual health or smoking cessation in schools or primary care, or stress management in psychiatric settings. So it is a skill that will prepare you for practice!

The key enemy to a good presentation is nerves! If you are not used to speaking in public, the very act of standing in front of an audience is a challenge in itself. The best way in which to reduce this problem is practice! Practise in front of your friends, family, colleagues at work, anywhere, and everywhere. This is a theory and practice-based technique linked to behavioural principles: the more we expose ourselves to feared stimuli and survive without harm, the more our nervous reactions will reduce (Hawton et al., 1989).

See Chapter 6 on behavioural principles for reassurance on this fact! You can also engage in positive and realistic thinking (again, see Chapter 6).

Remind yourself that you will not die, that the audience will not hate you and will probably be helpful and empathetic, that what you have to say is important or interesting (all good cognitive behavioural techniques), and that it will be a good step to developing your presentation skills so that next time you will be even better at it!

Organization and planning

What can reduce the success of a presentation is poor planning and organization. A useful checklist will help you to focus your planning for a streamlined presentation. This takes us through 'who, what, where, when, how, why'.

Who will be your audience? In nursing training, it will be either fellow students and your tutor or nursing colleagues on your practice placement. Qualified nurses may be presenting to nursing or multidisciplinary clinical colleagues in their workplace or to patient groups or students. The key factor here is gauging what they already know and how to pitch your descriptive material in the presentation: over their heads don't go but don't waste time explaining the obvious.

What is your topic? You may be presenting your research on a subject or feeding back from a workshop that you attended. The key element here is that you will need to ensure that you are familiar with the subject or at least plan the presentation to highlight the key areas. In structuring a presentation, keep the subject matter relevant and work toward the 'take-home message'. A tip that might help is to plan the presentation from the bottom up; identify the point for which you are aiming and work backwards from there. Ask yourself: what does the audience need to know in order to understand fully my key point?

Where are you presenting? Check out the environment, the equipment, where you will stand or sit. Will you be interrupted? Will there be noise? How can you limit these potential problems? Try to 'take control' of the environment. Don't just rely on someone else to do it. Move furniture, arrange your notes, close windows or curtains. Whatever. Take control.

'When' is related to 'where' in that the environment and your audience are likely to be affected by when the presentation takes place. Following the principle of 'take control', try to make sure that you have a specified time for your presentation. If it is on your practice placement, you need to let people know precisely when you will be presenting so that they will be there on time. There's nothing worse than waiting for people to turn up! Also, unless there is good reason to delay, start your presentation when you planned to. Don't wait for people to arrive or settle down. Once you have started, people will be quiet, and late arrivals will creep in apologetically. You are in charge!

How will you make your presentation? How long will it take, or how long have you got? This makes a huge difference to your planning. A short presentation means clear and relevant facts only—bullet points perhaps—a short introduction, and getting straight to the point. Longer presentations mean that you can introduce a bit more detail and even entertain your audience! A long presentation that contains streams of facts and constant overheads, for example, can be really tedious. Tell a few anecdotes that relate to the subject. Keep your audience interested by switching focus.

Why are you making this presentation? Focus on the main aim of the presentation. Is it to educate practitioners or students? Is it to pass a marked assessment? Is it to practise giving presentations? Is it to present group work or study material? Ask yourself: what is it I want to achieve? If it is a marked assessment, plan your presentation around the marking criteria. If it is to impart knowledge, focus on the key points that you want the audience to appreciate and remember. Planning towards an identified goal again is helped by bottom-up planning. Work from the goal back to the method of achieving it.

 See a sister book in this series, Holland and Rees (2010), for detailed advice on making presentations.

The key points for surviving presentations can therefore be summarized as:

- think positively and realistically;
- know your topic;
- plan;
- identify your goals;
- take control.

Conclusion

This chapter has focused on some core professional skills needed particularly for nursing care management and personal and professional development. Writing skills are needed to communicate patient care needs clearly to our colleagues, and in using care plans and patient records. We also need good writing skills in order to disseminate ideas and concepts in evidence-based practice to justify our care and demonstrate our professional development. As students, you will need to do this through writing formal assignments during your training. As qualified nurses, you will need to use these skills to demonstrate continuing professional development through post-registration training and course work, and to support your professional role in disseminating good practice and innovations to fellow professionals through publication. We also need formal verbal skills in order to disseminate learning and evidence-based practice to our colleagues through making presentations. We may also use presentation skills to deliver health promotion to patients and the general public. Student nurses may think that academic writing and presenting is not important to nursing after qualification—that these skills are only required in order to get through the pre-registration course. However, as has hopefully been highlighted, these skills are required of a qualified nurse to meet the demands of the NMC Code of Conduct (2008) and to practise as a competent nurse.

 To learn more about professional communication skills for student survival, please now go online to **www.oxfordtextbooks.co.uk/orc/webb**

You also can access more material on academic writing and presentations online at **www.oxfordtextbooks.co.uk/orc/holland**

Further reading

Burnard, P. (2004) *Writing Skills in Health Care*. Cheltenham: Nelson-Thornes.

Hart, S. (2010) *Nursing: Study and Placement Learning Skills*. Oxford: Oxford University Press.

Holland, K. and Rees, C. (2010) *Nursing: Evidence-based Practice Skills*. Oxford: Oxford University Press.

Murray, N. and Hughes, G. (2008) *Writing up Your University Assignments and Research Projects*. Maidenhead: McGraw-Hill Education.

Nursing and Midwifery Council (2009) *Record Keeping: Guidance for Nurses and Midwives*. London: NMC.

Northedge, A. (1990) *The Good Study Guide*. Milton Keynes: Open University.

References

Bedford, D. and Wilson, E. (2006) *Study Skills for Foundation Degrees*. London: David Fulton Publishers.

Brennan, G. and McSherry, R. (2007) 'Exploring the Transition and Professional Socialisation from Healthcare Assistant to Student Nurse', *Nurse Education in Practice*, 7: 206–14.

Chesser-Smyth, P. (2005) 'The Lived Experiences of General Student Nurses on their First Clinical Placement: A Phenomenological Study', *Nurse Education in Practice*, 5: 320–7.

Hart, S. (2010) *Nursing: Study and Placement Learning Skills*. Oxford: Oxford University Press.

Hawton, K., Salkovskis, P., Kirk, J., and Clark, D. (1989) *Cognitive Behaviour Therapy for Psychiatric Problems*. Oxford: Oxford Medical Publications.

Holland, K. and Rees, C. (2010) *Nursing: Evidence-based Practice Skills*. Oxford: Oxford University Press.

—— Jenkins, J., Solomon, J., and Whittam, S. (2008) *Applying the Roper Logan and Tierney Model in Practice* (2nd edn). Edinburgh: Churchill Livingstone.

Lauder, W., Roxburgh, M., Holland, K., Johnson, M., Watson, W., Porter, M., Topping, K., and Behr, A. (2008) *Nursing and Midwifery in Scotland: Being Fit for Practice*. Dundee: University of Dundee.

Mackintosh, C. (2006) 'Caring: The Socialisation of Pre-registration Student Nurses— A Longitudinal Qualitative Descriptive Study', *International Journal of Nursing Studies*, 43: 953–62.

Nursing and Midwifery Council (2008) *The Code: Standards of Conduct, Performance and Ethics for Nurses and Midwives*. London: NMC.

—— (2009a) *Guidance on Professional Conduct for Nursing and Midwifery Students*. London: NMC.

—— (2009b) *Record Keeping: Guidance for Nurses and Midwives*. London: NMC.

Roberts, D. (2010) 'First Steps into Practice', in S. Hart (ed.) *Nursing: Study and Placement Learning Skills*. Oxford: Oxford University Press.

Yallom, D. (1970) *The Theory and Practice of Group Psychotherapy*. New York: Basic Books.

PART 3

Advancing application of communication skills

PART 3

The final part addresses communication and interpersonal skills through application in specific clinical scenarios. While the material in this book does not aim to separate different fields of care, this part acknowledges that different clinical areas demand specific skills in interpersonal communication. Chapter 11 addresses the skills needed for short-term and immediate care. This could be acute psychiatric settings, accident and emergency (A&E) departments, or any setting in which the care needed is immediate, essential, and brief. Chapter 12 looks at the other end of the care spectrum: the long-term and chronic care setting. This acknowledges that nurse–patient relationships can be long-term and enduring, and have specific health goals such as developing self-care, managing the process of chronic ill health, and even palliative care. Chapter 13 extends the demands on the nurse role to communicating with children, young people, and families. These nurse–patient relationships demand flexibility in communication and interpersonal skills, demand sound application of developmental stages and family dynamics, and test all nurses to adapt their communication to meet the needs of different family members. Chapter 14 also presents specific communication challenges with patients or significant others who have cognitive impairments that limit their ability to communicate. Again, the nurse is challenged to be adaptive, supporting, and understanding, and to maintain a non-judgemental approach to the interpersonal relationship. Chapter 15 returns to health promotion in application to specific health needs and in specific clinical settings. This chapter outlines approaches in communication shown to be beneficial to health promotion and that the nurse especially is well placed to deliver. Finally, Chapter 16 encourages the reader to consider using communication and interpersonal skills in personal and professional development. It suggests strategies by which nurses can use and develop their communication and interpersonal skills to meet the requirements of both pre-registration and post-registration education and practice (Prep), and to structure continuing professional development in ways that are evidence-based and demonstrate skills development.

11

Communicating in immediate and short-term care situations

Anne-Marie Borneuf and Jacqui Gladwin

This chapter will help you to achieve competencies in:

- ➔ managing and diffusing challenging situations effectively;
- ➔ showing ability to communicate safely and effectively with people, providing guidance for others;
- ➔ being proactive and creative in enhancing communication and understanding;
- ➔ using appropriate and relevant communication skills to deal with difficult and challenging circumstances, such as emergencies and unexpected occurrences;
- ➔ selecting and applying appropriate strategies and techniques for conflict resolution and de-escalation in the management of potential violence and aggression;
- ➔ working confidently as part of the team and, where relevant, as leader of the team.

Introduction

Managing acutely ill or injured patients in an acute or critical care setting places particular demands on the therapeutic nurse–patient relationship and, as such, calls for high-order communication and interpersonal skills. Variables that pose particular challenges include a high turnover of patients alongside the potential for the rapid deterioration of health of the patient. We can add to these challenges anxiety levels of staff, patients, and their family members, and, indeed, the sudden alterations in the dynamics of the care team due to the number of patients requiring specialist care at a moment's notice. The diverse nature of the patient population will also require nurses to tailor their communication styles moment by moment to achieve effective and safe care delivery for all patients.

This chapter will address the specific communication challenges in acute care settings. In any acute setting, the nursing management of patients in acute pain, who are psychologically disturbed, emotionally distressed, angry, or fearful, relies on confident communication and self-management skills. In the emergency care setting, for example, team members need to coordinate their actions, follow set protocols, and transfer information to other professionals, while working in a high-pressure environment. This chapter aims to demonstrate some of the specific communication approaches and their application in acute care and to challenge the reader to apply knowledge covered in earlier chapters to this particular care setting. There are a range of learning activities throughout designed to assist you in developing your knowledge and applying your learning to practical situations.

The challenges to communication in acute care

Diversity of acute care settings

Why are acute care settings particularly challenging to communicating? Acute care settings are often fast-paced or intense environments. They include accident and emergency departments (A&E), intensive care, psychiatric acute and intensive care (PICU), neonatal ICU, and high dependency, as well as medical assessment, units.

Acute care settings can be difficult places in which to work. They deal with a range of patients of diverse backgrounds and cultures, different ages, including children, and a variety of acute physical or mental health conditions. Teams working within this environment will be made up of different professionals who need to communicate effectively in order to manage the volume of activity in the department and ensure the safety of patients and staff working within it. The nature of acute settings means that there will be a requirement to communicate across professions and agencies both within health care and outside it.

Patients who are admitted to acute care environments are often acutely or even critically ill, in pain, anxious, frightened, and often disorientated. They may have relatives in attendance who are also anxious and frightened.

In addition, particularly within A&E departments, there will be patients with a range of problems, both minor and major, and each group will have different communication needs. A key priority need for all, though, will be information and a calm, reassuring approach from the nurse caring for them.

Acute care settings can be very frightening. With the exception of intensive care units, most acute care settings are noisy and busy areas. The turnover and volume of patients can be high, coupled with the frequent interruption of emergency patient situations that need to be dealt with quickly. This can be extremely frightening for patients and their families, especially if they have limited experience of this type of environment. It can also be frightening for students who have not been exposed to patients with traumatic injuries or florid psychotic symptoms.

Pierre et al. (2007) discuss communication within acute and critical care areas and identify the following reasons why it is so complex in nature:

- uncertainty;
- information overload;
- time pressures;
- risk;
- multiple people involved;
- multiple goals and priorities.

The unique nature of acute care environments is such that all of the above factors combine to create challenging situations. Therefore, a nurse needs to possess effective communication skills that can be easily adapted and which are flexible enough to cope with the fast pace and diverse group of people with whom they will come into contact.

Managing patients who have difficulties communicating is always challenging for nurses, but even more so within an acute environment. Acutely ill patients often have complex needs and those who have been admitted as an emergency will need to be assessed and prioritized effectively and quickly in order to ensure that their needs are met.

Problems with language are often increased, as there may not be easy access to interpreters, especially out of normal hours, and patients may be too distressed to express themselves clearly or to take in verbal information.

Patients who present with a learning disability or a mental health problem may often become very agitated and distressed in an acute environment. They can become more difficult to manage or communicate with and the nurse must identify their needs quickly to reduce the patient's anxiety and fear, and to promote effective communication between themselves, the patient, and the carers or family.

....

⊕ Learning point 1

Identify and list some situations in which communication has been a challenge in an acute practice setting. Write down in your reflective diary what made these situations challenging.

....

Priorities for high-risk patients

In order to assess patients quickly and identify priorities for their care, nurses can enhance their communication skills by following procedures. For example, in A&E departments and acute admission units, nurses often use a model of 'triage' to identify and rule out any life-threatening problems. Triage models such as 'Manchester triage' (Manchester Triage Group, 2005) incorporate a system of flowcharts relating to specific conditions. The nurse then assesses the patient using the flowchart to establish their priority for treatment. If the patient is suffering from a life-threatening or high-risk condition, communication with the patient may not be possible and the nurse will usually identify the level of priority from the presenting physiological or behavioural signs.

For those patients presenting with lower-risk conditions, the nurse can focus his or her communication approach to assess the patient more fully and ask the patient a series of questions to confirm that he or she does not require immediate treatment. For psychiatric states, for instance, the assessment will address the patient's risk of harm to self and others. For a thorough assessment, this demands specialist interviewing skills, but in the first instance, risk can be ascertained by sensitive questioning and listening, guided by the use of risk assessment tools. The importance of effective history-taking should not be underestimated. Diagnosis is primarily made on the history that a patient provides and effective communication skills are essential to obtain a full and detailed history.

Impaired ability to communicate

Patients with acute conditions often have impaired ability to communicate. This may be temporary or permanent. A patient who has an acute stroke, for example, may suffer acute dysphasia, which will impair their ability to communicate verbally. Patients with traumatic injuries may also lose the ability to communicate verbally because of reduced consciousness level or damage to their hearing or speech functions.

The NMC (2008) clearly identifies within *The Code: Standards of Conduct, Performance and Ethics* that nurses have a role as an advocate for patients and, as such, must find ways to represent their views even if they have impaired communication.

> You must act as an advocate for those in your care, helping them to access relevant health and social care, information and support.
>
> You must make arrangements to meet people's language and communication needs.

The challenge for nurses in this environment will often be that they have limited knowledge of the patient and therefore may not be able to understand the subtle forms of communication that the patient may use. Family members may be vital in interpreting a patient's efforts to communicate and nurses must try to establish some form of communication with patients as early as possible. This concept is supported by Glennon and DeCoste (1997), who identify the importance of ensuring that patients with acute and critical care needs have their communication needs met and are supported to maintain communication with their carers and families.

Case study 1: Communicating with a patient who has had a stroke

Mr Jones, a 35-year-old man admitted following a stroke, is ventilated and mildly sedated and being nursed in an intensive care unit. He is able to communicate with staff and family using his eyes and his hands only.

➕ Learning point 2

Read Case study 1. What will the challenges be for ensuring that Mr Jones has his communication needs met, and how might the nurse support and develop his limited ability to communicate?

Suggested answer to Learning point 2

The nurse will suggest touch, eye contact, facial expressions, simple gestures, and non-verbal responding (tapping, blinking, etc.) to closed questions (requiring only yes/no answers). He or she will, ask family members to interpret the patient's gestures, as they know him best. For simple communication, picture boards can be used to indicate choices.

Intoxication

A significant challenge within acute areas may be patients or their relatives who are intoxicated with alcohol or drugs. The Institute of Alcohol Studies (2009) identifies that alcohol is a significant factor in patients who present as an emergency admission and estimate that approximately 35 per cent of patients attending A&E departments are doing so because of alcohol-related incidents.

Intoxication in patients in whatever form causes some degree of cerebral impairment (Brown and Cadogan, 2006), which may lead to an acute confusional state or an impaired ability to communicate or process information effectively. It is important to be clear about whether the person is intoxicated with leisure substances or has a medical condition. Possible causes of confusion and impaired functioning include metabolic disorders such as diabetes or hypoxia, or congenital or pathological causes such as learning disability, dementia, or psychosis.

Intoxicated patients or relatives, if not at risk, are thankfully most likely to become sleepy because of the sedating effect of alcohol and common street drugs. Management of service users when they are in a talkative or agitated state demands assertive management and a **closing-down** approach. This is the use of short answers, closed questions, and even ignoring irrelevant chatter or behaviour. Be careful not to encourage further unhelpful behaviour by responding to 'chatter' or inappropriate behaviour if you have other care priorities. See Practice example box 1 for an example from practice.

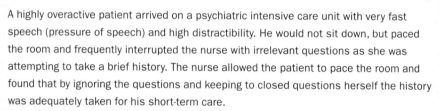

Practice example box 1: Using a 'closing-down' approach

A highly overactive patient arrived on a psychiatric intensive care unit with very fast speech (pressure of speech) and high distractibility. He would not sit down, but paced the room and frequently interrupted the nurse with irrelevant questions as she was attempting to take a brief history. The nurse allowed the patient to pace the room and found that by ignoring the questions and keeping to closed questions herself the history was adequately taken for his short-term care.

 Look back to Chapter 6 on operant conditioning, which shows how rewarding or ignoring certain behaviour can increase or diminish it.

Aggression

Patients or relatives who are intoxicated or confused may be aggressive towards the staff. The acute care environment can often precipitate or escalate aggression in individuals and the nurse should be aware of the potential for aggression in a range of patients. Emergency departments can often appear hostile and threatening environments to patients and relatives who may be in an emotionally charged state (Dolan and Holt, 2008). Acute or sudden illness will often be accompanied by great anxiety and fear for both patient and family. Nurses can use the environment and their communication skills to diffuse aggression through giving attention, information, reassurance, and removing the source of annoyance from the person—or the other way around! Nurses working in this area should also be aware of the challenges that the environment brings to situations and must have a risk-aware approach to maintaining their own and others' safety: for example, ensuring that you are always aware of where the exit route is, making sure the patient is never between you and the door, not getting backed into areas without an exit, making sure you don't have equipment (such as scissors, stethoscopes) sticking out of pockets or around the neck. Be aware of potential weapons and be alert to any patients or relatives who behave oddly or who you know have a previous history of violence against staff. Being aware and prepared is the greatest tool that a nurse has in this area of work when it comes to minimizing the risk of harm.

Chapter 7 gives specific details on de-escalation techniques and managing aggression.

Death

Sudden or unexpected death is one challenging situation that can be extremely difficult to manage for inexperienced and experienced staff alike. Many patients, both adults and children, who are admitted to hospital may deteriorate suddenly and die unexpectedly, or patients may be admitted as a cardiac arrest to A&E having collapsed in the street, home, or workplace or suffered serious life-threatening injuries. The shock and immense grief that is felt by relatives in this circumstance is often difficult to deal with even for the most experienced of nurses (Purves and Edwards, 2005). Situations like these require the nurse to remain calm and be able to communicate in a clear and effective way, remaining professional whilst being sympathetic and providing comfort.

Chapter 12 on chronic care illustrates two models for breaking bad news that apply equally to acute care. Best practice guidelines for breaking bad news in the acute setting include recommendations to meet accompanying relatives on arrival, to provide honest information, to use direct language such as 'dead' and 'dying' rather than 'passed away' to avoid confusion, to appoint 'relatives' nurses', and to have a designated area for imparting news and to allow witnesses into resuscitation (Harrahill, 2005; Purves and Edwards, 2005; Schubert and Chambers, 2005; Valks et al., 2005).

....

 Learning point 3

Look back at Practice example box 2 in Chapter 3. What aspects of the grieving process can you identify in this patient?

....

Suggested answer to Learning point 3

This lady is grieving before the event and certainly appears to be feeling guilty, but also anxious (wanting to talk to someone). We might anticipate anger too under the surface at being pressured into agreeing to the termination.

Multidisciplinary communication

There is often a need to communicate with other professionals within an acute setting. The handover of patients between professionals is extremely important. Patients may arrive by ambulance or with the police, social services, etc. The nurse's role is to ensure that they take an effective handover from the professional accompanying the patient. Equally, the nurse must then provide an effective handover of care from either the A&E department or the ward to theatre, or the intensive care unit. The acute nature of the area will often mean that the patient has undergone a substantial amount of assessment, investigation, and treatment. This care should be recorded accurately and then communicated to the receiving team. The practical application of this is covered in more detail in Learning point 4.

Confidentiality

In situations in which there is the possibility that patient confidentiality may have to be breached because of the need for child protection or because a crime has been committed, the nurse must ensure that all communications are recorded. If a nurse has to give evidence in a court of law, then they cannot claim privilege due to their professional position (Dolan and Holt, 2008).

 Learning point 4

See Practice example box 2. How would the nurses justify breaching confidentiality in this case in revealing to the police that this gentleman was still under the influence of alcohol? Can you find the relevant parts in the NMC Standards of Conduct (2008), and where should the nurses record their actions?

Practice example box 2: Limits of confidentiality

A gentleman with a Disulfiram implant (a medication designed to react negatively with alcohol) was admitted through A&E with a severe reaction to alcohol, including very high blood pressure. He had driven himself to A&E the previous evening and, on discharge in the morning, intended to drive home. He was advised that he was still intoxicated, but he insisted on getting into his car and driving away. The nurses contacted the police and reported his actions. He was stopped, breathalysed, and arrested for drink-driving.

Suggested answer to Learning point 4

The NMC Code (2008) states that nurses must:

Manage risk
- You must act without delay if you believe that you, a colleague or anyone else may be putting someone at risk

Respect people's confidentiality
- You must disclose information if you believe someone may be at risk of harm, in line with the law of the country in which you are practising

The nurses' actions should be recorded factually in the patient's notes (especially that he was advised not to drive) and, in accordance with many NHS trust policies, also reported on an incident form.

Developing communication skills

This section will address the communication skills required by nurses working in acute care when managing a range of patient issues. There are a range of situations that present as communication complexities and nurses may need to adapt their communication skills to be effective. Experiencing these situations helps to develop our abilities and ensure that we communicate effectively for future challenges we may face within this discipline.

Case management

Research has illustrated that interruptive communication seems to dominate in high-stress medical environments (Alvarez and Coiera, 2005). Try to reflect on the last time a patient or relative asked you a question or a query. How many times have you said 'I'll get back to you in a minute!' because you are busy dealing with the previous enquiry? Interruptions take place within the workplace all of the time. Take a look at case study 2.

Case study 2: Prioritizing needs

Mr Smith 89 is brought to A&E by ambulance from a nursing home. He is dehydrated and has a large pressure ulcer on his sacrum. He is disorientated and has a left-sided weakness due to a previous stroke. The paramedic hands the patient over, but a carer has not escorted him from the nursing home. The patient is extremely distressed and frightened. Mr Smith's daughter arrives and is very angry about the care that her father has received at the nursing home; she is also upset that he is in A&E and has not been admitted straight to a ward. She is confrontational and clearly distressed.

⊕ Learning point 5

Outline how you may deal with the above situation and identify the skills required for effective communication in this scenario.

Suggested answer to Learning point 5

As indicated earlier in this chapter, we have to take into account the obvious physiological barriers that affect Mr Smith's ability to communicate effectively, as well as receive and analyse information in relation to his clinical status. The patient is also without an escort, who may or may not have been able to provide more in-depth information that would allow the nurse a fuller holistic picture. This, in turn, would promote and optimize the assessment and prioritization of his nursing needs. It is clear that Mr Smith is frightened and distressed and the issues are exacerbated by an angry and distressed relative. Many patients are scared when they seek care, and fear may colour their interactions (Pytel et al., 2008). This scenario poses a significant challenge for the nurse dealing with this situation. It is easy to become overwhelmed because of the vast array of information, so let's go back to basics!

We need to draw on our nursing experience and the fundamental underpinning philosophy of nursing: the nursing process. In the first instance, we need to undertake a nursing assessment of the situation, and highlight and prioritize the key points. Whilst we are undertaking this assessment, we must ensure that we *talk* to the patient and *listen* to what information is being communicated back to us, by himself or his daughter. We will also have to *transmit* and *relay* information and may need to involve the multidisciplinary team members when implementing Mr Smith's care.

As with any interventions that are put in place, an evaluation of care must be undertaken and it is important that we do this effectively and safely. Therefore a variety of media resources may be required. It is important that, as nurses, we communicate in a way that the patient understands. Previous studies have identified several nurse-related communication barriers: stereotyping; poor articulation; and excessive use of medical terminology (Park and Song, 2005). Clinically, Mr Smith's neurological status is compromised; he needs nursing and medical interventions in place to address his clinical needs—in this case, hydration and pressure ulcer care and management needs. Not only must we involve Mr Smith in his care, but we must also involve his family and keep them informed as well, with the best information available. We might summarize the actions for Mr Smith's management as below.

- Reassure and orient the patient.
- Listen attentively to the relative and involve her in the patient's care.
- Enlist assistance of team members for medical assessment.
- Give simple explanation of events and interventions to both the patient and relative together.
- Empower the relative to assist rather than disrupt care-giving.

Dealing with conflict

Bach and Grant (2009: 95) suggest that 'Conflict can serve as an alarm to indicate that a relationship needs closer attention'. There are many reasons why conflict may occur within an acute or critical care setting and some have been highlighted above. Bizek and Fontaine (2009) indicate that anxiety can be alleviated with simple explanations. In 2003, the Department of Health (DoH) launched the Counter Fraud and Security Management Service (CFSMS) (DoH, 2003). The key aim of this strategy is to deliver a secure environment for those who use or work in the National Health Service (NHS), so that the highest possible standard of care can be made available to patients (DoH, 2003). Within this strategy, the Security Management Service (SMS) was set up in 2004 with a remit to facilitate implementation of a national conflict resolution syllabus to NHS trusts (SMS, 2004). Within this syllabus is a focus on communication skills for NHS staff when managing and resolving conflict. Examples of skills being taught include:

- identifying at least two forms of communication;
- identifying situations in which communication breaks down.

Acute care areas such as A&E departments have been highlighted as high-priority areas for receiving this training input (SMS, 2004). As nurses working within this discipline, we must ensure that de-escalation techniques are adopted, not only to promote our own safety, but also to ensure that a peaceful outcome is met without any injuries being incurred. Indeed, conflict resolution training should factor into any professional and personal development plans discussed by your clinical leads to ensure that your communication and interpersonal skills remain current.

 See Chapter 7 on de-escalation techniques and dealing with aggression.

Learning point 6

Can you identify two forms of communication that are likely to defuse an aggressive situation or to prevent such a situation? What rationale would you give for using these forms of communication in these situations? See Chapter 7 for possible answers.

Children and young people

Communicating with children or young people provides nurses in acute and critical care settings with a different set of challenges. You have to very quickly win over a child's trust, and build up a rapport and 'bond' with the child. Children will be very frightened, as clinical environments can look sterile, bright, and inevitably noisy. Furthermore, dependent on their age, children may find it difficult to express themselves effectively.

Equally, nurses need to take into account that a child's previous experience of hospital that may not have been favourable.

In 2005, the Department for Education and Skills (DfES) worked collaboratively with a variety of service users, employers, and worker interests to develop common core skills and knowledge for agencies who dealt with children and young people (DfES, 2005). The prospectus sets out the requirements into six areas of expertise, one of which is in relation to effective communication and engagement with children, young people, their families, and carers (DfES, 2005).

 Learning point 7

Look at Case study 3. Identify the communication skills required in this situation. How will you adapt or modify your communication skills to ensure that you maintain a high standard of care for Lucy and her mother? List the techniques you may use. Possible answers will be in the text below.

Case study 3: Communicating with a 2-year-old and parent

Lucy is 2 years old. She has fallen, sustaining a cut to her arm, and is distressed on arrival. She is accompanied by her mother, who is also upset, as Lucy was in her care at the time of the accident.

A child who is in pain and distressed will be difficult to assess and manage. There are many techniques that professional individuals can engage in when assessing and managing pain in children: for example, the use of distraction techniques, including toys, music, books, games and play.

In Case study 3, we need to take into account that Lucy *and* her mother are distressed. It will be important to ascertain Lucy's understanding of the situation. Every care must be taken to ensure the correct information is elicited from Lucy and her mother. Additionally, there will be pressure to act quickly to alleviate Lucy's pain. However, you must ensure any care that is given is done so in a safe and timely manner.

It is important to remember that children require a different set of skills, utilizing appropriate 'family-friendly' and indeed 'family-centred' care models that encompass holistically the needs of the child and their families or significant others. Nurses should also be mindful of safeguarding the interests of the child.

  See Chapter 13 for more on communicating with children and young people, and safeguarding their interests.

Patients with perceptual disturbance or confusion

Patients experiencing acute psychotic symptoms or disorientation are most likely to feel frightened by an unfamiliar environment and people they don't know. Such patients may lack understanding of what is happening around them or may have a quite erroneous idea of where they are, who the staff members are, and what people's intentions might be. People who are frightened and feel threatened are likely to become aggressive or withdrawn and uncooperative. Their understanding of verbal communication is often impaired because they may be distracted, have poor concentration, or not be able to process whole sentences. A communication priority for these patients is to *help them to feel safe*.

Earlier chapters have taken you through different communication methods and approaches, so you should be able to apply these principles to practice and give a rationale for each approach. Look at the list in Table 11.1 and see if you can identify some key actions that you could utilize with a patient with poor cognition and perceptual disturbance.

What patient behaviour would help you to evaluate the effectiveness of your practice in this situation?

There are lots of different approaches that you may have identified, but hopefully they will be those that aim to reduce distrust and improve the relationship between you and the patient.

Patients who cannot take in or respond to verbal reassurance and explanation will still be able to interpret the physical and human environment around them. When cognitive processing is impaired, people rely on emotional perception. If they feel fear, the environment will be interpreted as threatening. If they are helped to feel safe, the environment will be less scary.

 See Chapter 1 on the different theories of communication channels and Chapter 10 on de-escalation skills.

Table 11.1 Key actions by nurses for the patient with perceptual disturbance

Communication approach	To do	To avoid	Rationale
1. Body language			
2. Non-verbal style			
3. Verbal style			
4. Environment management			
5. Appearance			
6. Relationship building			

Table 11.2 Key actions by nurses for the patient with perceptual disturbance

Communication approach	To do	To avoid	Rationale
1. Body language	Open posture Keep at eye level Keep your distance	Touching Quick movements Close proximity	Gives non-threatening, even submissive messages
2. Vocal style	Quiet, reassuring tone, slow pace	Loudness, sudden or staccato speech	Avoid increasing nervous arousal
3. Verbal style	Give information & commentary on what is happening. Keep it simple.	Not speaking, even if patient is unresponsive.	Patient will be aware you are speaking to them. Will hear your tone of voice.
4. Environment management	Remove threats (or remove *from* threats). Keep feared objects out of sight.	Interruptions, security staff, technical equipmt, cameras, mobile phones, bleeps, sharps.	Reduce stresses. Aids relationship building. Electrical equipment is threatening to paranoid patients.
5. Appearance	Remove signs of authority. Smile. Wear jumper or cardigan over uniform (fluffy &cosy-looking).	Authoritarian or confusing clothes or accessories (keys, lapels, badges, male nurse tunics). Religious symbols (esp. with acutely psychotic patients).	Reduces risk of being confused with controlling authorities. Patient needs to maintain sense of control. Psychotic & disoriented patients will invent an explanation of their surroundings using human and environmental cues.
6. Relationship building	Active listening! Get person to talk, preferably about about themselves. Use familiar 'props', i.e. cup of tea, biscuits. Superficial self-disclosure.	Frequently leaving patient. Too many people with patient at any one time. Sending trusted relatives or friends away without good cause.	Demonstrates empathy & human contact. All aim to develop trust.

Sources: Based on Mason and Chandley (1999); Duxbury (2000).

Communication skills for emergency situations

An emergency situation, such as a cardiac arrest, a fire, or a patient being found injured, requires the nurse to act quickly and communicate effectively. A patient's condition can change suddenly and the nurse's role is to ensure that any sudden changes are detected and communicated quickly so treatment can be implemented. The Acute Illness Management Programme (AIMs) (Greater Manchester Critical Care Skills Institute, 2008) equips nurses of all branches with the skills to recognize potentially life-threatening signs of deterioration in patients, hopefully preventing them from suffering a respiratory or cardiac arrest that may be fatal.

Part of the AIMs programme focuses on communicating in an emergency and offers a framework—situation, background, assessment, response (SBAR)—for ensuring that the information that is relayed is effective and produces the required response from whoever it is being communicated to. This framework is utilized across the NHS for reporting incidents and emergency situations (Institute for Innovation and Improvement, 2008).

It provides a systematic approach to reporting information in an emergency and ensuring that the facts are communicated appropriately and effectively, preventing a delay in treatment for the patient or an inappropriate response to the emergency (see Table 11.3).

⊕ Learning point 8

Look at Case study 4. Using the above SBAR framework, identify the information that you will need to hand over to the doctor when you call them in order to ensure that they respond effectively and in the best interests of the patient.

Case study 4: Mrs James

Mrs James, aged 45, has been admitted to the medical assessment unit with pneumonia. On admission, she was dyspnoeic respiratory rate 36 and pyrexial temperature 38.5. You are asked by the staff nurse to complete some observations on her, but when you go to her bed, you find Mrs James to be restless and agitated. Her BP is 90/60 and her pulse is 110, respiratory rate is 40. She is responsive to voice, but is clearly confused.

As a student nurse, you call for help and the staff nurse asks you to go and phone the doctor.

Table 11.3 The principles of SBAR to be used when reporting an incident or emergency

Situation	Who you are Exact location The patient's name State the problem or identify the nature of the incident
Background	Give brief details relating to the patient history, i.e. date/time of admission, diagnosis, summary of treatment, any other relevant medical history
Assessment	State your assessment of the patient using the ABCDE* approach and include current vital signs, mental state, fluid balance, track and trigger score. Provide relevant and specific data that identify the exact condition of the patient
Recommendation	Explain what you need from the person to whom you are reporting Be specific about your request and the time frame Ask if there is anything else you can do before the other person arrives Document the call including date, time, and to whom you spoke

* See Table 11.6.

Table 11.4 Learning point 8: suggested answer

Situation	Who you are
	Medical assessment unit
	Patient: Mrs James
	Patient is confused
Background	Admitted with pneumonia, dyspnoeic on admission, no prior medical history and wasn't confused on admission
Assessment	She is breathing; her respiratory rate has increased from 36–40; her BP is 90/60 and her pulse is 110; temperature is 38.5; she responds to voice but is confused
Recommendation	You will ask the doctor to attend urgently to assess the patient
	You will ask if there is anything the doctor wishes you to do for the patient whilst you are waiting for them to arrive
	Ensure you document date, time, and to whom you spoke in the nursing notes

Teams involved in trauma resuscitations often wear tabards indicating their individual roles within the team. This process allows their roles to be easily identifiable to other staff or family members who come into the resuscitation room. In a stressful situation in which every second counts, it is vital that everyone in the team knows who is responsible for which element of the patient's assessment, care, and ongoing treatment to ensure that the patient has the best outcome possible.

Team communication in an emergency

When an emergency occurs, someone needs to take charge of the situation and direct the other people involved in that incident. There are no general rules about who that person should be as long as they manage the situation effectively and work within their scope of practice (NMC, 2008). Even junior nurses may have to take control of an emergency situation and manage it until someone more senior or more qualified arrives to help.

Teams are only effective if they have an effective leader and, in an emergency, it is paramount that the person who takes control is calm and in control of the situation. This will ensure that the other staff involved feel confident and assured that everything is under control. Effective resuscitations occur when all of those involved know exactly what their role is and what is expected of them.

Adair (1979), cited by Mullins (2004: 263), identifies three areas of need within a working team and suggests that the effectiveness of the team is entirely dependent on how effective the leader is at meeting these three areas of need (see Table 11.5).

In terms of working as a team in assessing and managing a critically ill or injured patient, the most effective team works simultaneously in a process known as 'horizontal organization' (Driscoll et al., 2003). For tasks to be performed simultaneously, there needs to be effective allocation of roles and responsibilities, as identified in Table 11.5. Each person within the team must understand what tasks need to be performed and in

Table 11.5 Adair's three areas of need in relation to effective teamworking in an emergency situation

1. Task function:
   - achieving the specific objectives of resuscitating the patient
   - planning the resuscitation and allocating roles within the team
   - controlling the resuscitation and monitoring performance of the team members ensuring a systematic approach is followed (ABCDE)
   - reviewing progress at various points through the systematic process

2. Team function:
   - maintaining morale throughout and reassuring the team members
   - ensuring standards are maintained (UK Resuscitation guidelines adhered to)
   - providing effective communication throughout the resuscitation and directing individuals to perform specific roles at appropriate times
   - ensuring that each member of the team is respected and valued

3. Individual functions:
   - providing feedback and debrief opportunity at the end of the resuscitation for the staff involved
   - ensuring any staff training or individual needs are identified and managed appropriately
   - providing information and support to the family of the patient
   - reconciling any conflict that may have arisen within the team if the resuscitation was problematic or unsuccessful in outcome

Source: Adair (1979), cited by Mullins (2004).

what sequence, and the role of the team leader is to oversee that the process occurs according to the specific protocol being used.

Using the example of a patient who has been involved in a road traffic collision who is unconscious on admission, the team will complete a systematic assessment of the patient using the ABCDE approach (see Table 11.6).

Nurses within the team will be assigned various roles associated with a specific part of the systematic assessment. The team leader will coordinate the assessment and collate all of the information received from the team relating to the status of the patient. Is the airway secure? What are their vital signs and their neurological status? Information will be gathered and communicated to other members of the healthcare team in order to instigate treatment, make referrals, or order investigations. The most important aspect of this kind of teamwork is that all of those involved will be communicating continuously whilst monitoring the patient or delivering care or treatment. The team will work

Table 11.6 Utilizing a systematic approach to patient assessment

A: Airway and cervical spine control
B: Breathing
C: Circulation
D: Disability
E: Exposure

together to achieve a common goal, which is essentially to do their best for the patient.

Situations such as these can be extremely stressful for all of those involved, including the relatives of the patient. Effective communication is required between the team leader and the nurse who is caring for the relatives so that they can be kept informed and involved in the decision-making process. Relatives are often encouraged, where appropriate, to remain with their loved one while the resuscitation is carried out. This can be stressful for them and the team, but can be beneficial for the relatives if supported appropriately throughout by the team.

Look back at case study 2. Here, we can see that involving the relative in the patient's care empowers the relative and distracts her from expressing her anger and interrupting the care team.

The resuscitation of children will almost always involve parents being with their child and this can be a very emotional experience for all involved. It is vital in these situations that the nurse remains with the relatives and is not involved in the actual resuscitation. Relatives may be traumatized by the situation that they observe and may have lots of questions, or none at all, and the nurse must be sensitive to their needs and their anxieties.

Case study 5: Mr Robertson

A 60-year-old man comes into the A&E dept following a cardiac arrest at home. His 24-year-old son James, who has learning disabilities, accompanies him and is extremely distressed. He wants to stay with his father, and so a nurse takes him into the resuscitation room and stays with him while the resuscitation team carry out the resuscitation.

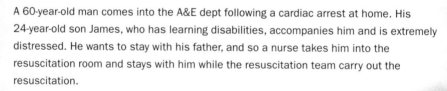

⊕ Learning point 9

Read Case study 5. Consider the effect that James being present in the room may have on the resuscitation team. How can the nurse support James throughout this process and what factors may need to be considered in relation to communication with him?

Suggested answer to Learning point 9

The nurse can support James by ensuring that he or she gives a full explanation of the resuscitation and what is happening to James' father, using simple terms and ensuring James understands (answering questions fully). Pre-empt the sequence of resuscitation so that you can prepare James for any invasive procedures. Attempt to get someone whom he knows to come to be with him to provide support. Ensure that he knows he can leave the room if he wants, offer refreshments, but stay with him at all times. Allow him to hold his father's hand when appropriate. The team needs to acknowledge that it is engaging in a witnessed resuscitation and that James may have difficulties comprehending questions or events.

There are a number of issues to be considered in relation to communicating in an emergency situation, either as an individual nurse or as a member of a team. The nurse must be able to respond quickly and identify the priorities for information-giving and ensure that the information relayed is acted upon to safeguard the interests of the patient.

Conclusion

This chapter has considered some of the complex and challenging issues that student nurses will inevitably face at some point in acute and critical care. Many of the issues require nurses to think, act, and communicate quickly with a wide variety of patients and professionals. Very often, it will be the nurse who is the starting point for any communication process that is required. As such, selection and justification of appropriate communication approaches are essential in order to promote patient safety and, where possible, facilitate a positive experience for the family and significant others.

 To find more resources to aid your learning, please now go online to **www.oxford textbooks.co.uk/orc/webb**. You will find video examples of the SBAR approach and communicating with confused patients.

Web links

Conflict Resolution
www.conflictmanagement.org
Counter Fraud and Security Management Service
www.nhsbsa.nhs.uk/security
Critical Care Skills Institute
www.gmskillsinstitute.nhs.uk/
Department for Children, Schools and Families: Every Child Matters
www.dcsf.gov.uk
Resuscitation Council
www.resus.org.uk/siteindx.htm
Royal College of Nursing Emergency Care Association
www.rcn.org.uk/development/communities/rcn_forum_communities/emergency_care
Royal College of Paediatrics and Child Health
www.rcpch.ac.uk/

References

Alvarez, G. and Coiera, E. (2005) 'Interruptive Communication Patterns in the Intensive Care Unit Ward Round', *International Journal of Medical Informatics*, 74: 791–6.

Bach, S. and Grant, A. (2009). *Communication and Interpersonal Skills for Nurses*. Exeter: Learning Matters.

Bizek, K. S. and Fontaine, D. K. (2009) 'The Patient's Experience with Critical Illness', in P. G. Morton and D. K. Fontaine (eds) *Critical Care Nursing: A Holisitic Approach* (9th edn). Philadelphia, PA: Lippincott, Williams & Wilkins.

Brown, A. and Cadogan, M. D. (2006) *Emergency Medicine: Emergency and Acute Medicine Diagnosis and Management* (5th edn). London: Hodder Arnold.

Counter Fraud and Security Management Service (2004) *Security Management Service (SMS): Protecting Your NHS—Conflict Resolution Training: Implementing the National Syllabus* (SMS/VAS/01/04). London: CFSMS.

Department for Education and Skills (2005) *Common Core of Skills and Knowledge for the Children's Workforce: Every Child Matters—Change for Children*. Nottingham: DfES Publications.

Department of Health (2003) *Counter Fraud and Security Management Service: Protecting Your NHS—A Professional Approach to Managing Security in the NHS*. London: DoH.

Dolan, B. and Holt, L. (2008) *Accident & Emergency: Theory into Practice* (2nd edn). London: Balliere Tindall Elsevier.

Driscoll, P. A., Gwinnutt, C. L., LeDuc Jimmerson, C., and Goodall, O. (2003) *Trauma Resuscitation: The Team Approach* (2nd edn). London: Bios Scientific Publishers.

Duxbury, J. (2000) *Difficult Patients*. Oxford: Butterworth-Heinemann.

Glennon, S. L. and DeCoste, D. C. (1997) *Handbook of Augmentative and Alternative Communication*. London: Delmar Singular.

Greater Manchester Critical Care Skills Institute (2008) *Acute Illness Management (AIM) Course Manual* (3rd edn). Manchester: AIM.

Harrahill, M. (2005) 'Giving Bad News Gracefully', *Journal of Emergency Nursing*, 31(3): 312–14.

Institute of Alcohol Studies (2009) *The Impact of Alcohol on the NHS: IAS Factsheet*. St Ives: IAS.

Manchester Triage Group (2005) *Emergency Triage* (2nd edn). London: BMJ Books.

Mason, T. and Chandley, M. (1999) *Managing Violence and Aggression: A Manual for Nurses and Health Care Workers*. Edinburgh: Churchill Livingstone.

Mullins, L. J. (2004) *Management and Organisational Behaviour* (7th edn). London: Financial Times Management.

National Health Service Institute for Innovation and Improvement (2008) *SBAR: Situation–Background–Assessment Recommendation*. Available at: www.institute. nhs.uk/quality_and_service_improvement_tools/quality_and_service_improvement_ tools/sbar_-_situation_-_background_-_assessment_-_recommendation.html (accessed December 2009).

Nursing and Midwifery Council (2008) *The Code: Standards of Conduct, Performance and Ethics for Nurses and Midwives*. London: NMC.

Park, E. K. and Song, M. (2005) 'Communication Barriers Perceived by Older Patients and Nurses', *International Journal of Nursing Studies*, 42: 159–66.

Pierre, M., Hofinger, G., and Buerschaper, C. (2007) *Crisis Management in Acute Care Settings: Human Factors and Team Psychology in a High-stakes Environment*. London: Springer.

Purves, Y. and Edwards, S. (2005) 'Initial Needs of Bereaved Relatives Following Sudden and Unexpected Death', *Emergency Nurse*, 13(7): 28–34.

Pytel, C., Fielden, N. M., Meyer, K. H., and Albert, N. (2009) 'Nurse–Patient/Visitor Communication in the Emergency Department', *Journal of Emergency Nursing*, 35(5): doi:10.1016/j-jen.2008.09.002.

Royal College of Paediatrics and Child Health (2007) *Services for Children in Emergency Departments: Report of the Intercollegiate Committee for Services for Children in Emergency Departments*. London: RCPCH.

Schubert, C. J. and Chambers, P. (2005) 'Building the Skill of Delivering Bad News', *Clinical Paediatric Emergency Medicine*, 6: 165–72.

Valks, K., Mitchell, M. L., Inglis-Simons, C., and Limpus, A. (2005) 'Dealing with Death: An Audit of Family Bereavement Programs', *Australian Intensive Care Units*, 18(4): 146–51.

12

Communicating with people with chronic and long-term health needs

Gary Witham

This chapter will help you to achieve competencies in:

- ➔ being proactive and creative in enhancing communication and understanding;
- ➔ using appropriate and relevant communication skills to deal with difficult and challenging circumstances, for example, conveying unwelcome news;
- ➔ promoting health and well-being, self-care, and independence through teaching and empowering people and carers to cope with their treatment and the consequences of their condition, including death and dying;
- ➔ discussing sensitive issues in relation to public health and providing appropriate advice and guidance to individuals.

Introduction

In England, one in three of the population (15.4 million people) lives with a long-term condition, and with an ageing population, this is set to rise by 23 per cent over the next twenty-five years (DoH, 2008). In Wales, population surveys suggest that 23 per cent of adults reported a long-term illness (WAG/NPHS, 2005), and in Scotland, from 2005 to 2006, 23.6 per cent of adults reported some form of long-term illness (Scottish Government, 2007). Those living with long-term conditions are intensive users of the NHS, using 52 per cent of all GP appointments and 65 per cent of all outpatient appointments (DoH, 2008).

Patients living with chronic illness learn to adapt and manage themselves in ways that meet their day-to-day needs. Their contact with healthcare professionals is often brief and so it is within this context that nurses may engage with this diverse patient group, as the following quote reinforces.

> Most patients with chronic illness will have approximately 4 appointments per year in an out-patient clinic where they will spend approximately 10 minutes per appointment; an hour a year seems a fair estimate of the duration of the direct contact between patient and . . . the health care system. This fairly simple arithmetic clearly demonstrates how it is almost impossible to underestimate the importance of how patients themselves have no choice but to incorporate their chronic illness into their daily lives.
>
> (Kaptein et al., 2003: 97)

Self-care and self-management are an integral part of UK government health policy (DoH, 2001; 2008; 2010). In supporting patients and facilitating this patient-centred approach, effective communication becomes a key component in patient care. The requirement to provide targeted information (DoH, 2006) appropriate to an individual's needs necessitates the establishment of professional relationships based on effective communication. The 'End-of-life Care Strategy' suggests that bereavement information and support should be available as part of end-of-life care provision and, in particular, recommends communication as an essential element of workforce training (DoH, 2008: 118). The National Service Framework for long-term conditions (DoH, 2005) and other guidance (DoH, 2010: 10) also highlight effective communication as an essential workforce requirement in supporting patients and carers.

In this chapter, we will explore the different ways in which to relate to people living with chronic illness. We will examine issues of self-care and behavioural change, eliciting patient concerns, handling bad or significant news, and dealing with loss and bereavement. Within the context of chronic disease, exchanging information, managing uncertainty, and the adoption of health-promoting behaviours are important issues.

Identifying patient concerns

Facilitating good self-care requires a relationship of trust that will sustain long-term clinical relationships and the provision of individualized health information and advice regarding access to reliable sources of information. The patient is the expert, therefore nurses need to be sensitive in providing support and advice about flexible and realistic interventions for people living with chronic disease. Identifying patient concerns, especially with many patients managing complex needs, is a vital component of nurse assessment.

Valuing patient experience can be difficult within a clinical consultation. Giving time to listen and identify the patient's main concerns allows the patient to share their experiences.

Look at Box 12.1, in which there is an exchange between a nurse and patient living with chronic obstructive pulmonary disease (COPD) during an assessment.

Box 12.1 Nurse–patient dialogue, part 1

Nurse: Hi Betty, have you been sleeping ok and are your bowels working?

Betty: Er, they're ok, thank you.

Nurse: You seem upset, is there anything wrong?

Betty: I've been thinking about the future. I've been coping well, but things are getting worse and I'm worried about what this all means.

Nurse: Don't worry; it's understandable that you're concerned, I think a lot of people in your shoes feel this way. Often, the worry goes once the treatment starts and you begin to feel better. I can get a doctor to give you information about the treatment, if that would help?

Betty: I don't really want to bother the doctor. Er, don't worry I'll be alright.

Nurse: I know it must be difficult. What does your husband feel about the situation?

Betty: Well, he's obviously concerned. I think it's difficult for all of us. I'm worried, but I've always been the strong one and I don't want to alarm the family.

Nurse: Oh, I see, do you have a big family?

Betty: Yes, I have three daughters, and four granddaughters. They're very good and live close to me.

Nurse: That's nice, to have that support around you. I suspect that's a great help, isn't it? I've just got to go and do something else, but can I quickly ask you if your appetite is ok?

Betty: Yes.

Nurse: Thanks, that's all the questions on my assessment form. I'll catch up with you later.

⊕ Learning point 1

Within the dialogue of Box 12.1, can you identify verbal behaviours and actions that prevent Betty from sharing her concerns?

Suggested answers to Learning point 1

Within the interview, you may have identified the following examples of behaviours that block open communication.

1. Closed questions ('Can I ask you if your appetite is ok?')

2. Multiple questions ('Have you been sleeping ok and are your bowels working?')

3. Switching the person ('What does your husband feel about that?')

4. Leading questions ('I suspect that's a great help, isn't it?')

5. Passing the buck ('I can get a doctor to give you information')

6. Minimizing or normalizing comments ('I think a lot of people in your shoes feel this way')

7. Premature reassurance ('Don't worry')

8. Premature or inappropriate advice ('Often, the worry goes once the treatment starts and you begin to feel better')

9. Overt blocking ('Oh, I see, do you have a big family?')

The next dialogue (Box 12.2) involves the same assessment, but the responses are handled differently.

Box 12.2 Nurse–patient dialogue, part 2

Nurse:	Hi Betty, How are you feeling?
Betty:	Er, well, I'm ok really.
Nurse:	You seem upset, is there anything wrong?
Betty:	I've been thinking about the future. I've been coping well, but things are getting worse and I'm worried about what this all means.
Nurse:	What are you worried about?
Betty:	I've coped well with my lung problems, but I'm getting more out of puff and I can't really do things I could do six months ago. Shopping's getting difficult. The doctor did say that there was not too much that could be done about it.
Nurse:	What did you understand by what she said?
Betty:	Well, it's obviously concerning, I don't know how long things are going to continue, I know I can't go on like this, I think it's difficult for all of us, I'm worried but I've always been the strong one and I don't want to alarm the family.
Nurse:	That sounds really difficult? (*Silence*)
Betty (*visibly upset*):	Yes.
Nurse:	Is it difficult being the strong one?
Betty:	Yes, I just can't do the cooking, shopping, or at times walk up the stairs. I don't think I can cope.
Nurse:	What does not coping mean to you?
Betty:	I'll have just let things go. I find it very difficult.
Nurse:	I can see, can you bear to tell me any other thoughts that you have had?
Betty:	I think how to talk to my husband about it all, he doesn't like to dwell on things.
Nurse:	So, can I check that I've understood: you are worried about what the future holds because your breathing is worse, this is affecting how you're coping at home with the shopping, cooking, and getting around, and you're worried how to talk to your husband?
Betty:	Yes.
Nurse:	Anything else worrying you?

Learning point 2

Can you identify verbal behaviours and actions that allowed Betty to share her concerns?

Suggested answers to Learning point 2

Within the interview, you may have identified the following examples of behaviours that encourage and facilitate open communication.

1. Open questions ('How are you feeling?')
2. Empathy ('That sounds really difficult?')
3. Open directive questions ('What did you understand by what she said?')
4. Negotiation ('Can you bear to tell me any other thoughts?')
5. Questions with a psychological focus ('Is it difficult being the strong one?')
6. Questions with cognitive focus ('Tell me any other thoughts')
7. Checking understanding and summarizing ('So, can I check that I've understood: you are worried . . .')
8. Clarifying psychological cues ('What does not coping mean to you?')
9. Screening questions to explore other concerns ('Anything else worrying you?')

Nurses need to be sensitive to patient cues within communication. Patient cues can be defined as follows.

> Words or phrases suggesting vague undefined emotions, verbal hints to hidden concerns, mention of psychological symptoms, neutral mention of an important life event and repetition of a previous neutral expression. Non-verbal cues include expression of emotion: crying or hints of emotion: sighing, frowning.
>
> (Del Piccolo et al., 2006)

Patients are much more likely to tell nurses of their concerns if the nurse asks questions with a psychological focus in the presence of a cue. In our scenario, for example, the nurse notices that Betty is upset and asks if there is anything wrong. The important element is to respond to that initial cue. A patient who needs to share a significant concern will often target a particular student or staff nurse rather than ask the first person who comes along. Therefore taking the question/cue seriously will often allow the trust necessary to explore the concern. There is evidence that picking up cues actually shortens consultation time (Butow et al., 2002).

In clarifying the patient's concerns, it is important to maintain a psychological focus, since evidence suggests that nurses' communication tends to be related to physical issues rather than an exploration of the patient's feelings (Kruijver et al., 2001). Many nurses may find it difficult to explore patient concerns for a number of reasons.

 Learning point 3

Can you think of the reasons why health professionals find exploring patient concerns difficult?

Suggested answers to Learning point 3

Some evidence suggests that, as nurses, we may fear that exploring issues with patients would take up too much time, that we may be faced with answering emotionally difficult questions, that we might get 'out of our depth' (Maguire, 1999; Friedrichsen and Milberg, 2006). Sometimes, our beliefs play a role: for example, that emotional problems are just a 'natural' reaction to advancing disease, that just talking is not going to fix anything, and that it's not really our role to explore these concerns. There may be issues of privacy in a busy ward or in someone's home with friends or family present. We may feel that we lack training or peer support and therefore actively avoid more meaningful interactions. We may also be afraid of overstepping the 'boundaries' of professional behaviour and getting 'too involved'.

 Learning point 4

Can you think of the reasons why patients may not talk about their concerns?

Suggested answers to Learning point 4

Some patients may feel that they would be a burden to the nurse and do not want to upset them. Others may feel that nurses are too busy and that other patients' needs are greater than their own concerns. Patients may also be sensitive to their environment; fear of getting upset on a busy ward with limited privacy may limit the disclosure of concerns. There may also be cultural and language barriers, or nurses may block patient cues and focus only on physical aspects of care. This, again, may prevent disclosure. This is an important issue since most NHS environments are focused on medical treatment rather than psychosocial support. The physical focus of the medical model of care, often associated with attempts at curing the ill patient, can make talk about 'feelings' very difficult for patients. People living with chronic disease may not fit into a system in which cure and medical treatment are always appropriate. However, they may still have important concerns that are not being addressed by health professionals.

Breaking bad or significant news

Breaking bad or significant news can be difficult. The reasons can be similar to talking about patient concerns: the fear of upsetting a patient, of not being able to 'handle' the situation, or of causing the patient harm. There is also the need for acceptance that, as a nurse, there are some situations in which we cannot make things 'better' and need to sit physically and sometimes emotionally with the patient through the conveying of difficult news. It is often the case that a doctor will break bad news, especially if it centres on treatment decisions, but it is also important to remember that it may be difficult for a patient to take all of the implications or information in at that one time point. Therefore you may be the person whom a patient will ask to 'unpack' the meaning of that information given.

Sometimes, doctors adopt a number of strategies to avoid the impact of breaking bad news. These strategies include lengthy information-giving or explanation, using complicated words, recommending another type of treatment, referring the patient to another department or suggesting discontinued treatment (Friedrichsen and Strang, 2003). These avoidance strategies make it difficult for patients to understand the implications of what is being said and lead to patient dissatisfaction with the breaking of bad news by doctors (Spiegel et al., 2009). Current practice in breaking significant news often increases the patient's unmet concerns and leads to increased anxiety (see Figure 12.1 for an illustration). Longer term, this can lead to higher emotional distress, associated anxiety, and depressive illness.

We will examine two models used for breaking significant news: the McMaster technique (see Figure 12.2) and the SPIKES model. The important elements in both are checking the patient's anticipation of the information that you will give them. Does the patient actually want the information? If you are unsure what the patient expects, give a warning shot first. It is better to give information in small chunks and in language that a patient will understand. After giving the information, look for cues of their emotional response. How does the patient feel about what was said? What is their understanding? This part is important in responding to the emotional impact and patient concerns with the breaking of significant news. Towards the end of the discussion, it can be helpful to summarize the main points and clarify that this understanding is shared by the patient. At this stage, a plan can be negotiated with the patient to address their concerns and expectations and to offer the appropriate support. It is important to offer written information to back up the verbal information given and to include relevant contact numbers.

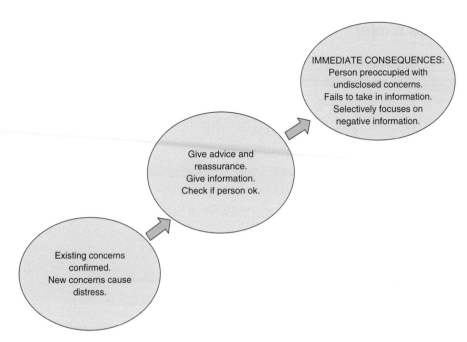

Figure 12.1 An example of current practice in breaking significant news

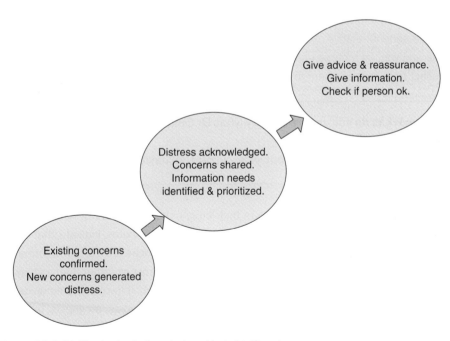

Figure 12.2 McMaster technique in breaking significant news

SPIKES model

Communication guidelines for breaking bad news in the USA are incorporated in the Education for Physicians on End-of-Life Care (EPEC). This is a six-step approach based on the SPIKES model: setting, perception, invitation, knowledge, empathy, and strategy/summary (Buckman, 2005; Wittenberg-Lyles et al., 2008).

First step: prepare for the interaction (setting)

Second step: assess knowledge base (perception—ask-before-you-tell principle)

Third step: gauging/negotiating the amount of information that the patient wants (invitation)

Fourth step: delivering bad news (knowledge)

Fifth step: physician response to bad news (empathy)

Sixth step: summary involving discussing the follow-up plan

The setting is an important component of sharing bad news, and in working with medical colleagues, it may be left to the nurse to identify the appropriate area to talk to patients and/or relatives. It can often be the first non-verbal trigger that significant information is to be shared and therefore can be a warning sign to patients/relatives that important information is to be exchanged. After the initial medical consultation is over, the patient/relative may have many questions. These can occur over a longer time frame and you, as a nurse, may be the first point of contact for the patient. Remember to reflect back to the patient to ascertain their understanding of the information.

> Nurse: What do you understand by what Dr Smith told you?
>
> or:
>
> Nurse: What do you know about your current situation?

Never assume that the patient knows their prognosis, or is aware of new significant information about their condition (even if nursing/medical notes indicate that a discussion has taken place). The patient may not have processed certain information and breaking significant news can be better viewed as a process rather than a focus on one central piece of information or consultation. Sometimes, it involves communication 'clean-up' with patients who have not shared honest diagnosis/prognosis talk with previous doctors (Wittenberg-Lyles et al., 2008).

Patients or relatives may ask the same questions of different health professionals. It is important for trust and consistency to be honest and open about the level of information you can give. If you are unsure of the answers, say so and, if appropriate, ask the person why they are asking that particular question. This can help you to understand the reasons why patients/relatives may be checking the consistency of the information given and allow you to further 'unpack' the issues and offer support.

....

 Learning point 5

> What are the reasons why patients sometimes do not acknowledge the reality of significant events or situations?

....

Denial

Denial can be associated with improved psychological functioning and can be helpful if the denial is an active strategy: for example, realizing that one has cancer, but choosing not to let that diagnosis control one's life by ignoring the illness and creating a positive outlook. Denial can relate to poorer psychological functioning by adopting passive strategies: for example, refusing to believe it has happened or hoping for a miracle (Vos and de Haes, 2007). A patient who has been given significant news, such as a poor prognosis, may not be ready to process that information. It may be too difficult to explore or imagine. The function of denial is to protect the patient against intolerable distress. Denial of the reality of death can generate difficulties for the patient or relative to work through important emotional and practical aspects of living with a life-limiting condition. The subsequent 'unfinished business' can lead to a more complicated bereavement process. When supporting a patient in complete denial, it is important to acknowledge the protective nature of this mechanism and that direct confrontation may not be the best approach. It is a powerful psychological defence unlikely to be broken by sensitive probing or exploration.

If the denial is not complete, then it may be appropriate for the health professional to reassess their denial status—to explore this area to open up discussion. In order to gauge the level of denial, one can try challenging any inconsistencies in the patient's or relative's story.

> Nurse: You told me that the surgery wasn't significant, but you have been recovering for three months and may have more treatment?

A nurse can also check if the denial is total by seeing if there is a 'window' on the denial.

> Nurse: I wonder if there was a time you felt that things were not going to be OK?
> Nurse: Can you possibly share those feelings?
> Nurse: Can you bear to go any further?

Collusion

The relative

Relatives will sometimes try to protect themselves and the patient from the impending loss related to end-stage illness. This can involve not disclosing information about the prognosis to a patient and requesting that health professionals collude in this by withholding the truth. This can affect the trust between nurse and patient and lead to communication difficulties. Certain subject areas can become 'off-limits', restricting the dialogue of important issues at the end of life. In dealing with collusion, the first step is to talk with the relative responsible for the collusion. How are they coping with the present situation? Is it taking an emotional toll? If they give you any cues, try to establish the extent of the strain. Avoid minimizing the situation or answering your own questions, since the person may feel torn between an awareness of the impact of the disease and a strong wish to avoid facing it and maintaining the pretence. The nurse could then check if the collusion is affecting the relative's relationship with the patient. This may establish if it is affecting the communication between them and the subsequent impact on the colluder. It is important to identify why the relative feels that collusion is in their relative's interest and to gauge the strength of those beliefs (without judging their rationale). The nurse can summarize the cost to the colluder and ask permission to check out the patient's awareness of the present situation. Establish the 'ground rules' with the relative, noting that, if the patient has no insight into their current situation, you will not give them new information.

The patient

The second step would be to talk to the patient and check their understanding of the situation. How do they interpret what is happening to them and how do they feel about it? You may find that the patient often has more awareness than the relative thinks they do and this gentle probing can sometimes lead to more open communication.

Where both parties are trying to protect each other from distress, this intervention can subsequently allow them to explore their feelings.

If you can then negotiate an open discussion with the relative and patient, as a third step, you can then recap on what has been discussed, acknowledge the distress, and check if they wish to talk either alone or with you present. More open communication can be encouraged by the relative and patient identifying each concern and working through it by dialogue.

Dealing with loss and bereavement

Loss and bereavement are difficult for nurses to negotiate since we cannot make things 'better'. We may need to navigate through the intense personal experience of loss in a cathartic approach.

    See Chapter 3 for Heron's six-category intervention analysis on cathartic interventions.

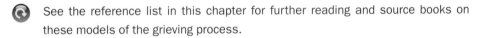 Learning point 6: Reflection

Think of a time in your clinical practice in which a patient was dying or had died.

- How did it make you feel?
- Did you find it easy to speak with family and friends about the death?
- How did you or other staff communicate with the friends and family of the patient that died?

In Box 12.3, Joan Didion describes her personal experience of grief at the sudden loss of her husband. It highlights the isolation and intensity of loss experienced by the bereaved and the attempt to make sense of loss in the narrative of their lives. A question many recently bereaved people ask is: 'Am I going mad?' Talking of the normality of such reactions as Didion's can be very supportive to the bereaved.

Box 12.3 Joan Didion's personal experience of grief at the sudden loss of her husband

Grief turns out to be a place none of us know until we reach it. We know that someone close to us could die. We might expect to feel shock. We do not expect this shock to be obliterative, dislocating to both body and mind. We might expect to be prostrate, inconsolable, crazy with loss. We do not expect to be literally crazy, cool customers who believe that their husband is about to return and need his shoes. Nor can we know ahead of the fact—and here lies the heart of the difference between grief as we imagine it and grief as it is—the unending absence that follows, the void, the relentless succession of moments during which we will confront the experience of meaninglessness itself.

(Didion, 2005: 188)

There are many theoretical models of the grieving process, such as Bowlby and Parkes (1970), who identify four main stages in the grief process, Kubler-Ross (1970), in her seminal work *On Death and Dying* in which she identifies five stages, and Worden (1991), who examines four 'tasks' of mourning.

See the reference list in this chapter for further reading and source books on these models of the grieving process.

Walter (1996) challenges these grand narratives. He describes the journey of the bereaved as one of trying to construct a narrative that incorporates the dead person within the structure of their lives and that will continue to endure through time. The construction of a biography is vital to the incorporation of the memory of the dead into the bereaved person's continuing life. This process is developed, according to Walter, by conversation with others who knew the deceased. There is no 'closure' and 'resolution of grief'. Therefore it is important for health professionals to give the grieving person the opportunity to talk about their loved one and to describe the meaning and impact that the dseceased had in their lives. This is a difficult process, as Mallon (2008: 15) comments.

> There are no easy formulas for dealing with grief and bereavement. Each person has to live with it, live through it and grow through it. There are no fixed person times for its duration, despite theories of time-bound grief models, nor are there certainties about when or if understanding or acceptance will occur. Responding with sensitivity and care and holding the emotions of the bereaved as they travel through their grief are essentially healing aspects of our work.

There may be other factors that affect grief and the grieving process. The person's previous experience of death, the nature of the relationship (attachment), the circumstances of the death, and the social support network will all have an impact. In terms of our role as a nurse, it can be difficult to sit with the pain of grief from the patient's significant others, as well as deal with our own feelings and emotions. If we have built up a relationship with the patient, it can be hard not to be overwhelmed by the stressful event. It is important to remember that just your presence can be valued, since it provides someone who will listen, who has known the patient and family, and who can acknowledge their grief. If there is ongoing contact with relatives, it can put any feelings of guilt they may have into words—for example, 'Could I have done anything differently?'—and provides consolation in their loneliness (Milberg et al., 2008). In terms of your own feelings and emotions, it is important to acknowledge them and it can be helpful to share those feelings with colleagues in the clinical environment in which you work. By 'unpacking' the situation, it can be a way in which to acknowledge the tragic, stressful event and gives you the opportunity to talk about anything in particular that was significant for you.

Ambiguous loss: dementia

Loss and bereavement can also be seen in terms of accepting the changes that occur when living with chronic and long-term conditions. The changes in family roles in the presence of chronic illness can disrupt social functioning: for example, a family member living with dementia. The term 'ambiguous loss' (Boss, 1999) can often be described in this situation in which there exists unfinished business in which the family of a person living with dementia has to adjust to 'losing' its family member (in terms of cognitive/psychological functioning) before death. Health professionals need to offer time, and engage with people encountering the continuing loss of a loved one.

In communicating with someone living with dementia, it is important to acknowledge the importance of body language and non-verbal cues. Language may be affected as the person becomes increasingly unable to interpret the world in a way that makes sense to them. This can lead to misunderstandings and communication difficulties that can be frustrating for both the person living with dementia and those around them. Therefore tense, agitated facial expressions or movements may upset the person trying to understand what you want to communicate. Remaining calm, giving your full attention, and remaining below their eye level rather than standing above them may create a safe environment in which feelings may be expressed, even in the absence of language. When speaking, use simple, short sentences, allowing time for the person to process what has been said. Try not to ask the person to make complicated decisions that could cause confusion or frustration. If the person's conversation is not based in reality, try to respond in a way that does not cut off dialogue, or is too grounded in reality. For example, if a person states that she needs to go home to look after the baby, acknowledge that once she was a mother with a small baby and ask her about that time in her life.

Self-care and behavioural change

Cognitive behaviour therapy

Let's now look at a common approach to managing chronic disease: **cognitive behaviour therapy** (CBT). Cognitive behaviour therapy examines the cause and effect within ourselves related to the decisions that we make. Specific behaviours can relate to four interactive elements: physical sensation; behaviour; thoughts; and emotions. How these elements interplay can affect a person's way of dealing with a situation. For example, Tim has chronic back pain, but wants to go swimming. On the day, his back pain is particularly bad and he is unable to get out of the house. Tim may think that his day has been spoilt, so his emotional reaction will be negative; physically, he may experience loss of energy and increased pain, and his *behaviour* may become restless and aimless. Alternatively, if Tim can plan a more achievable activity, then the emotional reaction of being unable to swim can be modified by thoughts about achieving another goal, so producing a physical response of improved energy, leading to behavioural changes to achieve the new goal. Tim's response is generated from the meaning that he attaches to the circumstances in which he finds himself.

The style of communication often involves note-taking within an interview setting. Educating the patient in the cognitive behavioural approach is important and engaging the patient in self-care is an important patient-centred aspect of CBT. Goal/contract-setting provides a framework, highlighting the methods to be used by the therapist and the commitment by the patient in applying them. The sessions often remain structured and involve agenda review, homework feedback, a discussion of the next topic from treatment plan, and homework setting.

In terms of the evidence base and chronic illness, CBT can be effective in improving the quality of life of patients living with cancer compared to no psychological intervention or receiving supportive counselling (Greer et al., 1992; Moorey et al., 1998). It can be effective in cardiac rehabilitation to reduce anxiety and depression (Linden, 2000), as well as to support people to adjust in coping with multiple sclerosis (Thomas et al., 2006). It can also offer an improved outcome for people with chronic pain (Henschke et al., 2010).

 See Chapter 6 for further explanation of CBT and explanation of negative thinking patterns.

Motivational interviewing

Motivational interviewing (MI) can be defined as 'a client-centred, directive method for enhancing intrinsic motivation to change by exploring and resolving ambivalence' (Miller and Rollnick, 2002). The essential elements of MI are to attempt to change patient ambivalence, which can be a barrier to health behaviour change.

Case study 1: Example of a clinic review

David is 50 years old and lives with his wife. He has a busy life, working long hours in a stressful insurance company. He is overweight and has a poor diet. A lifelong smoker (twenty a day), Peter was diagnosed with COPD two years ago after persistent breathing difficulties. He attends clinic for a review every six months, but feels he is getting more breathless.

Case study 1 outlines a typical case scenario of chronic illness associated with behaviour. There are obvious areas that would make David's COPD worse—principally, smoking and being overweight. He has been told that changes to his lifestyle, such as a healthier diet, gentle exercise, and reducing his smoking, would make a huge difference to his health, but it does not make a difference to his behaviour.

⊕ **Learning point 7**

Why do some patients make lifestyle changes while others do not?

Suggested answer to Learning point 7

Many people feel that there are too many barriers to making changes and focus only on the negative aspects of behaviour change rather than the benefits. This results in

ambivalence to change. Instead of viewing the patient as an individual who does not want to change, MI is concerned with focusing on what the patient wants and how to achieve that goal. It selectively elicits and reinforces the patient's own arguments for change. It therefore encourages 'change talk': the benefits of changing behaviour or the costs of not changing. Three core communication skills central to MI are as follows.

Asking: What are the patient's goals? Get to know them and develop a relationship with the person.

Informing: Give the patient options and check out their understanding.

Listening: Respect the patient's wishes and offer help appropriately.

The communication skills used in MI are, for example, making summaries, reflective listening both to show empathy and lead patients to 'change talk', and also open questions. Use of open questions and reflection avoids the question-and-answer dialogue associated with closed questions that can often restrict communication between health professionals and the patient. It also avoids the 'righting reflex' whereby a nurse tries to fix things through information or advice and gets into a confrontational argument with the patient. In motivational interviewing, it is better to **roll with resistance** by accepting that behaviour change is generated by the patient and not the health professional.

Motivational interviewing is not a technique or tool, but is a clinical skill grounded in an interpersonal relationship with the patient and derives from a more humanistic approach. It is a guiding style for developing intrinsic motivation to change (Rollnick et al., 2008). The important principles can be described by the acronym 'RULE'.

- Resist the righting reflex.
- Understand your patient's motivations.
- Listen to your patient.
- Empower your patient.

The evidence for MI is predominately in the treatment of drug and alcohol misuse, but since it has been applied within general health care, it is becoming increasingly popular (Cummings et al., 2008, Everett et al., 2008).

 You will find more detail on behaviour change and applying motivational interviewing in Chapter 15.

Conclusion

This chapter encourages you, as a nurse, to consider the communication issues prevalent in supporting patients living with chronic illness. It highlights the need to work, non-judgementally, with patients' own motivations in changing behaviour. This is applicable when working in either an acute or community-based environment. It also identifies difficult areas in communication, such as working with patients who have received significant news, and issues of bereavement and loss. One of the key aspects of communication is to identify patients' concerns. Patients living with chronic illness are 'experts' in living with many competing health issues. Nurses need to take seriously the patient's own narrative in how to cope with ill health and how to support them when accessing and receiving health care.

 To find more resources to aid your learning, please now go online to **www.oxfordtextbooks.co.uk/orc/webb** See the video 'Handling bad news' to see the skill in practice.

Web links

Try this continuing care website for more on motivational interviewing: **www.motivationalinterview.org**

Further reading

Dart, M. A. (2010) *Motivational Interviewing in Nursing Practice: Empowering the Patient.* London: Jones and Bartlett Publishers International.

Hudson, R. (2003) *Dementia Nursing: A Guide to Practice.* Abingdon: Radcliffe Publishing.

Jeffrey, D. (2006) *Patient-centred Ethics and Communication at the End of Life.* Abingdon: Radcliffe Publishing.

Perry, K. N. and Burgess, M. (2002) *Communication in Cancer Care.* Oxford: Blackwell Publishing.

References

Boss, P. (1999) *Ambiguous Loss.* Cambridge, MA: Havard University Press.

Bowlby, J. and Parkes, C. M. (1970) 'Separation and Loss within the Family', in E. J. Anthony and C. J. Koupernik (eds) *The Child in His Family.* Chichester: Wiley.

Buckman, R. A. (2005) 'Breaking Bad News: The SPIKES Strategy', *Commonly Oncology*, 2(2): 138–42.

Butow, P. N., Brown, R. F., Cogar, S., Tattersall, M. H., and Dunn, S. M. (2002) 'Oncologists' Reactions to Cancer Patients' Verbal Cues', *Psycho-oncology*, 11: 47–58.

Carrier, J. (2009) *Managing Long-term Conditions and Chronic Illness in Primary Care: A Guide to Good Practice.* London: Routledge.

Corbin, S. and Rosen, R. (2005) *Self management for Long-term Conditions.* London: King's Fund.

Cummings, S. M., Cooper, R. L., and Cassie, K. M. (2008) 'Motivational Interviewing to Affect Behavioural Change in Older Adults', *Research on Social Work Practice*, 19(2): 195–204.

Del Piccolo, L., Goss, C., and Bergvik, S. (2006) 'The Fourth Meeting of the Verona Network on Sequence Analysis: Consensus Finding on the Appropriateness of Provider Responses to Patient Cues and Concerns', *Patient Education and Counseling*, 60: 313–25.

Department of Health (2001) *The Expert Patient: A New Approach to Chronic Disease Management for the 21st Century.* London: DoH.

—— (2005) 'National Service Framework for Long-term Conditions'. Available at: www.dh.gov.uk/en/Publicationsandstatistics/Publications/PublicationsPolicyAndGuidance/DH_4105361 (accessed March 2010).

—— (2006) *Our Health, Our Care, Our Say: A New Direction for Community Services.* London: DoH.

—— (2008) *Raising the Profile of Long-term Conditions Care: A Compendium of Information.* London: DoH.

—— (2010) *Improving the Health and Well-being of People with Long-term Conditions: World-class Services for People with Long-term Conditions—Information Tool for Commissioners.* London: DoH.

Didion, J. (2005) *The Year of Magical Thinking.* London: Fourth Estate.

Everett, B., Davidson, P. M., Sheerin, N., Salamonson, Y., and Digiacomo, M. (2008) 'Pragmatic Insights into a Nurse-delivered Motivational Interviewing Intervention in the Outpatient Cardiac Rehabilitation Setting', *Journal of Cardiopulmonary Rehabilitation and Prevention*, 28(1): 61–4.

Friedrichsen, M. and Milberg, A. (2006) 'Concerns about Losing Control When Breaking Bad News to Terminally Ill Patients with Cancer: Physician's Perspective', *Journal of Palliative Medicine*, 9: 673–82.

—— and Strang, P. M. (2003) 'Doctor's Strategies When Breaking Bad News to Terminally Ill Patients', *Journal of Palliative Medicine*, 6: 565–74.

Greer, S., Moorey, S., and Baruch, J. D. R. (1992) 'Adjuvant Psychological Therapy for Patients with Cancer: A Prospective Randomised Trial', *British Medical Journal*, 304: 675–80.

Henschke, N., Ostelo, R. W. J. G., van Tulder, M. W., Vlaeyens, J. W. S., Morley, S. J., Assendelft, W. J. J., and Main, C. J. (2010) 'Behavioural Treatment for Chronic Back Pain', *Cochrane Database of Systematic Reviews*, 7/CD002014. DOI: 10.1002/14651858.CD002014.pub3. http://onlinelibrary.wiley.com/o/cochrane/clsysrev/articles/CD002014/pdf_abstract_fs.html

Kaptein, A. A., Scharloo, M., Helder, D. I., Kleijn, W. C., van Korlaar, I. M., and Woertman, M. (2003) 'Representations of Chronic Illness', in L. D. Cameron and H. Leventhal (eds) *The Self-Regulation of Health and Illness Behaviour*. London: Routledge, 97–118.

Kruijver, I. P. M., Kerkstra, A., Bensing, J. M., and van de Weil, H. B. M. (2001) 'Communication Skills for Nurses during Interactions with Simulated Cancer Patients', *Journal of Advanced Nursing*, 34(6): 772–9.

Kubler-Ross, E. (1970) *On Death and Dying*. London: Tavistock.

Linden, W. (2000) 'Psychological Treatments in Cardiac Rehabilitation: A Review of Rationales and Outcomes', *Journal of Psychosomatic Research*, 48: 443–54.

Maguire, P. (1999) 'Improving Communication with Cancer Patients', *European Journal of Cancer* (December), 35(14): 2058–65.

Mallon, B. (2008) *Dying, Death and Grief: Working with Adult Bereavement*. London: Sage.

Milberg, A., Olsson, J. A., Olsson, M., and Fredrichsen, M. (2008) 'Family Members' Perceived Needs for Bereavement Follow-up', *Journal of Pain and Symptom Management*, 35(1): 58–69.

Miller, W. R. and Rollnick, S. (2002) *Motivational Interviewing* (2nd edn). New York: Guilford Press, 25.

Moorey, S., Greer, S., and Bliss, J. (1998) 'A Comparison of Adjuvant Psychological Therapy and Supportive Counselling in Patients with Cancer', *Psycho-oncology*, 7: 218–28.

Rollnick, S., Miller, W., and Butler, C. (2008) *Motivational Interviewing in Health Care*. New York: Guilford Press.

Sage, N., Sowden, M., Chorlton, E., and Edeleanu, A. (2008) *CBT for Chronic Illness and Palliative Care: A Workbook and Toolkit*. Chichester: John Wiley and Sons.

Schofield, N. G., Green, C., and Creed, F. (2008) 'Communication Skills of Healthcare Professionals Working in Oncology: Can They Be Improved?', *European Journal of Oncology Nursing*, 12(1): 4–13.

Scottish Government (2007) *Characteristics of Adults in Scotland with Long-term Conditions: An Analysis of Scottish Household and Scottish Health Surveys*. Available at: www.scotland.gov.uk/Publications/2007/10/29093311/0 (accessed October 2010).

Spiegel, W., Thomas, Z., Maier, M., Vutuc, C., Isak, K., Karlic, H., and Michsche, M. (2009) 'Breaking Bad News to Cancer Patients: Survey and Analysis', *Psycho-oncology*, 18(2): 179–86.

Thomas, P. W., Thomas, S., Hillier, C., Galvin, K., and Baker, R. (2006) 'Psychological Intervention for Multiple Sclerosis', *Cochrane Database of Systematic Reviews*, 1/CD004431. DOI: 10.1002/14651858.CS004431.pub2. www2.cochrane.org/reviews/en/ab004431.html.

Vos, M. S. and de Haes, J. C. J. M. (2007) 'Denial in Cancer Patients: An Explorative Review', *Psycho-oncology*, 16: 12–25.

Walter, T. (1996) 'A New Model of Grief: Bereavement and Biography', *Mortality*, 1(1): 7–25.

Welsh Assembly Government/National Public Health Service, Wales (WAG/NPHS) (2005) *A Profile of Long-term and Chronic Conditions in Wales*. Cardiff: WAG.

Wittenberg-Lyles, E. M., Goldsmith, J., Sanchez-Reilly, S., and Ragan, S. L. (2008) 'Communicating a Terminal Prognosis in a Palliative Care Setting: Deficiencies in Current Communication Training Protocols', *Social Science and Medicine*, 66: 2356–65.

Worden, J. W. (1991) *Grief Counselling and Grief Therapy: A Handbook for the Mental Health Practitioner* (2nd edn). London: Routledge.

13

Communicating with children and young people and their families

Caroline Ridley, Val Helsby, and Kathy Crew

This chapter will help you to achieve competencies in:

- ➲ being accepting of differing cultural traditions, beliefs, UK legal frameworks, and professional ethics when planning care with people and their families and carers;

- ➲ communicating effectively and sensitively in different settings, using a range of methods and skills;

- ➲ being proactive and creative in enhancing communication and understanding;

- ➲ acting professionally and autonomously in situations in which there may be limits to confidentiality, for example, public interest and protection from harm;

- ➲ providing safe and effective care in partnership with people and their carers within the context of people's ages, conditions, and developmental stages;

- ➲ making effective referrals to safeguard and protect children and adults requiring support and protection;

- ➲ working with people to provide clear and accurate information.

Introduction

All health professionals will have contact with children and young people and all have a duty of care to ensure their safety across the range of settings in which they work. A young person may be an informal carer, or dependent on the care of someone with a serious mental, physical, or behavioural disability. Similarly, children and young people are encountered in clinical areas as patients, dependants, and visitors.

The variety of ways in which children and young people live, learn, and play, and the transition into different types of family group, for many children create new challenges and opportunities. Nursing the child frequently means nursing the family, as the needs of children are inextricably linked to the needs of their carers. Communication with these users of healthcare services is not always straightforward and involves nurses in both acute and primary care settings being willing and able to listen, explain, empower, consult and negotiate, empathize, challenge, reward, and stimulate (Department for Education and Skills, 2004). Whilst some of these skills and related issues are discussed more specifically within particular sections of this chapter, they are transferable skills that can be equally applied across the other sections described.

Getting involved

Nurses working in the specialist fields of child health are ideally placed to meet their complex needs. However, *all* nurses have a duty of care to provide general care and to recognize difficulties early, to make timely and appropriate referrals to other agencies, and to encourage, promote, and support optimum health (DfES, 2004). To do this successfully, nurses need to have a basic knowledge of child development and an understanding of the risk factors that can lead to health breakdown. Developing a confident working knowledge in these areas will serve to ensure that any communication you have with children and young people is productive and in their best interests.

⊕ Learning point 1

Consider the different communication needs of children/young people in the age groups (see Table 13.1) and list the different ways in which a nurse may communicate effectively with these different age groups.

Table 13.1 Communicating with different age groups

Age of child	Different ways a nurse may communicate effectively
Infant	
Toddler	
Pre-school age	
Primary school age	
Adolescent	

Suggested answers to Learning point 1

Different ways in which a nurse may communicate effectively with different age groups are set out below.

Infant	Touch, facial expression, singing, baby-face vocalizing
Toddler	Simple language, touch, physical role-modelling and demonstrating, enactment
Pre-school age	Verbal, picture books, play modelling and enactment, cartoons, video
Primary school age	Verbal, pictures, diagrams, written (simple), video, complex physical role-modelling and enactment
Adolescent	Verbal, written, video, texting, email, leaflets, books, websites.

Inclusive communication with children/young people

Communicating effectively

Effective communication with children and young people requires nurses who are prepared to build empathy, to work in partnership, and to demonstrate common core skills and knowledge of issues including confidentiality, ethics, and respect (DfES, 2005a). According to the Department of Health's National Framework for Children, children and young people are not always treated with sensitivity or courtesy and have rights that are not always understood or respected (DoH, 2003). The nurses' professional Code calls for nurses to '*listen* to people in their care and *respond* to their concerns and preferences' (NMC, 2008), yet young people themselves have identified a range of barriers to effective use of services including a lack of information and expertise, as well as a failure by health professionals to respect their views (RCN, 2009). The National Children's Bureau Public Health Reference Group (Brady, 2008) emphasized the importance to young people of professionals listening to their views and not just doing it because it 'looks good', and the Consultation Paper *Youth Matters* (DfES, 2005b) also highlighted young people's desire to be heard: 'People should listen to us more. They never do, they always do what they want anyway' (DfES, 2006: 13). See Practice example box 1 for an example of active listening in practice.

Practice example box 1: Active listening in A&E

During a hospital assessment with a 15-year-old girl, accompanied by her father, the doctor got negative answers to the 'ever smoked' and 'have you had a drink' questions. Once the father went to get a coffee, the doctor explained to the girl that the questions aimed to assess the risk to the patient and were not a judgement on her character. The doctor explained that such a history would indicate the need for TEG stockings in surgery to avoid thrombosis. When asked again, the girl gave a history of smoking and heavy drinking.

Creative communication

Motivated nurses might consider how interactive technology (IT) and the use of other 'new media' communication tools could be used to enhance discourse and contact with children/young people. Digital TV and more widespread Internet access have changed the ways in which children and young people live and learn. Increasing numbers of children and young people own or have access to mobile phones (Ipsos Mori, 2005) and guidance from the RCN (2006) provides useful information and advice for nurses who might want to use text messaging when working with children/young people in practice.

Traditional forms of written communication may impede those with restricted physical access or reading from full and meaningful engagement. It is estimated that 10 per cent of the population have dyslexia (Dyslexia Action, 2009). These particular children/young people might benefit from alternative ways of communicating, such as an increased emphasis on visual imagery. For children/young people with attention deficit hyperactivity disorder (ADHD), try to give them individual attention in a relaxed environment. Communicate with them on a one-to-one basis and avoid talking to other children at the same time. Children/young people with autistic spectrum disorder will present with a varying degree of communication difficulty, but a common problem across the spectrum is their difficulty relating to others. Be aware of your non-verbal signals, such as your posture, facial expression, pitch, and tone of voice.

Electronically mailed information means that they can access it at a time and place suited to them and in a way specifically suited to their particular learning needs. Children/young people who use non-verbal communication might require interpreters or signers to ensure full participation in any consultation and those with learning/behavioural difficulties such as autism and ADHD might benefit from the inclusion of their family, primary carers, or advocacy services.

⊕ Learning point 2: Inclusive communication

Not all children/young people with a hidden communication difficulty, such as dyslexia, may choose to disclose their disability to you. What strategies might you employ that would optimize any contact these children/young people have with you and your service?

Suggested answer to Learning point 2

- Spend time getting to know the child/young person. Making time reflects your interest in them and makes it more likely that they will share any difficulties with you. Reassure them about confidentiality.

- Be proactive. Don't be afraid to ask direct questions such as: 'Do you have any particular preferences regarding communication? Would it be easier for me to write to you with future appointments or to call or text you?'

- Support written information with verbal/visual/practical explanations. Avoid jargon or complex language. Ask the child/young person if they would like anyone to be present during your consultation.

- Create an atmosphere that facilitates disclosure. A poster on the wall about dyslexia, for example, may signal your department's recognition of the condition. It is legitimate to refer to 'some other' children/young people who have told you that they have had difficulty reading information given to them. This may reduce any feelings of isolation.

Fraser Guidelines and 'Gillick competence'

Age may be a determinant in assessing a child or young person's competence, but it is not always a reliable indicator of their ability to make informed and independent decisions regarding health advice and treatment. 'Fraser Guidelines' support the objective assessment of an individual's level of competence relating to contraceptive advice and treatment (*Gillick v West Norfolk and Wisbech AHA and DHSS*, 1985), but the test for 'Gillick competence' can be applied in all settings in which decisions have to be made related to a child's assessment of competence (Wheeler, 2006). Children under the age of 16 may be deemed 'Gillick competent' if they are able to:

- understand the reasons for and nature of any treatment that is offered;
- understand the principal benefits and risks of treatment and available, and alternative courses of action;
- understand the consequences of any refusal to have treatment;
- make a choice free from coercion or pressure.

....

➕ Learning point 3: Assessment of 'Gillick competence'

Consider an occasion within your own practice on which the test for 'Gillick competence' might be applied. What questions would you need to ask the child/young person and how would you document the consultation? With whom within the multi-professional team might you need to consult in order to deliver the best possible care for your patient?

....

Suggested answer to Learning point 3

- Explain issues clearly, free from unnecessary jargon. Make time for questions and consideration of the issues before they make their decision. Suitable questions to ask may include inviting the child/young person to repeat instructions for taking medication, and asking them to tell you what might happen if they do not comply with the preferred choice of treatment and about any possible side effects of treatment.

- You should document clearly in writing what you have discussed with your patient, including the questions that you have asked and the child/young person's responses: for example, 'the condition was explained to the patient and they were able to describe the condition and reasons for treatment' (RCN, 2008: 12).

- Liaison with other professionals caring for the patient such as a paediatrician, teacher, or social worker will help you to make a well-informed decision and any consultations should be recorded with details of what was agreed and by whom.

Communicating with children/young people at home

The environment is an important factor in shaping communication (Hargie and Dickson, 2004) and the Department of Health (2001) have called for children's and young people's health care and treatment to be delivered in settings that cause minimal disruption to their ordinary home life. Within the home setting, the balance of power between professional and patient means children/young people may feel less threatened and the patient may feel more able to talk honestly and openly about matters of importance to them (Shaw, 2009).

Trust between the nurse and patient is built by a commitment to respect an individual's cultural norms and values. Within the home setting, the unique ways in which a child/young person and their family live can be open to scrutiny and judgement. Engagement with children/young people requires a degree of humility, and nurses have to learn to accept that others' values and beliefs are as valid and important as theirs are to themselves: 'Many people have a natural prejudice in favour of their own cultural heritage and upbringing' (Hugman, 2009: 128).

Young carers

Nurses working with children/young people at home should be mindful of those young carers looking after family members at home. Whilst community nurses are more likely to be involved with families where a member has a long-term illness, many children who care 'remain hidden in the community' fearful of professional intervention that may threaten their home life and routine (Aldridge and Becker, 1993: 460). Department of Health (2008) guidance reminds healthcare professionals of the detrimental effects caring can have on young carers' physical and emotional health and calls for whole-family support in these circumstances. Box 13.1 lists some practical ways in which you might communicate effectively with young carers.

Box 13.1 Dealing with young carers

- Be alert to children/young people who are carers and approach the issue with sensitivity and understanding.
- Encourage young carers to talk to you about their responsibilities so that appropriate support packages might be employed. Children/young people may need to be told that they have a choice in whether or not to take on a caring role.
- Every young carer's situation is unique. Listen to what the young carer wants or needs. With their permission, make referrals to other agencies as necessary.
- Encourage young carers to engage with opportunities to enhance their own health and well-being.
- Children should not be used as interpreters in health settings as this places them in a difficult and prematurely adult role (British Psychological Society, 2008). In the family home, this may be unavoidable, however, it is important to remind families that a professional interpreter can be made available to them and familiarize yourself with local arrangements.
- Keep lines of communication open. When your role with the family ends, take steps to ensure the young person is in contact with others who can help, such as Connexions, their Local Young Carers Forum, or charitable organizations such as the Children's Society.

Methods of communication in community settings

The home visit may be the first time that the nurse and child/young person meet, and how the initial contact is made to arrange the meeting can affect the ensuing relationship. Warmth and friendliness can be conveyed through the language you use in the letter or phone call, and the tone of your voice might help to break down a perception of the nurse as authoritative and interfering rather than empowering and supportive. Letters to children/young people may be opened by adults with or without parental responsibility and not everyone can read well. A telephone call or text message may be more appropriate. Might you be introduced via a colleague already working with the child/young person and whose trust is established? Remember, families may be apprehensive at the thought of your visit, especially if you are calling because of challenging issues such as teenage pregnancy or suggested abuse.

Once a mutually convenient appointment has been arranged, it is useful to ask yourself the following questions before your visit.

- **Is the visit really necessary?** Time is a valuable resource and should not be abused or wasted.

- **Is the purpose of your visit clear?** Do you have enough background information to guide your planning and determine clear aims and objectives?

- **Where can you obtain appropriate and necessary background information?** Remember to follow the procedures and legislation related to matters of confidentiality for your particular job role. There should be no 'hidden agenda' and the child/young person, and their carers should feel equally prepared and ready for your visit.

- **How old is the child/young person you are visiting?** Failure to address different levels of maturity between children can undermine the nurse's attempt to form a rapport (Thompson, 2009). Can the child/young person communicate effectively themselves or is the nurse reliant on information from the parent or carer? Wherever possible, communicate directly with the child/young person even if they are relatively young (Berry, 2007). What difference will this make to your planning? Will you, for example, need to request a private space to facilitate a young person's right to confidential advice and treatment?

- **Have you considered the impact of the family dynamics?** Parents/carers should almost always be expected to know their children best (DfES, 2004), but family tension and relationship complexities will influence any communication that you have with your patient. For example, a child who is fearful of their parent may remain silent and withdraw from the consultation. Younger teenagers may want their parents involved, but older teenagers may not (Berry, 2007). The observant nurse will be attuned to non-verbal signals that offer clues about how a child/young person might really be feeling. See Practice example box 2 for an example from practice. It is important that you record information accurately to 'support patient care and communications' (NMC, 2009).

- **What is the relationship between the carer and the child/young person?** Observe eye contact between the child/young person and their carer. Do they seem anxious and too willing to please? Are they checking that their responses are met with approval? Do they contribute freely to the conversation or are they more restrained?

- **Who has parental responsibility and who should be involved in the consultation and kept informed?** In the child/young person's home, you will have less control over the physical environment. You may need to exercise negotiation skills in order to request that particular individuals leave the room or make a polite request that interruptions to your consultation are minimized.

Practice example box 2: Reading non-verbal communication

A family consisting of both parents, two boys (aged 12 and 8), and an older girl (aged 14), had been convened for a family therapy session. The discussion between the parents and the older boy became quite heated, and it was noted that the younger boy then went to look out of the window. In doing so, he had created a barrier of the backs of the chairs between himself and the heated discussion. This was a significant indicator of his own distress at the family's problems, but he was not empowered to express this distress openly.

 See Chapter 7 for more on overcoming communication difficulties in the domiciliary visit.

Communicating with the child/young person in hospital

The environment as a barrier

A hospital can be a strange place to a child or young person. There are staff in uniform, unusual smells, unfamiliar noises, scary medical equipment, and an unfamiliar cot or bed.

All of these may precipitate stress, anxiety, and fear. Nurses working in hospital settings are ideally placed to consider the environment in which they work. Creating an atmosphere of warmth and friendliness on a ward or clinic may seem obvious, but communication is further enhanced through less obvious measures such as low reception desks so that children can see the faces of staff involved in their care, easy wheelchair/pushchair access, clear signposting, and provision of private areas for those in need (NHS Estates, 2003).

Family-centred care

Promoted as an ideal model of care for meeting the needs of hospitalized children/young people, Smith et al. (2002: 20) define family-centred care (FCC) as 'the professional support of the child and family through a process of involvement, participation and partnership underpinned by empowerment and negotiation'. This fits well with the Children's Hospital Standard (DoH, 2003), which makes explicit reference to a need for hospital services to be centred around the needs of children and their families. The Bristol Royal Infirmary Inquiry (COI Communications, 2001) found that hospital facilities frequently failed to address the differing needs of children/young people at different ages, treating them all as 'mini-adults' rather than as discrete groups with particular and specific needs. Children who are frightened by pain or illness may be further disadvantaged by having to communicate their concerns to strangers (Elliott, 2009). Staff working in hospitals must be willing to listen to children/young people and to provide information that is factual, objective, and non-directive (DoH, 2003). Evidence has revealed that children are more compliant and better able to endure treatment if they have been involved in decision-making and empowered to retain a sense of control over the situation (Runeson, 2002). Sick children/young people have a compelling desire for health professionals to give them honest, clear, and in-depth information (Smith and Callery, 2005). In Young et al.'s (2003) study of communication about cancer in childhood, parents found that communication with their children became more honest and open as they became less 'controlling' and communicated more as 'partners' as the illness and treatment progressed.

Managing complex communication

Nurses utilizing active listening skills will be attuned to non-verbal and verbal signals that offer clues to a child/young person's readiness to engage in conversation. Asking questions of you may indicate their interest or concern. Eye contact may be a clue to a child's desire to be heard, and defensive body language may suggest tension or fear. See Practice example box 3 for an example of active listening skills in practice.

Practice example box 3: Active listening skills on a medical ward

A shy teenage girl's frequent vomiting was puzzling everyone on the medical team. Major medical and behavioural factors had been ruled out. Having resolved to give up and discharge her, a junior doctor asked her if there was anything that the girl wished someone had asked her during her stay in hospital. The girl replied that she had recently lost her grandmother of whom she was very fond, but that nobody had asked her to talk about things like that.

 See Chapter 4 for detailed explanation of active listening skills.

Children/young people may commonly use euphemisms or 'slang' language to describe their feelings, their conditions, or problems, and when referring to body parts. They may feel more relaxed using their own language, particularly if the issue that they are discussing is embarrassing or highly personal. Whilst it is important to communicate with them in a way that they understand, it is also important that you, as the health professional, seek clarification over language with which you are unfamiliar or simply do not know.

Communicating through play

Play is a fundamental aspect of healthy childhood. Play provides valuable information about a child's cognitive development and language ability and can be helpful in conveying information and facilitating questions, as well as helping children to express fears and anxieties. Mathison and Butterworth (2001) refer to three forms of play, all of which require skilled communication to engage the child.

- **Normative**, or everyday, play in hospital helps to recreate the familiar, serves to distract children, and enhances feelings of security.
- **Educative** play enables the transfer of information to the child.
- **Therapeutic** play can be used to help children to make sense of their illness and may support better understanding of a procedure or treatment.

Activities normally enjoyed by children when they are well can often be adapted for situations when they are unwell, and finding activities that they can enjoy helps to normalize a situation and demonstrates a nurse's interest in, and care for, them (Elliott, 2009). Play should be age-appropriate and a range of activities should be considered.

- **Babies** enjoy toys that serve to engage and distract, such as mobiles and colourful visual imagery. The use of music may be comforting. The tone and pitch of the nurse's voice will impact on a baby's behaviour and emotional state.

- **Toddlers** can be strong-willed as they develop their 'sense of self'. Toddlers respond to nurses who are patient, friendly, and willing to engage and explain. Through the use of dolls and teddies, a nurse can demonstrate a procedure and help the toddler to 'see' and 'feel' what might happen. The nurse can observe the toddler's reaction to better understand their concerns. Toddlers are sensitive to both verbal and non-verbal cues and attuned to their surroundings, so the effect of a nurse's language and behaviour towards both the toddler and their family should be considered.

- **Pre-school children** can express their feelings through drawing and painting. They are often sociable and friendly. Imaginative and 'pretend' play may offer clues to what they are feeling (Dunn, 2004). Educative play through the use of stories, for example, can help the pre-school child to better understand what will happen. It is important to build trust, and nurses must be honest when explaining any procedures or treatments (Sepion, 2009). The nurse–young patient relationship can trigger pertinent questions and strengthen professional bonds.

- **Primary-aged children** in hospital should be invited to engage with health professionals about what is going to happen. They are usually able to articulate their needs well. School-aged children can answer questions and have the right to be included in conversations about their illness and treatment. Writing poems, verses, and cards can also provide insight into a child's thoughts and facilitate communication with those about whom they care most.

Young people in hospital require careful consideration. Those interviewed in Kelsey and Abelson-Mitchell's (2007) study exploring their perceptions of their involvement in health care reported satisfactory experiences when staff exercised the following communication traits:

- spoke directly to them seeking relevant information;
- accommodated their specific needs, thereby demonstrating listening skills support and attention;
- made sure that language was understandable and avoided technical jargon;
- made them feel comfortable and were kind and empathic.

Poor experiences were associated with the following communication traits and triggered feelings including frustration, worry, and lack of trust:

- did not focus on *them*—for example, speaking directly to their parent;
- emphasized the power difference through behaviours such as 'siding' with parents or asking questions that they were not able to understand;
- were not honest;
- demonstrated through non-verbal signals their lack of interest in them, such as looking at their notes during a consultation.

Learning point 4: Transition from child to adult services

The transition from child to adult services can be challenging for young people with long-term conditions such as arthritis. Consider communication strategies that might alleviate stress and anxiety at this time.

Suggested answer to Learning point 4

- Find out the young person's concerns. The parents could also be asked this.

- Work out questions with the young person and parents that will need to be answered. Do this separately. Suggest to the young person that they rehearse with you or their parents what they want to say to or ask of the adult team, so that they become more confident in their communication with someone they know first.

- Arrange a personal introduction and visit to adult services. Plan with the young person when they will meet the adult team with their parents, and without their parents and with a friend. Provide a list of key professionals in both child and adult services who may be contacted if problems arise.

- Plan with the young person to start taking on more responsibilities for self-care and self-medicating.

- Suggest to the young person the of a diary in which they can record their self-care, unexpected issues, and feelings.

Further useful information and guidance for staff on the use of play can be found in guidance from the National Association of Hospital Play Staff (2003).

Engagement with parents and siblings in hospital

Parental anxiety due to the hospitalization of their child may serve to decrease the amount of involvement that some parents feel able to commit to in caring for their sick child (Coyne, 1994). Parents are usually the experts on their child, yet they may feel disempowered in the hospital setting, which increases their own anxiety. Evidence demonstrates that parents often feel excluded from the decision-making processes (Hummelinck and Pollock, 2006) and report feeling anxious when observed by nurses (Darbyshire, 1994). Whilst older children may have different wishes to those of their parents, skilled nurses will be mindful of the need to support both parties if optimum outcomes for the child/young person are to prevail. Being approachable, with a willingness to answer questions, and making time to talk with parents are important and nurses should be alert to the misunderstandings that can originate from the use of medical jargon.

Family-centred care attends to the needs and influence of siblings. Craft and Craft (1989) found that siblings of sick children were often neglected and it is easy for the needs of a very ill child to dominate the thoughts of parents in a way that ignores the less-pressing needs of a well brother or sister. Appropriate and thoughtful explanation to a sibling can facilitate positive outcomes for all children in the family (see Practice example box 4).

Practice example box 4: Family-centred care in health visiting

A mother is preoccupied with her six-week-old baby who has persistent colic. She is breastfeeding and still recovering from a complicated labour and birth. Her toddler son is confused and upset at the change of circumstances at home and is missing the attention he normally gets from his mother. He associates crying and screaming with the receipt of affection and begins throwing violent temper tantrums. When his mother acknowledges his feelings, includes him in the care of the baby and makes time to play/read/eat/rest with him during quieter moments in the day, his behaviour improves and the family is more relaxed.

The vulnerable child/young person

Knowing what the child or young person expects from any interaction that you have with them is important, as is your responsibility to explain your role and any limitations clearly. This is particularly important when children and young people are considering disclosing sensitive or highly personal information, such as abuse. Particular groups of children and young people have been identified as more susceptible to poorer health outcomes and deserving of professionals' heightened awareness (DoH, 2004). These include those experiencing psychological or social disadvantage, looked-after children, and those with family care responsibilities. They may be less able to approach health professionals and it is vital that nurses do not miss valuable opportunities for contact. Recognizing potential communication barriers and responding in a timely and appropriate manner increases the likelihood of improved health outcomes and a positive relationship with health professionals.

Table 13.2 A brief checklist to help to reduce potential communication barriers

Communication barrier	Considerations for nurses
Uniform and appearance	Is it really necessary? Is it intimidating? Is the nurse distinctly recognizable? If you are wearing regular clothing: is your status/name clearly visible? Are you carrying on your person medical equipment, e.g. a stethoscope?
Administrative systems	Do you have a formal appointment system? Can you be more flexible? How about drop-in centres located within schools, colleges, and the community?
Demeanour	Are you interested, approachable, and friendly? Have you said hello? Have you used the patient's preferred name? Have you introduced yourself to them? Do you look as if you have time to listen? Are you prepared to drop everything for an important disclosure? Never underestimate the courage it takes for children/young people to come forward. This might be your only chance to offer support.
Non-verbal signals	Eye contact; an important channel of communication, demonstrates warmth, interest and concern, and builds trust. Do you smile? It helps to break down barriers and builds trust. Posture: the way you walk, stand, and sit conveys powerful messages.
Setting	Does the setting feel safe and welcoming? Is it child- or young person-friendly? Do you have a suggestions/comment box?
Verbal communication	Think about the language you use. Do you avoid technical/medical jargon? How do you check that information you give is understood? Asking the child/young person to repeat information is a simple way to check understanding. How clearly do you speak? The success of verbal communication is influenced by the tone, pitch, and rhythm of your voice. What if you don't know something? It is better to be honest and invite the young person to speak to someone else or for you to find out on their behalf.
Confidentiality policies/ guidelines	Do you have a confidentiality policy that reflects professional and legislative practice and guidance? 'Absolute confidentiality' cannot always be guaranteed (DoH, 2004) and if you believe there is a risk to the health, safety, or welfare of a child/young person, that is serious enough to outweigh their right to privacy. In all other circumstances, nurses are duty-bound to uphold a child/young person's right to confidential advice and treatment. Children/young people want clarity over confidentiality procedures (DoH, 2004). Is your confidentiality policy clearly stated and prominently placed in your workplace?

Communication barriers

Whether you are in a child or adult placement setting, Table 13.2 shows a brief checklist to help you to consider how you can reduce potential communication barriers that might exist.

The teenage parent

Teenage parents have been identified as a particularly vulnerable group. They endure poorer child health outcomes, poorer emotional health and well-being, and poorer economic well-being compared with older parents (DCSF, 2007).

Teenage parents have spoken of healthcare professionals who are sometimes judgemental and unresponsive to their particular needs, making them less likely to attend for antenatal care (DCSF, 2007). They have reported feeling 'singled out' and 'being checked up on', and young fathers have reported feeling unwelcome and ignored, with resultant disengagement from consultations and appointments (DCSF, 2007). Young people generally report feeling intimidated by both 'service' and 'service providers' and are concerned about issues relating to confidentiality and trust (Croghan et al., 2004; DCSF, 2009). When first-year undergraduate nursing students were asked in Leishman's (2004) study what might reduce the *risk* of teenage pregnancy, responses included:

- not being judgemental;
- not telling young people off or talking down to them when they seek advice;
- being an educator and providing information at an appropriate level that can easily be understood.

These thoughts are mirrored elsewhere (DfES, 2006) and the list below offers further information to support you when working with teenage parents.

- **Show them respect.** Teenage parents can be confident, capable, and caring. Respectful communication includes not making assumptions or relying on stereotypes (Thompson, 2009).
- **Listen actively.** Listen carefully to what they have to say. Paraphrasing helps to establish empathy and provides an opportunity for the young person to confirm or adjust what they have said (Moss, 2008).
- **Observe carefully.** Uncommunicative teenage parents may give clues to their emotional state through non-verbal language such as poor eye contact or busying themselves with their child during a consultation. Offer more time and use closed questions to reduce their stress and anxiety (Lloyd and Bor, 2004).
- **Be non-judgemental.** Avoid making assumptions about their situation or behaviour.
- **Empower.** Empowered teenage parents are enabled to make appropriate decisions and take responsibility for their own actions. Avoid fault-finding and be 'open, positive empathic and supportive' (DeVito, 2009: 300).
- **Respect confidentiality.** 'You're Welcome' quality criteria (DoH, 2005) help providers of healthcare services to make services young-person-friendly. Teenage parents have a right to a confidential service and the principles include a need for professional teams to have a shared understanding of their confidentiality procedures.

- **Be flexible.** Teenage parents may need to access services outside of the school, college, or work setting, and will respond more appropriately if they are offered flexible services and appointment times.

 Learning point 5

Go back to Learning point 1. Can you now add more communication methods to the list?

Conclusion

This chapter has introduced you to the diverse communication needs of children/young people in a range of settings in which contact may be made. The health and well-being of every child and young person is important, and healthcare professionals who are motivated to develop and practise skilled communication techniques will facilitate the development of meaningful relationships that address these needs now and into the adult years.

 To find more resources to aid your learning, please now go online to **www.oxfordtextbooks.co.uk/orc/webb**. You will find video material relating to communicating with children/young people in 'Children's nurse interview', 'Communicating with young children', and 'Challenging communicators'.

Further reading

Dogran, N., Parkin, A., Gale, F., and Frake, C. (2009) *A Multidisciplinary Handbook of Child and Adolescent Mental Health for Front-line Professionals* (2nd edn). London: Jessica Kinsley.

Hubbuck, C. (2009) *Play for Sick Children: Play Specialists in Hospitals and Beyond*. London: Jessica Kingsley.

Jones, D. P. H. (2003) *Communicating with Vulnerable Children: A Guide for Practitioners*. London: DoH.

Kumin, L. (2004) *Early Communication Skills for Children with Down's Syndrome: A Guide for Parents and Professionals* (2nd edn). Bethesda, MD: Woodbine House.

Levevre, M. (2010) *Communicating with Children and Young People: Making a Difference*. Bristol: Policy Press.

MacGregor, J. (2008) *Introduction to the Anatomy and Physiology of Children: A Guide for Students of Nursing, Child Care and Health* (2nd edn). Abingdon: Routledge.

Reid, G. (2009) *Dyslexia: A Practitioner's Handbook* (4th edn). Chichester: Wiley Blackwell.

Sheridan, M., Sharma, A., and Cockerill, H. (2007) *From Birth to Five Years: Children's Developmental Progress* (3rd edn). New York: Routledge.

Smith, P. (2010) *Understanding Children's Worlds: Children and Play*. Chichester: Wiley Blackwell.

Spohrer, K. E. (2006) *Supporting Children with Attention Deficit Hyperactivity Disorder* (2nd edn). London: Continuum International Publishing Group.

Teare, J. (ed.) (2008) *Caring for Children with Complex Needs in the Community*. Oxford: Blackwell.

Trigg, E. and Mohammed, T. A. (eds) (2006) *Practices in Children's Nursing: Guidelines for Hospital and Community* (2nd edn). Oxford: Churchill Livingstone.

Winter, K. (2010) *Building Relationships and Communicating with Young Children: A Practical Guide for Social Workers*. Abingdon: Routledge.

References

Aldridge, J. and Becker, S. (1993) 'Children as Carers', *Archives of Disease in Childhood*, 69: 459–62.

Berry, D. (2007) *Health Communication Theory and Practice*. Maidenhead: Open University Press.

Brady, L. M. (2008) *National Children's Bureau: Young People's Public Health Reference Group. Pilot Project—Final Report*. Available at www.york.ac.uk/phrc/YPPHRG_ FR_1.08.pdf (accessed October 2009).

British Psychological Society (2008) *Working with Interpreters in Health Settings: Guidelines for Psychologists*. Available at www.ucl.ac.uk/clinical-psychology/ traininghandbook/sectionfiles/Appendix_6_BPS_guidance_on_working_with_ interpreters.pdf (accessed May 2010).

COI Communications (2001) *The Inquiry into the Management of the Care of Children Receiving Complex Heart Surgery at the Bristol Royal Infirmary*. Available at www. bristol-inquiry.org.uk/final_report/index.htm (accessed November 2009).

Coyne, I. T. (1994) 'Parental Participation in Care: A Critical Review of the Literature', *Journal of Advanced Nursing*, 21(4):716–22.

Craft, M. J. and Craft, J. L. (1989) 'Perceived Changes in Siblings of Hospitalized Children: A Comparison of Sibling and Parent Reports', *Child Health Care*, 18(1) (Winter): 42–8.

Croghan, E., Johnson, C., and Aveyard, P. (2004) 'School Nurses: Policies, Working Practices, Roles and Value Perceptions', *Journal of Advanced Nursing*, 47(4): 377–85.

Darbyshire, P. (1994) *Living with a Sick Child in Hospital: The Experience of Parents and Nurses*. London: Chapman & Hall.

Department for Children Schools and Families (2007) *Teenage Parents Next Steps: Guidance for Local Authorities and Primary Care Trusts*. London: DCSF/DoH.

—— (2009) *Healthy Lives, Brighter Futures: The Strategy for Children and Young People's Health*. London: DCSF/DoH.

Department for Education and Skills (2004) *Every Child Matters: Change for Children*. London: DfES.

—— (2005a) *Common Core of Skills and Knowledge for the Children's Workforce*. London: DfES.

—— (2005b) *Youth Matters: Green Paper*. London: DfES.

—— (2006) *Youth Matters: Next Steps—Something to Do, Somewhere to Go, Someone to Talk to*. Available at www.dcsf.gov.uk/everychildmatters/Youth/youthmatters/youthmatters/ (accessed September 2009).

Department of Health (2001) *Seeking Consent: Working with Children*. London: DoH.

—— (2003) *Getting the Right Start: National Service Framework for Children—Standard for Hospital Services*. London: DoH.

—— (2004) *Best Practice Guidance for Doctors and Other Health Professionals on the Provision of Advice and Treatment to Young People Under 16, on Contraceptive, Sexual and Reproductive Health*. London: DoH.

—— (2005) *You're Welcome Quality Criteria: Making Health Services Young People Friendly*. London: DoH.

—— (2008) *Carers at the Heart of 21st-century Families and Communities: A Caring System on Your Side—A Life of Your Own*. London: DoH.

DeVito, J. A. (2009) *The Interpersonal Communication Book* (12th edn). London: Pearson Education.

Dunn, J. (2004) *Children's Friendships: The Beginnings of Intimacy*. Oxford: Blackwell.

Dyslexia Action (2009) *About Dyslexia. What is Dyslexia?* Available at www.dyslexiaaction.org.uk/Page.aspx?PageId=1 (accessed September 2009).

Elliott, B. (2009) 'Communicating with Children, Young People and Families in Healthcare Contexts', in A. Dunhill, B. Elliott, and A. Shaw (eds) *Effective Communication and Engagement with Children and Young People, Their Families and Carers*. Exeter: Learning Matters.

Gillick v West Norfolk and Wisbech AHA (1985) AC 112. Available at www.hrcr.org/safrica/childrens_rights/Gillick_WestNorfolk.htm (accessed November 2009).

Hargie, O. and Dickson, D. (2004) *Skilled Interpersonal Communication: Research, Theory and Practice* (4th edn). London: Routledge.

Hugman, B. (2009) *Healthcare Communication*. London: Pharmaceutical Press.

Hummelinck, A. and Pollock, K. (2006) 'Parents' Information Needs about the Treatment of Their Chronically Ill Child: A Qualitative Study', *Patient Education and Counseling*, 62(2): 228–34.

Ipsos Mori (2005) *Young People and Mobile Phones: Nestlé Social Research Programme*. Available at www.ipsos-mori.com/researchpublications/researcharchive/poll.aspx?oItemId=707 (accessed November 2009).

Kelsey, J. and Abelson-Mitchell, N. (2007) 'Adolescent Communication: Perceptions and Beliefs', *Journal of Children's and Young People's Nursing*, 1(1): 42–9.

Leishman, J. (2004) 'Childhood and Teenage Pregnancies', *Nursing Standard*, 18(33): 33–6.

Lloyd, M. and Bor, R. (2004) *Communication Skills for Medicine* (2nd edn). Edinburgh: Churchill Livingstone.

Macdonald, E. (2004) *Difficult Conversations in Medicine*. Oxford: Oxford University Press.

Mathisen, L. and Butterworth, D. (2001) 'The Role of Play in Hospitalisation of Young Children', *Neonatal, Pediatric and Child Health Nursing*, 4(3): 23–6.

Moss, B. (2008) *Communication Skills for Health and Social Care*. London: Sage.

National Association of Hospital Play Staff (2003) *Guidelines for Professional Practice*. Available at www.nahps.org.uk (accessed November 2009).

National Health Service Estates (2003) *Improving the Patient Experience: Friendly Healthcare Environments for Children and Young People,* London: HMSO.

Nursing and Midwifery Council (2008) *The Code: Standards of Conduct, Performance and Ethics for Nurses and Midwives*. Available at www.nmc-uk.org/aDisplayDocument. aspx?documentID=5982 (accessed September 2009).

—— (2009) *Record Keeping: Guidance for Nurses and Midwives*. Available at www. nmc-uk.org/aDisplayDocument.aspx?DocumentID=6269 (accessed October 2009).

Royal College of Nursing (2006) *Use of Text Messaging Services: Guidance for Nurses Working with Children and Young People*. London: RCN.

—— (2008) *Adolescence: Boundaries and Connections—An RCN Guide for Working with Young People*. London: RCN.

—— (2009) *Mental Health in Children and Young People: A Toolkit for Nurses Who Are Not Mental Health Specialists*. London: RCN.

Runeson, I. (2002) 'Children's Participation in the Decision-making Process During Hospitalization: An Observational Study', *Nursing Ethics*, 9(6): 583–98.

Sepion, B. (2009) 'Communicating with Children and Young People', in L. L. Childs, L. Coles, and B. Marjoram (eds) *Essential Skills Clusters for Nurses Theory for Practice*. Chichester: Wiley-Blackwell.

Shaw, A. (2009) 'Engaging with Children, Young People, Families and Carers at Home and in Other Settings', in A. Dunhill, B. Elliott, and A. Shaw (eds) *Effective Communication and Engagement with Children and Young People, Their Families and Carers*. Exeter: Learning Matters.

Smith, L. and Callery, P. (2005) 'Children's Accounts of Their Pre-operative Information Needs', *Journal of Clinical Nursing*, 14(2): 230–8.

——, Coleman, V., and Bradshaw, M. (eds) (2002) *Family-centred Care: Concept, Theory and Practice*. Basingstoke: Palgrave.

Thompson, N. (2009) *People Skills* (3rd edn). Basingstoke: Palgrave Macmillan.

Wheeler, R. (2006) 'Gillick or Fraser? A Plea for Consistency over Competence in Children', *British Medical Journal*, 332 (8 April), 807.

Young, B., Dixon-Woods, M., Windridge, K. C., and Heney, D. (2003) 'Managing Communication with Young People Who Have Potentially Life-threatening Chronic Illness: Qualitative Study of Patients and Parents', *British Medical Journal*, 326: 305.

14

Communication and the cognitively impaired patient

Duncan Mitchell

This chapter will help you to achieve competencies in:

- ● communicating effectively and sensitively in different settings, using a range of methods and skills;
- ● being proactive and creative in enhancing communication and understanding;
- ● assessing and responding to the needs and wishes of carers and relatives in relation to information and consent;
- ● acting collaboratively with people enabling and empowering them to take a shared and active role in the delivery and evaluation of nursing interventions;
- ● making effective referrals to safeguard and protect children and adults requiring support and protection.

Introduction

One of the recurring themes of this book is that people are individuals and need to be treated as such. Whilst this seems a rather obvious point, its failure in practice leads to many, if not most, communication problems. This chapter examines the general approach that nurses need to take when nursing people with cognitive impairments. It will focus on the needs of service users who have some form of cognitive impairment that requires specific communication skills in response. It will explore the nature of mental impairment and offer some golden rules that nurses need when nursing people with cognitive impairments. It will use specific conditions as examples and introduce you to some guidance that will help you to adapt your skills to working with people with specific conditions.

Why does cognitive impairment present a communication problem for nurses?

Adults and children with some form of cognitive impairment are just as likely as anyone else to access a broad range of health services, particularly children with learning difficulties (Kerzman and Smith, 2004). Patients may have a range of communication difficulties, from having no speech at all, to having difficulty understanding complex language or concepts. Some people will have a permanent impairment due to an acquired brain injury, or a developmental impairment such as autism or Down's Syndrome. Some patients may have a temporary impairment due to an acute illness or toxic state, such as an infection and high temperature, or lack of oxygen, both of which can cause confusion. People with serious mental illnesses may also have altered and fluctuating abilities to understand because the illness interferes with functional thinking, concentration, and attention.

School nurses will have experience with children with learning difficulties and autistic spectrum disorders who often present with styles of communication that their families and education carers have adapted to, but which present a barrier to health professionals. It can be useful in general care settings for nurses to strive to understand and adopt the communication styles used by family and carers, because these are not only effective, but are also familiar to the patient and reduce anxiety and improve recovery (Kerzman and Smith, 2004; Sellars, 2006; Balandin et al., 2007). In many fields of care, nurses will encounter patients with acquired cognitive impairments such as dementia or stroke, whose communication abilities are likely to be limited by disorientation, poor short-term memory, and emotional lability (being prone to strong and fluctuating emotions).

What are cognitive impairments?

To understand terms that seem complicated, it is usually necessary to break them down into manageable sections. So, to help with understanding of the term 'cognitive impairment', each word will be defined before looking at the term itself.

- **Cognitive:** the noun for this word is cognition and this means 'the mental processes by which knowledge is acquired' (Martin, 2002: 144). For example, if one is given a message by someone else, it is cognitive skills that will determine the understanding of that message.
- **Impairment:** this means a damaging or weakening of a function or process.

So, put together, the two words mean a damaged or weakened ability to understand information. It is really important to understand that this is about knowledge, not about emotion. For example, you might have heard a phrase like 'just because I'm slow, it doesn't mean that I don't have feelings'. See case study 1 for a short patient example that has been split up to identify the cognitive impairment.

Case study 1: A young man with learning disabilities in A&E

Mark, a young man with learning disabilities, arrives at A&E having been involved in a road traffic accident. He was hit by a car and has a badly damaged right leg (physical injury).

He is confused because he is in shock (natural response).

However, even when he isn't in shock, he finds it difficult to understand things quickly, especially when events are unexpected or unfamiliar. Mark cannot understand what happened to him and what might take place in the hospital (cognitive impairment).

He is in a lot of pain and is very frightened and upset (natural response).

Later in this chapter, we will come back to this example to see why it is so important to be able to understand that some people have cognitive impairments. First, let's have a look at the range of the things that might involve cognitive impairment.

⊕ Learning point 1

Make a list of the sort of things that you think might involve a cognitive impairment.

Suggested answers to Learning point 1

There are a range of conditions that might be included in your list. The following are some examples, but are by no means the only ones:

- learning disability, sometimes also known as 'learning difficulty', 'developmental disability', 'intellectual disability';
- dementia, usually but not always affecting older people;
- brain damage following an accident;
- brain damage following stroke;
- some mental health conditions;
- drug/alcohol use.

This list is a simple one and each condition can be split into all sorts of different aspects. Some of the conditions are short-term and others are longer-term or permanent. This chapter is not designed to give you information about each condition. This would be a book in itself. For example, if we were to look just at learning disability, the definition is far from fixed and covers a very wide range of people. At one extreme are people who need support with basic needs such as eating and drinking, toileting and dressing, and, at the other extreme, people who have difficulty in their learning but require few, if any, specialist services. An estimate of the number of people with learning disabilities made in 2004 by the Institute of Health Research at Lancaster University was 985,000, with 224,000 being known to social services (Emerson and Hatton, 2004).

Basic assessment of cognitive impairment

Nurses in all fields of practice are expected to be able to make assessments of patient need and, of course, this includes communication ability. Nurses are sometimes worried that this means that they are required to make specialist assessments of the wide range of conditions that they come across in their field of practice: this is not the case. Nurses need to be able to identify whether someone has an understanding of what is being communicated to them. If there is a problem, then nurses need to be able to examine and adapt their own communication method (remember the models in Chapter 1—that communication works at least two ways). Nurses then need to know when to refer for specialist help.

Case study 2 is from the code of practice of the Mental Capacity Act 2005.

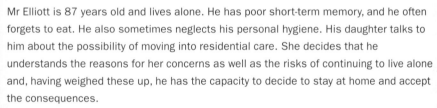

Case study 2: Example of capacity issues from the Code of Practice of the Mental Capacity Act 2005

Mr Elliott is 87 years old and lives alone. He has poor short-term memory, and he often forgets to eat. He also sometimes neglects his personal hygiene. His daughter talks to him about the possibility of moving into residential care. She decides that he understands the reasons for her concerns as well as the risks of continuing to live alone and, having weighed these up, he has the capacity to decide to stay at home and accept the consequences.

Two months later, Mr Elliott has a fall and breaks his leg. While being treated in hospital, he becomes confused and depressed. He says he wants to go home, but the staff think that the deterioration in his mental health has affected his capacity to make this decision at this time. They think he cannot understand the consequences or weigh up the risks he faces if he goes home. They refer him to a specialist in old-age psychiatry who assesses whether his mental health is affecting his capacity to make this decision. The staff will then use the specialist's opinion to help their assessment of Mr Elliott's capacity.

(Dept of Constitutional Affairs, 2007: 57)

In this example, staff believe that there may be an issue about Mr Elliott's cognitive ability and his capacity to make a decision. The Mental Capacity Act 2005 is very clear that professionals have to assume that people have capacity to make decisions unless they have reasons to believe otherwise. It is the individual communication skills of nurses that will help them to decide whether people have capacity to make decisions, as well their ability to communicate with individuals.

 Learning point 2

> In Case study 2, consider what might give you cause to think that Mr Elliott's mental health is deteriorating? In what sort of ways do you think you would communicate with Mr Elliott to help with your assessment?

Suggested answer to Learning point 2

It is most likely that staff have noticed that Mr Elliott's memory has deteriorated. This might be his short-term or his long-term memory, or possibly both. The signs may have been that Mr Elliott was slow to recognize someone he knew, forgot that he had had a meal, or did not know where he was. He may be struggling to find the correct words for common objects, or perhaps get his words mixed up.

To help to assess Mr Elliott, the staff will have to spend time with him and try to look at everything he is saying rather than isolate some elements that might seem confusing. Any perceived pressure might lead Mr Elliott to feel that he is being tested by the staff. It is important to speak clearly and listen carefully, and not to ask the same question in lots of different ways. Remember that your assessment at this point is to find out whether there is a need to ask for a specialist assessment.

When talking to people, remember that some questions seem very strange and it is not always easy to remember simple things. If someone were to ask you what you had for your meal last night, would you remember immediately?

It is common for nurses to have to make quick assessments when they first meet people. Whilst patients may have notes that tell you about underlying conditions, this may not always be the case. In fact, many nurses say that they have insufficient information about cognitive impairments and have to make decisions about the help that people might need.

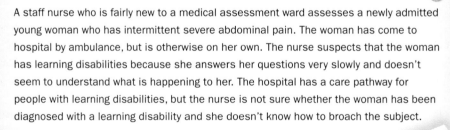

Case study 3: The knowledge of healthcare staff

A staff nurse who is fairly new to a medical assessment ward assesses a newly admitted young woman who has intermittent severe abdominal pain. The woman has come to hospital by ambulance, but is otherwise on her own. The nurse suspects that the woman has learning disabilities because she answers her questions very slowly and doesn't seem to understand what is happening to her. The hospital has a care pathway for people with learning disabilities, but the nurse is not sure whether the woman has been diagnosed with a learning disability and she doesn't know how to broach the subject.

Learning point 3

What sort of things would you ask a person to find out whether he or she has a learning disability?

Suggested answer to Learning point 3

There is no absolute list for this sort of informal assessment, but, in order to know whether someone has a learning disability, the questions in Box 14.1 will help. They are from the Royal College of Nursing's guidance for nursing staff about the health needs of people with learning disabilities.

Box 14.1 RCN Guidance on learning disabilities for nursing staff (RCN, 2006: 3)

- Ask the person if they have learning disabilities.
- Does the person have a social worker, care manager, or key worker?
- Did the person go to a special school or attend mainstream school with special support?
- Does the person go to a day centre?
- Has the person ever been seen by learning disability staff or lived in a learning disability hospital?
- Can the person read or write?
- Can the person tell the time?
- Does the person have difficulty in communicating?
- Can the person remember certain everyday facts about themselves (where they live, their birthday)?

Of course, you would not be expected to ask the whole list of questions. Some of them would be part of a standard assessment (such as date of birth). Some of them would be very difficult to answer for the woman when she is in pain. However, they would help you to understand whether someone is cognitively impaired due to learning disability.

The nurse's role in assessment is therefore important in helping to understand whether people are cognitively impaired and whether specific communication techniques are needed. It is important to remember that an impairment does not define everything about an individual, nor, as will be seen in the next section, does it provide a model for communication.

Communication with people with cognitive impairments

There are some golden rules in communication with people with cognitive impairments.

- Always address the patient first, and if you need to speak to a relative or carer, then keep coming back to the patient.
- Never assume that someone doesn't understand what you are saying.
- Remember that it takes at least two people to communicate—it may be the way in which you are giving the message that stops someone understanding.
- Make sure that you have the person's attention.
- Never blame the patient for not understanding—showing your impatience could also add to the problem.
- Always find out if the person uses any communication aids.
- Always use very clear language and avoid idioms such as 'under the weather'.
- Remember that many people want to please others and will give answers even if they don't understand the question.
- Always treat people with respect.

These rules are not exhaustive and you may want to add to them yourself. You will certainly need to add other communication approaches learnt from this book. You may think that some of these are common sense—they should be, but if they were always practised, then people would not need to be constantly reminded about them. You might also think that some or all of them apply to all patients, not only those who are cognitively impaired. In this, you would be quite right.

There is one further golden rule that requires a little more explanation—that is: avoid assuming that a physical symptom is part of someone's cognitive impairment. This is sometimes known as **diagnostic overshadowing** and, according to the Disability Rights Commission, is common when treating people with mental health problems and learning disabilities. It is also likely to be a feature of the care of other people with cognitive impairments. The Disability Rights Commission (2006: 69) explained that:

> Many of the people who took part in our consultation referred to problems in communication with healthcare staff. This could be a failure by staff to listen or understand and a tendency to attribute heath problems to a person's learning disability and/or mental health problem. This tendency, known as 'diagnostic overshadowing' was reported to us particularly by people with mental health problems. However, people with learning disabilities and their families also reported that when they told health professionals about changes in their physical well-being, they were sometimes explained as behavioural but turned out to be caused by pain or a significant physical illness.

Many people with learning disabilities are supported by other people. Sometimes, these are family members; sometimes, they are paid members of staff. It is sometimes really important to involve such people in care. In its examination of hospital care for people with learning disabilities, Mencap (2007: 19) found that:

> Parents and family members can often provide vital information that can help doctors and nurses to decide on appropriate treatments for people with a learning disability. But there appears to be a tendency among healthcare professionals to discount this information, or not even to consult family members in the first place. It is often assumed that they are over-emotional, irrational and uninformed. By disregarding the views and information that family members provide, doctors can make diagnoses, leading to premature, avoidable deaths.

There is sometimes a tension between both protecting confidentiality and keeping the person at the heart of decision-making and involving family members and other carers. Some people may not want their families involved in some aspects of their care and it is always important to have informed consent. However, many people would see their involvement as natural and it is often families and carers who know most about the people for whom they care (Kerzman and Smith 2004; Thurman et al., 2005).

Consent

One of the issues that often confuses nurses is whether they can give treatment to a patient who cannot give clear consent. Sometimes, this is when a patient cannot give written consent; sometimes, they appear to withhold consent by their actions (such as shying away from having an injection). This is usually an issue of communication and involves sensitive talking and listening.

Case study 4 is another example from the Mental Health Act 2005 Code of Practice.

The Code of Practice for the Mental Capacity Act is concerned with much more than capacity to consent to treatment, but it helps to provide the framework that nurses need when communicating with people with cognitive impairments. In the case study, the nurse knows that it takes time to help her patient to understand a procedure and to consent to it.

Priorities for care

Now, we are going to return to the first short case study of this chapter. Look again at the example of Mark, in case study 1. Some of the care that Mark needs will be exactly the same as that needed by anyone else with a similar injury. His injury will need to be assessed and a decision made about whether treatment is urgent.

Case study 4: An example of consent issues from the Mental Health Act 2005 Code of Practice

Luke, a young man, was seriously injured in a road traffic accident and suffered permanent brain damage. He has been in hospital several months, and has made good progress, but he gets very frustrated at his inability to concentrate or do things for himself.

Luke now needs surgical treatment on his leg. During the early morning ward round, the surgeon tries to explain what is involved in the operation. She asks Luke to sign a consent form, but he gets angry and says he doesn't want to talk about it.

His key nurse knows that Luke becomes more alert and capable later in the day. After lunch, she asks him if he would like to discuss the operation again. She also knows that he responds better one-to-one than in a group. So she takes Luke into a private room and repeats the information that the surgeon gave him earlier. He understands why the treatment is needed, what is involved, and the likely consequences. Therefore Luke has the capacity to make a decision about the operation.

(Dept of Constitutional Affairs, 2007: 37)

 Learning point 4

Think about how Mark's cognitive impairment might affect his response to initial assessment and treatment. What are the ways in which you would communicate with Mark?

Suggested answer to Learning point 4

Mark's cognitive impairment means that he may not see the connection between his accident and being in hospital. He may confuse being in hospital with other times at which he has had treatment. It is likely that he will take a long time to understand information and that the pain that he is experiencing will make this even more difficult for him.

It is important to remember the golden rules. Speak to Mark directly: he will understand some of what you are saying and you can ask him questions to check his understanding. Mark may have limited speech, but you can use touch to communicate, especially if trying to locate areas of pain, and, of course, if it is possible, find out if Mark uses any communication aids. Give Mark plenty of time to absorb information and don't give him lots of information or ask lots of different questions at once. Do many of the things that you would do with any other patient; in particular, be reassuring and calm. There will need to be an assessment of Mark's mental capacity to consent to treatment, and if Mark is unable to consent, then the team will need to consider a best-interests decision.

For further reading, see the Mental Capacity Act 2005 Code of Practice available at: **www.dh.gov.uk/prod_consum_dh/groups/dh_digitalassets/@dh/ @en/documents/**

Whilst Mark's cognitive impairment is unlikely to change, the shock will diminish, as will his being frightened and upset. It is therefore important that assessment of understanding continues during and after treatment.

Communication techniques for people with severe cognitive impairment

Sometimes, we may have a patient who is unable to speak or who is unable to comprehend their environment or the people around them. This may be due to an altered state of consciousness, such as a comatose patient, someone in an acute or chronic confused state due to poor memory retention or impaired concentration, or someone very distracted by impaired thought processes and interference from acute psychological symptoms. As mentioned earlier in this chapter, many people with communication difficulties may rely on communication aids. These can be physical aids such as picture cards or techniques such as Makaton, a simple sign language commonly used in the UK that uses gestures or pictures for simplified communication (Sellars, 2006). More complex techniques such as augmentative and alternative communication (AAC) may be used in specialist education and care areas (Graves, 2000), and it may be worth finding out about an individual patient's needs and abilities from their usual carers regarding common and useful techniques that can be used that the person will understand.

People with specific cognitive impairments are likely to have functional strengths that can be used for communication and understanding. Elderly dementia patients, for example, often have varied levels of impairments in different cognitive areas. Hall (1988) identified four different areas of impairment common in dementia patients:

- **intellectual loss**—memory, attention, sense of time;
- **affective/personality loss**—raised anxiety, emotional blunting;
- **planning loss**—loss of functional thinking; can't plan or problem-solve;
- **low stress threshold**—inability to tolerate stress or frustration, emotional lability (easily provoked to anger, crying, laughing).

These different areas of impairment mean that the person may have strengths in one, but not another. So, a patient with an impaired memory may still understand on an emotional level and so understand kindness—or anger—and learn to trust or distrust a person, even when they don't know who that person is.

Rantz and McShane (1995) made a study of nursing home staff who worked with chronically confused patients and found four nursing interventions that improved communication and understanding and so reduced patient anxiety and distress:

- **interpreting reality**—use of familiar objects in the patient's environment such as photos, mementos;

- **maintaining normality**—having a routine that can be understood by the patients on a behavioural level;

- **meeting basic needs**—for exercise, reducing boredom, and social activities;

- **monitoring for signs of distress**—good observation skills, using the individual patient's ways of communicating distress such as agitation, crying, withdrawal, reluctance, or changes in behaviour.

Sometimes, simply being with someone, holding their hand, or simply spending time with them can communicate an idea of trust and togetherness. Even a person who does not know who the nurse is will gain an emotional relationship with them. This is referred to as 'transference' and describes a situation in which one person emotionally relates to another as if they were someone else and a previous relationship appears to be re-enacted in the patient–nurse relationship (Burnard, 2005). See case study 5 for an example.

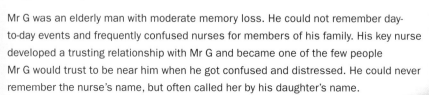

Case study 5: Transference for patient with cognitive impairment

Mr G was an elderly man with moderate memory loss. He could not remember day-to-day events and frequently confused nurses for members of his family. His key nurse developed a trusting relationship with Mr G and became one of the few people Mr G would trust to be near him when he got confused and distressed. He could never remember the nurse's name, but often called her by his daughter's name.

In this example, Mr G appears to have used emotional memory to understand his relationship with his key nurse. He has unconsciously transferred his memories of his daughter to someone who 'reminds him' of his daughter on an emotional level. This kind of relating is common in many intense counselling and psychotherapy relationships, but also occurs apparently quite easily with people whose intellectual abilities are impaired or suppressed and unable to 'interfere' with the emotional aspect of a relationship (Bateman and Holmes, 1995).

Conclusion

This chapter has introduced you to communication with people who have cognitive impairments. You now know about different cognitive impairments and some of the ways in which they affect communication. You now have some golden rules about nursing people with cognitive impairments. The key to working with people with cognitive impairments is to treat people individually and with respect, and to add lessons from this chapter to those that you have learnt from the rest of this book.

 To find more resources to aid your learning, please now go online to
www.oxfordtextbooks.co.uk/orc/webb. You will find videos 'The confused patient', 'Specialist dementia nurse interview', and 'Nurse Consultant in acute psychosis interview', all of which are linked to this chapter. You can also view 'Challenging communicators', linked to Chapter 13, for more on communicating with people with autism and attention disorders.

Further reading

Bowers, L., Brennan, G., Winship, G., and Theodoridou, C. (2009) *Talking with Acutely Psychotic People*. http://citypsych.com

Department of Constitutional Affairs (2007) *Mental Capacity Act Code of Practice.* London: DCA.

Hoe, J. and Thompson, R. (2010) 'Promoting Positive Approaches to Dementia Care in Nursing', *Nursing Standard*, 25(4): 47–56.

Nind, M. and Hewett, D. (2005) *Access to Communication: Developing the Basics of Communication with People with SLD* (2nd edn). London: David Fulton.

Stevenson, L. and Chapman, A. (2008) *Hearing the Voice: Improving Communication with People with Dementia*. Sterling: Dementia Services Department.

Web links

Communication and mental health
http://citypsych.com
www.starwards.org.uk
Makaton
www.makaton.org/

References

Balandin, S., Hemsley, B., Sigafoos, J., and Green, V. (2007) 'Communicating with Nurses: The Experiences of 10 Adults with Cerebral Palsy and Complex Communication Needs', *Applied Nursing Research*, 20: 56–62.

Bateman, A. and Holmes, J. (1995) *Introduction to Psychoanalysis: Contemporary Theory and Practice*. Hove: Brunner-Routledge.

Burnard, P. (2005) *Counselling Skills for Health Professionals* (4th edn). Cheltenham: Nelson Thornes.

Department of Constitutional Affairs (2007) *Mental Capacity Act Code of Practice*. London: DCA.

Disability Rights Commission (2006) *Equal Treatment: Closing the Gap—A Formal Investigation into Physical Health Inequalities Experienced by People with Learning Disabilities and/or Mental Health Problems*. London: DRC.

Emerson, E. and Hatton, C. (2004) *Estimating Future Need/Demand for Supports for Adults with Learning Disabilities in England*. Lancaster: Institute for Health Research, Lancaster University.

Graves, J. (2000) 'Vocabulary Needs in Augmentative and Alternative Communication: A Sample of Conversational Topics between Staff Providing Services to Adults with Learning Difficulties and Their Service Users', *British Journal of Learning Disabilities*, 28(3): 113–19.

Hall, G. (1988) 'Care of the Patient with Alzheimer's Disease at Home', *Nursing Clinics of North America*, 23: 31–46.

Kerzman, B. and Smith, P. (2004) 'Lessons from Special Education: Enhancing Communication between Health Professionals and Children with Learning Difficulties', *Nurse Education in Practice*, 4(4): 230–5.

Martin, E. A. (2002) *Oxford Concise Medical Dictionary*. Oxford: Oxford University Press.

Mencap (2007) *Death by Indifference*. London: Mencap.

Rantz, M. and McShane, R. (1995) 'Nursing Interventions for Chronically Confused Home Residents', *Geriatric Nursing*, 16: 22–7.

Royal College of Nursing (2006) *Meeting the Health Needs of People with Learning Disabilities: Guidance for Nursing Staff*. London: RCN.

Sellars, G. (2006) 'Learning to Communicate with Children with Disabilities', *Paediatric Nursing*, 18(9): 26–8.

Thurman, S., Jones, J., and Tarlton, B. (2005) 'Without Words: Meaningful Information for People with High Individual Communication Needs', *British Journal of Learning Disabilities*, 33(2): 83–9.

15

Engagement, motivation, and changing behaviour

Maxine Holt and Lucy Webb

This chapter will help you to achieve competencies in:

- ➡ actively helping people to identify and use their strengths to achieve their goals and aspirations;
- ➡ using appropriate strategies to empower and support patient choice;
- ➡ promoting health and well-being, self-care, and independence through teaching and empowering people to cope;
- ➡ discussing sensitive issues in relation to public health and providing appropriate advice and guidance to individuals, communities, and populations;
- ➡ working within a public health framework to assess needs and plan care for individuals, communities, and populations;
- ➡ supporting people in making appropriate choices and changes to eating patterns;
- ➡ discussing in a non-judgemental way how diet can improve health and the risks associated with not eating appropriately.

Introduction

This chapter builds on the health promotion strategies addressed in Chapter 8 by considering how the underpinning theories support the delivery of health promotion and behaviour change in practice settings.

When we consider health promotion interventions, one important feature of the process is identifying and understanding the attitudes, beliefs, and values that our patients have regarding their health and well-being. Ideally, exploration of these variables should be done with the patient or groups that we are working with. Once we have identified these, we can then tailor our interventions to meet their motivation needs to change behaviour. First, we need to consider the theories behind health beliefs.

Theories behind health beliefs

The health belief model

An established theoretical model of health beliefs is by Rosenstock (1966) and Becker (1974). The theory underpinning the health belief model is that the perceived threat of disease serves as a motivator for the patient to take action. In other words, it is about communicating to patients that behaviours such as smoking, lack of exercise, and poor diet may lead to coronary heart disease and stroke, in an effort to motivate the patient to modify such behaviours and reduce their risks of disease (see Figure 15.1).

The health belief model can be an effective framework within which nurses can evaluate patients' health behaviour and deliver interventions. Nurses can use this model effectively for health promotion for breast-cancer screening (Medina-Shepherd and Kleier, 2010), smoking cessation (Schofield et al., 2007), mapping and improving sexual health behaviour (Browes, 2006), and treatment choice for obesity (Armstrong et al., 2009).

The model in Figure 15.1 is based on the individual's beliefs of how they consider themselves to be.

Perceived susceptibility ('am I going to get the disease?')

Most of the time, people tend to think that they are less likely to develop a health problem compared to other people. Therefore, some people do not think that health

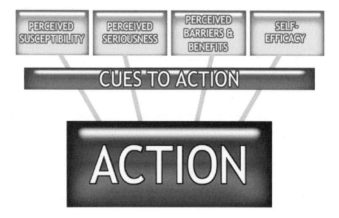

Figure 15.1 The health belief model

information is relevant to them. An example of this is health promotion campaigns on the increasing risks of HIV transmission amongst heterosexuals.

> Nurse: Jenny, here is the prescription for the contraceptive pill. You have mentioned that you don't have a steady partner at the moment, so I would really like to advise you that it's better also to use condoms to protect you against a number of sexually transmitted diseases including HIV.
>
> Patient: Oh, I don't need to worry: things like that don't happen to people like me.

Perceived seriousness ('how bad would it be?')

Some patients believe that it is better to leave things alone at the moment and perhaps return to thinking about it in the future.

> Nurse: Sam, your blood pressure is a little on the high side. We need to think how we might help to reduce this. I wonder if you might consider losing some weight, as there is significant evidence that losing even 10 per cent of your weight helps to lower your blood pressure. What do you think?
>
> Patient: I'll give it some thought maybe, but perhaps later when I get back from my holiday or after Christmas maybe. Besides, my dad was fat and lived to a ripe old age, and his mother was thin and she died in her 50s. Anyway, nurse, when your time's up, that's it. You've got to go sometime.

Perceived barriers and benefits ('will it be easy to get something done about it? What will it cost me?')

Here, the person weighs the pros and cons. It is based on the fact that the person must believe that a change in behaviour will benefit them. These costs are weighed up not just in financial terms, but in terms of other areas of their lives.

> Nurse: Reducing your lithium medication when you're so stressed, Joe, is putting you at risk of becoming manic.
>
> Patient: I know, but the stress is down to the amount of work I have to get through right now and being just a bit high helps me get through it quickly.

Self-efficacy ('Is it possible for me to do something about it? What are the things that might stop me?')

Patients will consider whether the time is right for them and the possible negative outcomes.

> Nurse: Mary, we have discussed the fact that if you carry on smoking 30 a day you are at risk from developing smoking-related diseases. Do you think you could consider how you might stop smoking using one of the therapies we have discussed?
>
> Patient: I'm not sure I can do it. I know, you see, that the minute I give up I will put loads of weight on and I don't want that.

Cues to action: take action ('ok, I am ready to make a change')

This model proposes that some patients need cues in order to change some health-related behaviour, such as a change in their appearance, a death of a close family member, a comment from a close friend or relative or significant other. As nurses, we can sometimes be the significant other. Once this happens, the patient is ready to make a change based on having the correct information and an improved motivation to change (see case study 1).

Case study 1: Giving information to facilitate change

Alan is staff nurse on a paediatric ward caring for Jimmy, who is seriously ill with measles. Jimmy's mother visits every day after dropping her other two children off at the nursery. She tells Alan that none of her children have been immunized against measles as she doesn't believe in immunizations anyway. After getting to know her, Alan asks about her concerns regarding vaccination, and he is able to allay some of her fears. He asks whether she would now consider having her other two children immunized to protect them from the terrible effects that the disease has had on Jimmy. She agrees and he arranges an appointment for her in the local clinic.

As nurses, we have a responsibility to communicate the need for our patients to consider healthier lifestyles to prevent disease. Understanding our patients' beliefs about their health and well-being is an important factor in communicating health promotion. It enables the patient to feel valued and listened to. The health belief model is not a model that can predict behaviour or identify those factors that are important in influencing behaviour change. However, it does enable us to consider overall the complex range of factors that influence a person's health behaviour.

 Learning point 1

Think back over your placement experiences so far and about some of the patients for whom you have recently cared. Can you use the main aspects of the health belief model to identify the range of factors that may have influenced their health behaviour?

- **Perceived susceptibility:** Am I going to get the disease?
- **Perceived seriousness:** How bad would it be?
- **Perceived barriers and benefits:** Will it be easy to get something done about it? What will it cost me?
- **Self-efficacy:** Is it possible for me to do something about it? What are the things that might stop me?
- **Cues to action:** take action—OK, I am ready to make a change.

If you were to meet these patients on placement again, how might you respond differently in conversations you had?

One of the identified barriers to more effective use of the health belief model is that, while nurses are in a good position to deliver health promotion, they feel uncomfortable translating their knowledge into practice, Across six Western countries, Lally et al. (2008) found that only 50 per cent of oncology nurses considered discussing smoking with their cancer patients. Schofield et al. (2007) similarly found older smokers unable to sustain healthy changes in their smoking habits, and considered lack of sustained encouragement from health professionals to be a key factor. This evidence suggests that the model helps nurses to identify patient behaviour change problems, but that they still need to change their use of health promotion to make sustainable changes in their patients.

The behaviour change model

Another useful model is offered by Prochaska and Di-Clemente (1984; 1986; 1992). The model considers how patients make health-related behavioural decisions, the stages they go through, and how they move from one stage to another. The model focuses on *how* people change rather than *why*. The model is based on sequential stages:

1. pre-contemplation;
2. contemplation;
3. preparation to change;
4. action for change;
5. maintenance;
6. relapse.

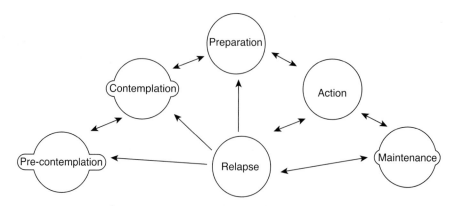

Figure 15.2 The behaviour change model

The model is characterized very much like a revolving door and the length of time spent in each stage varies. Throughout each stage, people are occupied in different physical and mental processes (see Figure 15.2).

Pre-contemplation

A patient in the pre-contemplative stage does not intend make any change to their health behaviour in the foreseeable future. Patients may be in this stage because they are uninformed or not really interested about the consequences of their behaviour, or they may have tried to change in the past and been unsuccessful.

> Patient: Sorry, nurse, but, before you start about my smoking, I've tried nicotine gum, but it didn't work for me. Nothing really works for me, so I just have to face it, I will always be a smoker. Anyway, my dad was a smoker and lived to a good age.

Contemplation

Patients here are thinking about their health and lifestyle behaviour and intending to do something about it, usually in a given time scale, and can often stay in this stage for a very long time or may never actually move forward at all.

> Patient: I am sick of being out of breath all the time and I know it's smoking that's causing it. I'd like to do something about it, but don't know what.

Preparation to change

This is the stage in which the patient is intending to take action in the immediate future. Again, this may be measured in time: for example, 'in the next month'. Some patients with whom we work may already have made a move to words taking action, such as joining a gym.

> Patient: I have thought about cutting down on my cigarettes, but I think I need some help to do this. I have heard about nicotine patches. Do you think they will help me?

Action for change

This is the stage in which patients have made specific obvious changes in their health behaviours and lifestyles within the past six months. This stage involves clear and realistic time-planned goals that are supported by others to ensure success.

> Patient: I feel so much better. I haven't had a cigarette for three weeks now and that nicotine gum you suggested has really helped. It's difficult though and sometimes, after tea, I really crave one.

Maintenance

Patients in the maintenance stage are working to prevent relapse and a return to their old health and lifestyle behaviours. The new health behaviour therefore becomes a normal pattern. Many patients find this a difficult stage and many people relapse and revert back to any of the above stages.

> Patient: It's been a year now since I smoked. It feels good when someone says are you a smoker and I say no. It's difficult sometimes, but I get tempted less and less and if I do, I immediately get on with doing something to take my mind off it like we discussed.

Relapse

A patient may relapse to an earlier stage. It is important that we provide positive support and do not allow the patient to consider themselves as having failed, but encourage them to review their action plans and recognize that relapse is a part of the process of change.

> Patient: Oh, I feel so annoyed with myself! I was doing so well and then I went to a party and an old friend offered me a cigarette and I just took it to be sociable. Before I knew it, I had smoked three and then bought a packet on the way home. I am back to square one now. It's hopeless.

Prochaska et al. (1994) modified the model and added a further stage described as 'termination or final stage' in which people experience no temptation to return to their old behaviour patterns.

The behaviour change model in action

Let us consider how both of the above models can be applied to our work in communicating with patients about health issues. It is useful to have a guide on how to get started, and Ewles and Simnett (2005) and Rollnick et al. (2007) provide us with some tips on how to do this (see Figure 15.3).

Using the case scenarios from the previous page, let's consider each of the steps (in Figure 15.3, labelled A–D) in working with a patient from the pre-contemplation stage through the whole cycle and how we communicate with patients to effect change.

Step A

Nursing is a very busy job, but it is important that we do not just skip over or ignore this stage, as it is in the early interaction that the nurse–patient relationship is formed. It is at this stage that the patient gains the first impression of us as professionals and how interested we are in them as individuals. It is difficult, sometimes, to rectify this at a later date. In getting to know the patient, we need to ensure that we are in the correct environment. A patient's bedside on a noisy ward or a busy waiting room may not be the best place in which to initiate a discussion with a patient. The physical setting is therefore important and being able to add other interesting materials that communicate health issues, such as posters, leaflets, and reading materials, may prompt cues for discussing change. We need to get to know the patient, what their beliefs and knowledge about their health and well-being are, and whether they are ready to change. One useful way of getting to know the patient is by using narratives or stories: for example, getting the patient to talk about what a typical day is like for them.

When using this approach, the nurse asks the patient to take them through a journey of their typical day in relation to a health behaviour or health problem. In other words, the patient is painting a picture that we can use to try to better understand the patient. The following is a scenario about a patient called John, whose heavy smoking is contributing to his chest problems and breathlessness.

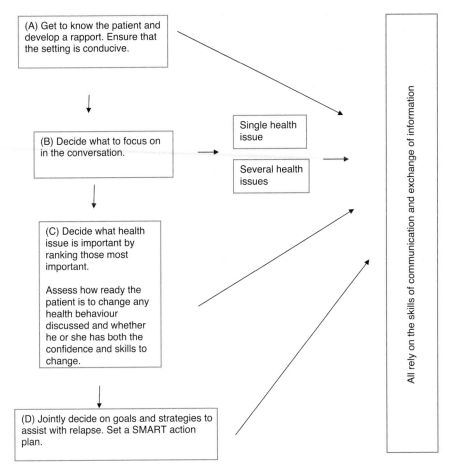

Figure 15.3 The behaviour change model in action (adapted from Ewles and Simnett, 2005, and Rollnick et al., 2007)

The pre-contemplation patient

Nurse: Hello, John, my name is Nurse Jones and I am hoping to help you with why you have come here today—particularly the problem you're having with your chest.

Patient: Sorry, nurse, but before you start about my smoking, I've tried nicotine gum in the past, but it didn't work for me. Nothing really works for me, so I just have to face it: I will always be a smoker. Anyway, my dad was a smoker and lived to a good age.

Nurse: OK, John, I understand, but perhaps we'll just begin by getting to know each other a little. Maybe you could tell me what a typical day is like for you with your chest from when you get up in the morning. How does that sound?

As nurses, the skill that we need to apply here is one of listening and following the story and only interrupting if really necessary and with very simple questions. Rollnick et al. (2007) suggests that you will know that you have got the balance right if you are only doing 10–15 per cent of the talking.

Step B

Some patients will have a number of health behaviours that they want to discuss and this can make it difficult for both the nurse and the patient to know where to start.

> Nurse: John, it seems that there are a number of things you are concerned about. These are your chest, weight, and that you cannot get out and exercise. Perhaps we can look at which ones are most important to you and begin there? How about we list the problems that cause you problems in your day-to-day life and you put them in order of importance?

Step C

The skill here is that the nurse does not rush into the discussion, but ascertains what is (are) the most important issues that the patient can focus on at that time. It is important to note that a patient may only be able to focus on one behaviour change at a time. Also, it is worth remembering that a change in one health behaviour may have a positive effect on another, which can act as a powerful motivator.

> Nurse: I know that you have had a poor experience with nicotine gum in the past, John, and this has put you off thinking about how you might give up smoking. How about we begin by looking at this again and seeing how we might help you to consider giving up smoking? If we can improve your chest, it will help you to get out and about and exercise more, which will help with your weight loss. How does that sound?

Once you have begun to talk about health behaviour with the patient, it is important to assess how ready they are to change their health behaviour(s). Patients may feel willing, but not actually have the confidence to change. Rollnick et al. (2007) propose adopting a curiously approach to this, rather than a question–answer approach.

> Nurse: OK, John, because of what you initially said when we first talked about the nicotine gum, I am unsure *how* you feel at the moment about stopping smoking and how important is it to you. Can we chat about this for a moment and then we can decide what to do next?

From contemplation to preparation

> Patient: I am sick of being out of breath all the time and I know it's smoking that's causing it. But now you have explained to me the different things that I could use to try to stop smoking, and that I can get help with this, I think I may be able to give it another go. Especially if it will help me to lose weight as well. So I have decided that I am definitely going to quit smoking after my holiday next month.
>
> Nurse: That's great and sometimes it's a good idea to have something to focus on. How about we set a date to follow this up when you get back from your holiday?

It is important to remember that we can apply the model of behaviour change to any nursing setting and that patients may present to us at any stage in the cycle. For example, the patient and nurse scenario above could occur on a hospital ward, outpatient department, or in a community setting. The key is that a follow-up opportunity has been discussed and arranged, with all of the necessary details communicated to those involved, so that, when the patient returns, both can continue to work through the process of moving the patient to the next stage. Once the patient has a real commitment to change, then we need to discuss with them strategies for achieving goals and coping with relapses.

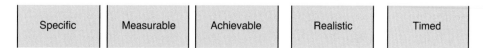

| Specific | Measurable | Achievable | Realistic | Timed |

Figure 15.4 SMART principles

Step D

Once the patient has a clearer view of the need for behaviour change and the benefits, it is important to discuss how they are going to achieve their goal(s). One of the techniques used in motivational interviewing using SMART principles (Figure 15.4).

In our case, John has set a goal to quit smoking after his holiday and, on returning, has managed to cut down on the number of cigarettes he smokes in a day. At present, the prospect of a whole life without smoking may be overwhelming for John, but a day without smoking may seem far more realistic. The key is to build up goals from this.

> Nurse: Hello, John, I hope you enjoyed your holiday? I understand that last time you were considering stopping smoking once you returned from your holiday. Shall we look at how we can help you with this?
>
> Patient: Well nurse, I have managed to cut down on my cigarettes, but not given them up completely. I think I need some help to do this and I have heard about nicotine patches. Do you think they will help me?
>
> Nurse: That's already a great start, John, well done. What we need to do is to enable you to reduce the number of cigarettes you smoke even further now and I think that it might be a good idea to try nicotine patches. Let's set some small goals at first, so that it doesn't seem impossible. How about trying to cut down again by three cigarettes a day for the first week? Then, in two weeks' time, see how the patches help with a short-term goal of a whole day without smoking? Remember that, as you reduce your smoking, you will also see the benefits in your breathing, which will help you to get out and walk a bit more to increase your exercise.

Notice the SMART principles in this example. Decisions and goals agreed between the patient and the nurse are specific, measurable, achievable, realistic, and timed.

Maintenance

Devising coping strategies is important for success, as many people have to cope with a number of difficulties until their new changed behaviour becomes the norm. Patients will adopt a variety of coping strategies and these should be explored with the patient, as they may have very individual ideas and ways of doing this. Examples would include:

- changing routines;
- finding substitutes.

> Patient: I feel so much better. I haven't had a cigarette for four months now and that nicotine gum you suggested has really helped. It's difficult, though, and sometimes, after tea, I really crave one.
>
> Patient: It's been a year now, nurse, since I smoked. It feels good when someone says are you a smoker and I say no. It's difficult sometimes but I get tempted less and less, and if I do, I immediately get on with doing something to take my mind off it like we discussed.

Relapse

The experience that patients undergo when changing health behaviour(s) can be life-changing for them. However, many do not exit the cycle the first time around and they relapse back to their old unhealthy habits. Indeed, Prochaska and Di-Clemente (1983) found that, in the case of smokers, many had to take three journeys through the whole process before they were successful. It is important that we communicate to our patients their success and encouragement when things do not go to plan.

> Patient: Oh, I feel so annoyed with myself! I was doing so well and then I went to a party and an old friend offered me a cigarette, and I just took it to be sociable. Before I knew it, I had smoked three and then bought a packet on the way home. I am back to square one now. It's hopeless.
>
> Nurse: It's okay! It's inevitable that you will slip back from time to time. We are all human! The important thing is to realize that you have been able to not smoke for such a long time, and you will be able to improve on this.

This section has tended to focus on working with an individual; the same principles can be applied to working with groups or communities. The National Institute for Health and Clinical Excellence (NICE) offers a useful booklet for professionals, with key points and examples of how to apply change on a larger scale. This can be found at the following web page.

 www.nice.org.uk/media/D33/8D/Howtochangepractice1.pdf

Applying behaviour change skills in different settings

We've seen how people can be at different stages of engaging in the process of health behaviour, and that the professional has a role at every stage of the process. There are some specific communication skills that the professional can adopt to help people in this process, especially those who are not engaged in change or who are disheartened by perceived failure.

Motivational interviewing

Motivational interviewing (MI) was developed by two psychologists, Miller and Rollnick, in the 1990s particularly to tackle the motivation problems of people with alcohol dependency (Miller and Rollnick, 1995). There used to be an assumption among clinicians in this field that alcohol dependency treatment works for those who want to change, but that if someone isn't motivated to stop drinking, no treatment in the world will work! So, for Miller and Rollnick to develop a technique of interviewing people that develops motivation was quite a step forward. Motivational interviewing has been demonstrated to work in many trials now—particularly, the Project Match study for alcohol dependency (Project Match Research Group, 1998), HIV and sexual health (Dunn et al., 2001; Burke et al., 2003; Wolfers et al., 2009), accident risk among adolescents (Johnson et al., 2002), and cancer and diabetes (Wahab et al., 2008; Leak et al., 2009). In general, it is often recommended for conditions that have poor treatment adherence such as addictions, bulimia, obesity, and psychosis, but potentially it can be used for any situation in which poor treatment adherence or engagement is a problem. It is also shown to be effective in a range of applications when delivered by nurses with some skills in its use (Brodie et al., 2008; Brodie and Inoue, 2009), but evidence also suggests that, where nurses lack skills in communication to motivate patients, opportunities are missed to effect improved patient care (Hambly et al., 2009; Lai et al., 2010). This evidence suggests that nurses taking on the health promotion role need to be equipped with communication skills that support motivation and behaviour change.

Motivational interviewing uses the principles of the Prochaska and DiClemente's behaviour change model, as illustrated above, and fuses it with four principles taken from cognitive behavioural therapy (CBT) and Rogerian counselling. The nurse's intervention is pitched at the stage at which the patient is in the model, and adopts two specific principles to target the motivation stage of the patient.

CBT—cognitive dissonance

Cognitive dissonance is a phenomenon identified in cognitive psychology whereby anyone feels psychologically uncomfortable when in a state of ambivalence—that is, when their behaviour and their values, attitudes, or beliefs don't match. The principle of cognitive dissonance is that something has to change to relieve the person of that psychological discomfort: either they change their behaviour or they change their beliefs. For example, a woman who continues to drink excessively and discovers that her children are being harmed by her drinking behaviour will either have to stop drinking to stop feeling guilty or will develop beliefs and excuses for her behaviour.

> Patient: It's an illness that I have no control over.
>
> Patient: My dad was a drinker and it didn't do me any harm when I was growing up.

Using MI, the nurse targets the belief system to develop and enhance the discomfort, or 'dissonance'. This is called developing the **discrepancy** between behaviour and values.

Rogers's core principles of person-centred counselling

It sounds a bit cruel just to make someone feel uncomfortable about their behaviour, but such therapeutic communication needs to be delivered in an ethical way—that is, person-centred. So the relationship is based on Rogerian principles of expressing empathy and genuineness, working with the person to develop their self-efficacy, and avoiding confrontation.

Boxes 15.1 and 15.2 outline the four principles of MI and specific techniques identified by Miller and Rollnick for practice application.

Box 15.1 Miller and Rollnick's four principles of MI in practice

1. Express empathy—use reflective listening skills to demonstrate understanding of the person's problems and dilemmas in a non-judgemental way.
2. Develop discrepancy—between the person's deeply held values and their current behaviour.
3. Roll with the resistance that inevitably occurs—don't be confrontational or get into an argument.
4. Support and promote self-efficacy—help the person to believe they can effect change for themselves.

Box 15.2   Specific techniques in MI

1. Strive to understand the person's point of view and experiences, and make it clear to them that you accept their unique condition.
2. Focus on statements that encourage change and don't focus on negative and stable statements: 'I can't change—there's no point trying.'
3. Ask questions that elicit statements (self-statements) of problem recognition and desire to change: 'If you were to stop drinking now, what would your life be like in five years' time?'
4. Match your questions to the person's stage of change—don't jump ahead of the patient.
5. Support and promote self-efficacy—help the person to believe they can effect change for themselves.
6. Constantly refer back to the patient's freedom of choice and ability to choose their own path.

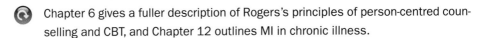 Chapter 6 gives a fuller description of Rogers's principles of person-centred counselling and CBT, and Chapter 12 outlines MI in chronic illness.

Anyone in health care can use MI skills when faced with patients with poor compliance and poor prognosis. Often, such patients are seen as 'heart-sink' patients, because nurses become frustrated with trying to persuade them to change their behaviour. Such patients may be good candidates for MI.

Let's look at some of the new skills mentioned above. There are examples of others in Chapter 6. The techniques must, of course, be based on an empathetic and cooperative style of relationship-building.

How to develop discrepancy

A person with a serious health problem due to their behaviour or lifestyle is often in denial about the reality of their situation. They have already closed their minds to the facts and developed defences, such as a set of beliefs, that protect them from feeling uncomfortable. Just telling someone won't get very far, as they have been told enough times before; it is up to the interviewer to highlight the reality of their situation. We can highlight some of the negative points whenever the opportunity presents, and create those opportunities by getting the person to state them for themselves. This is called eliciting a **self-statement**. See the example in Box 15.3.

Box 15.3   A sexual health nurse is interviewing a sex industry worker

Patient:	I suppose I would like to know whether I'm HIV positive or not.
Nurse:	What's stopping you?
Patient:	Well, because they might say I am HIV positive!
Nurse:	And what would be bad about that?
Patient (*laughs*):	Well, it would mean I'm going to die, wouldn't it?

Notice how the nurse gets the patient to make the statement about this fear herself, even though the answer is easy to anticipate. That way, the person is 'owning' her own values rather than having them thrust upon her in a confronting way.

This style of questioning is called **Socratic questioning**, whereby the nurse persists in asking even obvious questions in order to get the person to make the obvious statements of fact or belief themselves.

 See Chapter 4 for more on Socratic questioning.

Roll with resistance and avoid argumentation

Direct advice and confrontation with someone who is ambivalent about change will simply create resistance and defensiveness (see Box 15.4).

Box 15.4 Creating resistance

Nurse: Have you thought about cutting down on your smoking? It will help to reduce your blood pressure.

Patient: Yes, I've tried, but frankly, I enjoy smoking. It helps me to relax and that probably reduces my blood pressure too.

Nurse: But you could relax in other ways. In the long term, your blood pressure will reduce if you stop smoking.

Patient: Yes, I know smoking is bad for me in all sorts of ways. But quitting isn't as easy as you make it sound.

Nurse: What about trying nicotine patches?

Patient: Yes, but . . .

This interviewer has got into an argumentative dialogue with this patient and the patient is responding with lots of statements about why he won't stop smoking.

Look at the next example (Box 15.5).

Box 15.5 Rolling with resistance

Nurse: I guess you've tried cutting down your smoking?

Patient: Oh yes, but as soon as I feel stressed or go out socially, I want a cigarette.

Nurse (*avoiding a confrontational question*): What do you think makes you smoke in those situations?

Patient: Just habit, I suppose, but when I'm stressed I don't care about my health.

Nurse (*in response to the negative stance by the patient*): I can see on those occasions it is hard. Let's look at when you find it easier.

Here, the nurse has spotted that they are about to fall into an oppositional relationship, so he agrees with the patient about it being hard (because it is!) and moves toward talking about success instead of failure. This will also highlight the patient's sense of self-efficacy—what he *can* do.

So the relationship is about 'being on the same side' as the patient in making changes, rather than being in a professional–patient relationship and resorting to advice and persuasion. Evidence indicates that treatment dropout is higher when the professional adopts a dictatorial style (Stott and Pill, 1990).

Resistance in the patient can be spotted by the development of:

- arguing;
- interrupting;
- denying;
- ignoring.

The key to dealing with resistance is to recognize it and move away from the topic or shift the focus, ensuring that the patient knows it is about their choice. We can then go back to the topic once we feel that the time is right and the patient is much more open to discussion. Rollnick et al. (2007: 34) offer a useful checklist for us to adapt and use to check that all is going well and we are getting it right.

- The nurse is speaking slowly.
- The patient is doing much of the talking and is actively talking about behaviour change.
- The nurse is listening carefully and directing the interview at appropriate stages.
- The patient is 'working hard', with evidence of realization of issues and asking the nurse for advice and information.
- The process presents as both the nurse and the patient putting the pieces of a jigsaw together to reveal the full picture.

Support self-efficacy

The main aim of MI is to promote the patient's perception of their own abilities to make changes. A good strategy to adopt when meeting any resistance is to acknowledge and empathize with the patient's view, and to focus on the achievement the patient has made, even if it seems small. A resistant patient turning up for a clinic appointment is often a positive sign of motivation and hope, and can be explored (see Box 15.6).

Box 15.6 Encouraging self-efficacy

Patient: I can't alter the way I am, I'm just fat and that's that.

Interviewer: You sound really fed up about it, but I think you are already making changes by coming here. You've made a very positive start.

Notice how the nurse emphasizes that the patient has done something positive, implying that the patient is already making choices about change. The nurse could have emphasized how much attending clinic will help the patient—but that takes the power to change away from the patient, suggesting that it is the clinic that will make the difference. Instead, the nurse gives the message that the patient will make the difference by choosing to attend the clinic and using the help on offer.

Brief intervention

With pre-contemplative patients, it is hard to get as far as even discussing the problem without meeting instant resistance and disinterest. However, there is another evidenced technique that we can employ that aims to move someone toward contemplation of change. This is called brief intervention therapy (BIT).

Brief intervention aims to raise the patient's awareness of the problem and reduce any misconceptions. It adopts a similar strategy to MI by avoiding confrontation and helping the patient to 'own' their beliefs by eliciting self-statements. Look at the example in Box 15.7.

Box 15.7 Brief intervention

An underage teenage girl presents at A&E with alcohol poisoning. She indulges in heavy binge-drinking most weekends. Her understanding of her risk is epitomized by her statements.

Patient:	Everyone I know drinks like I do, there's nothing wrong with them. I'm young and fit, my body can cope.
Nurse:	I see you are due for a liver scan in a bit. Do you know what that's for?
Patient:	Just to check that my liver's OK, I guess.
Nurse (*looking serious*):	Well, it's a bit more than that really. There may be liver damage, judging by your level of alcohol intake. A female of your age is particularly vulnerable to liver damage.

The nurse in Box 15.7 is being quite dramatic, but not unrealistically so, and not 'preaching'. The message being given is that this person in particular is at specific risk of liver damage. This indirectly challenges the patient's existing beliefs of being invulnerable at her age and in comparison with others.

Brief intervention is about sowing seeds of doubt or hope, giving people 'food for thought', and making even a small change to how he or she views his or her situation and behaviour. When someone presents with an acute problem, it is very often a good opportunity to highlight the reality of their behaviour. However, it is more effective if it is personalized—the message is: it is *you* who are in hospital/clinic, *you* who is having immediate treatment, and *you* who has chosen this course of action.

Another strategy in BIT is to elicit a statement about what the person would like to change if they could. A person who believes that they are predestined to fail can still have dreams or have a wish list. See Practice example box 1 for a real example of BIT with a female heroin user.

Practice example box 1: Working with a drug-using sex worker

Nurse: If you had a magic wand, what would you change?

Patient: Oh, I'd go back in time and not start taking heroin.

Nurse: If you could do that, what would you have done instead?

Patient: I'd have gone to college and perhaps been a nurse or something, instead of a prostitute.

Nurse: Going to college sounds like something you could do in the future.

Patient: But I've ruined my life already.

Nurse: Not yet. You're still alive. Some of your friends aren't. They have ruined their lives. You haven't.

With BIT, the seeds sown often need to be left to take effect. The health professional has no control over what people do with the intervention given during the short opportunity that presents. But evidence indicates that BIT can be the first prompt that gets someone to think about things, seek more information, and perhaps approach health services for support (Watson, 1992; Freemantle et al., 1993).

⊕ Learning point 2: Self-assessment

Test yourself on what you have learnt about MI and BIT by trying the multiple-choice questionnaire.

1. Motivational interviewing:
   a. is about confronting the person about their health risk behaviour.
   b. is only relevant for drug and alcohol problems.
   c. requires the health professional to be specially trained.
   d. should be delivered with a person-centred approach.
   e. was found to be less effective than ordinary CBT by the project MATCH study.

2. Strategies in motivational interviewing include:
   a. directly challenging the patient's beliefs.
   b. agreeing with the patient at all times.
   c. looking for arguments.
   d. taking on the role of the expert professional.
   e. looking out for resistance.

3. Brief intervention therapy:

    a. is a form of psychotherapy.

    b. is complicated to deliver.

    c. aims to elicit negative statements from the patient.

    d. aims to elicit hopeful statements from the patient.

    e. aims to show the patient how their beliefs are wrong.

4. In practising MI or BIT, the practitioner needs to:

    a. encourage the patient to make choices.

    b. challenge the patient's defences.

    c. tell the patient when they are wrong.

    d. advise the patient how to behave more healthily.

    e. teach the patient how to change.

Answers to Learning point 2

1 (d); 2 (e); 3 (d); 4 (a)

Conclusion

Modern nursing is not just about caring for the sick patient. Nurses are now health promoters and expected to help patients to improve and maintain healthier lifestyles. To do this, we need the communication skills that encourage people to engage in healthier behaviour. Encouraging patients to change their health behaviour can be a challenge, especially when we consider the many factors that contribute to why patients adopt unhealthy lifestyles and behaviour. Using a theory to guide our communication with patients about their health beliefs and health behaviours is useful as it enables us to work with patients in a logical way and to plan interventions with them that target their individual needs. As nurses, we need to be aware of the impact that our position can have on our patients' ability to consider healthy behaviours, and use this in a way that facilitates and encourages healthy behaviours. This process requires effective communication skills if we want to achieve positive outcomes for our patients.

 See the Online Resource Centre video interview 'Communication for behaviour change' in which motivation skills are applied.

To find more resources to aid your learning, please now go online to **www.oxfordtextbooks.co.uk/orc/webb**

Further reading

Ewles, L. and Simnett, I. (2005) *Promoting Health: A Practical Guide* (5th edn). Edinburgh: Balliere Tindell Elsevier.

Holloway, A. and Watson, H. (2002) 'Role of Self-efficacy and Behaviour Change', *International Journal of Nursing Practice*, 8(2): 106–15.

Miller, W. R. and Rollnick, S. (1995) *Motivational Interviewing: Preparing People to Change*. New York: Guilford Press.

References

Armstrong, S., Anderson, M., Le, E., and Nguyen, L. (2009) 'Application of the Health Belief Model to Bariatric Surgery', *Gastroenterology Nursing*, 32(3): 171–8.

Becker, M. H. (1974) 'The HBM and Preventative Health Behaviour', *Health Education Monographs*, 2: 354–68.

Browes, S. (2006) 'Health Psychology and Sexual Health Assessment', *Nursing Standard*, 21(5): 35–9.

Burke, B., Arkowitchz, H., and Menchola, M. (2003) 'The Efficacy of Motivational Interviewing: A Meta-analysis of Controlled Clinical Trials', *Journal of Consulting and Clinical Psychology*, 71: 843–61.

Dunn, C., Deroo, L., and Rivara, F. (2001) 'The Use of Brief Interventions Adapted from Motivational Interviewing across Behavioural Domains: A Systematic Review', *Addiction*, 96: 1725–42.

Ewles, L. and Simnett, I. (2005) *Promoting Health: A Practical Guide* (5th edn). Edinburgh: Balliere Tindell Elsevier.

Freemantle, N., Gill, P., Godfrey, C. et al. (1993) *Brief Interventions and Alcohol Use: Are Brief Interventions Effective in Reducing Harm Associated with Alcohol Consumption?* Effective Healthcare, 7. Leeds: Nuffield Institute for Health.

Lally, R., Chalmers, K., Johnson, J., Kojima, M., Endo, E. et al. (2008) 'Smoking Behaviour and Patient Education Practices of Oncology Nurses in Six Countries', *European Journal of Oncology Nursing*, 12(4): 372–9.

Leak, A., Davis, E., Houchin, L., and Mabrey, M. (2009) 'Diabetes Management and Self-care Education for Hospitalized Patients with Cancer', *Clinical Journal of Oncology Nursing*, 13(2): 205–10.

Medina-Shepherd, R. and Kleier, J. (2010) 'Spanish Translation and Adaptation of Victoria Champion's Health Belief Model Scales for Breast Cancer Screening: Mammography', *Cancer Nursing*, 33(2): 93–101.

Miller, W. R. and Rollnick, S. (1995) *Motivational Interviewing: Preparing People to Change*. New York: Guilford Press.

Prochaska, J. O. and Di-Clemente, C. C. (1983) 'Towards a Comprehensive Model of Change', in W. R. Miller and N. Heather (eds) *Treating Addictive Behaviours: Process of Change*. New York: Plenum.

—— and Worcross, J. C. (1992) 'In Search of How People Change: Applications to the Addictive Behaviours', *American Psychologist*, 47(9): 1102–14.

——, Norcross, J. C., and Di-Clemente, C. C. (1994) *Changing for Good*. New York: William Marrow & Co.

Project MATCH Research Group (1998) 'Matching Alcoholism Treatments to Patient Heterogeneity: Project MATCH Three-year Drinking Outcomes', *Alcohol Clinical Experimental Research*, 22: 1300–11.

Rollnick, S., Mason, P., and Butler, C. (2007) *Health Behaviour Change: A Guide for Practitioners*. Edinburgh: Churchill Livingstone Elservier.

Rosenstock, I. (1974) 'The HBM and Preventative Health Behaviour', *Health Education Monographs,* 2: 354–68.

Schofield, I., Kerr, S., and Tolson, D. (2007) 'An Exploration of the Smoking-related Health Beliefs of Older People with Chronic Obstructive Pulmonary Disease', *Journal of Clinical Nursing*, 16(9): 1726–35.

Stott, N. and Pill, R. (1990) '"Advise Yes, Dictate No": Patients' Views on Health Promotion in the Consultation', *Family Practice*, 7(2): 125–31.

Wahab, S., Menon, U., and Szalacha, L. (2008) 'Motivational Interviewing and Colorectal Cancer Screening: A Peek from the Inside Out', *Patient Educaton and Counseling*, 72(2): 210–17.

Watson, H. E. (1992) 'A Study of the Effectiveness of Brief Intervention for Problem Drinkers in an Acute Hospital Setting', Unpublished dissertation. Glasgow: University of Strathclyde.

Wolfers, M., de Wit, J., Hospers, H., Richardus, J., and de Zwart, O. (2009) 'Effects of a Short Individually Tailored Counselling Session for HIV Prevention in Gay and Bisexual Men Receiving Hepatitis B Vaccination', *BMC Public Health*, 9: 255.

16

Communication for personal and professional development

Lucy Webb

This chapter will help you to achieve competencies in:

- ➔ demonstrating, through reflection and evaluation, commitment to personal and professional development and lifelong learning, as applicable to communication skills;
- ➔ using professional support structures to learn from experience and make appropriate adjustments to communication skills;
- ➔ using professional support structures to develop self-awareness, challenge own prejudices, and enable communication within professional relationships so that care is delivered without compromise;
- ➔ having insight into own values and how these may impact on communication interactions with others.

Introduction

Communication is now one of the key practice standards in the NMC's revised standards for pre-registration education (NMC, 2010). During a pre-registration course, students will undertake academic projects at different levels in Years 1, 2, and 3, as well as attending placements in many different settings while achieving increasingly complex levels of competency. These experiences will require escalating communication skills—with each term and year, students build upon their existing knowledge and encounter new situations that demand new practical responses. It is therefore necessary for students to be continuously aware of their personal and professional development as it applies to their communication skills. We have all made mistakes and had negative experiences from which we have learnt, as well as thrilling new experiences in which we have excelled. It is no different in nursing.

Not only does this continual process of learning, trying, adapting, reviewing, and learning again take place in pre-registration nursing, but it also continues throughout our careers as nurses. It is expected that newly qualified nurses will continue to develop professionally and maintain their skills and knowledge throughout practice. This chapter aims to give a brief introduction to some of the ways in which students can continue to develop and qualified nurses can apply communication skills in order to meet the requirements of continuing professional development (CPD).

Personal and professional development

Pre-registration nurse training is recognized as a process that changes the person. Mackintosh believes that nurse students:

> become accultured to the values, norms and expectations of the profession . . . to such a point that the individual not only recognises the identity of the profession, but recognises this professional identity within themselves.
>
> (Mackintosh, 2006: 954)

Mackintosh is describing the process of professional socialization that changes the student professionally and personally. Concern was expressed that traditional nurse training held nurses in a task-oriented form of practice in which nurses were doctors' assistants and the medical profession took clinical responsibility for patient care (Bishop, 2001). Modern nursing, under the framework of clinical governance (see Box 16.1), can be seen to have facilitated the development of nursing as a profession toward greater autonomy, responsibility, and accountability, with a focus on evidence-based, up-to-date practice (Sackett et al., 1996; Bishop, 2001; Scott, 2001).

Box 16.1 Clinical governance aims

. . . to provide a service that will continually improve the overall standard of clinical care, reduce variations in outcomes and ensure clinical decisions are based on the most up-to-date evidence.

(Scott, 2001: 40)

For students entering the nursing profession, the emphasis on autonomous practice, accountability, lifelong learning, and professional development may seem, at times, at odds with their experience of the culture in practice. Mackintosh found some students' experiences were disillusioning when they encountered nurses who were uncaring or unprofessional. As one student stated in Mackintosh's study: 'They've lost the reason why they do the job, and it's just a ways and means of earning money, and they're used to working in that field' (Mackintosh, 2006: 957). Clinical governance and the focus on personal and professional development aims to overcome the problems of the depreciation of skills among trained professionals, who can otherwise become outdated, unmotivated, and, as a consequence, deliver an increasingly poor standard of care. This process is focused not just on post-qualified nurses, but also on students themselves, so that, during the training period, students become socialized into the nursing profession, both personally and professionally, with the motivation, skills, and attitude to engage in ongoing learning and the continuing development of their practice.

Two of the key mechanisms that aim to help students to engage in professional and personal development, and that are facilitated specifically by communication skills, are probably the student–mentor relationship and the use and practice of reflection. So let's look at the first of these.

The student–mentor relationship

The practice mentor allocated to students is responsible for guiding the student's learning and supporting the student to facilitate the student's achievement of the learning outcomes (Hart, 2010). The mentor does not do the 'teaching' in practice, but supports the student to gain access to learning opportunities. This relies on a positive working relationship between the student and the mentor, and key to this is communication (Cavanagh, 2002). The student–mentor relationship is a complex one, especially when a student is struggling, because, for one reason, the mentor role itself is one of role confusion (Bray and Nettleton, 2007). The Nursing and Midwifery Council (NMC, 2008b) stipulates that a nurse mentor should:

- facilitate learning in practice;
- support and supervise students;
- assess their achievements.

Hence, a mentor has to be a student support and the assessor, as well as a practising nurse. This is described as having to be 'three selves' (Orland-Barak, 2002) and as being pulled in different directions by different demands. There is a danger that the student–mentor relationship can be dysfunctional (toxic mentoring), in which the mentor creates dependency on the part of the student and restricts the student in exercising self-directed learning (Morton-Cooper and Palmer, 2000). This suggests that the relationship is based on an asymmetrical power base in which the mentor is too controlling and the student too compliant.

Learning point 1

Look back at Chapter 3 and the section on transactional analysis. Which type of ego states do you think would be involved in a student–mentor relationship in which a mentor became authoritarian and the student dependent? What strategies could the student use to change a 'toxic mentoring' relationship to one of mutual relating? What might happen if nothing changes in this relationship?

Suggested answer to Learning point 1

The imbalance in toxic mentoring could be a 'critical' or 'nurturing parent' with a 'compliant child'. The student could attempt to put the relationship onto an adult–adult footing by responding to the mentor's parent state from an 'adult' ego state. This might involve simple subtle changes or, if that doesn't work, having a frank and open discussion with the mentor as two adults to solve the relationship problem. If nothing changes in this relationship, either the student will remain a dependent, compliant 'child' and not get as much valuable learning from the placement as he or should could have, or, if frustration sets in, the student may become a 'rebellious child' and take an opposing stance to the mentor. This is likely to lead to confrontation or withdrawal and the relationship will break down.

Students have described a good mentor as friendly, patient, accessible, and, particularly, nurturing (Wilkes, 2006). However, being a 'knowledgeable friend' (Bennett, 2002) has been seen as a negative experience perhaps because of this multiple role of being a supporter and the assessor. Wilkes (2006) advises that the student–mentor relationship needs to be a professional one that attends to clearly defined boundaries, good planning from the outset of the placement, and is based on partnership and mutual respect. Mentors are expected to understand the student's experience, but equally, if the student can understand the mentor's experience, a relationship of partnership and mutual respect is more likely to develop.

Hart (2010) suggests that students have a wealth of learning opportunities on every placement, but need to engage with the staff available to get the most out of these situations.

Box 16.2 **Student comment on learning in practice**

'Be enthusiastic . . . because if you don't look like, or say that, you want to learn and see things, then the staff and your mentor won't think of you when opportunities arise. Also, if you do miss opportunities, then talk to your mentor (be diplomatic of course) and ensure that next time you don't miss the opportunities. You really must push yourself out there, and not expect mentors to constantly spoon-feed your opportunities.'

(Hart, 2010: 144)

See Hart (2010) for more on the mentor's role in student nurse education and training.

Reflective practice

This brings us on to reflective practice, a vital component of personal and professional development for the student and the qualified nurse. Reflection is reliant on good communication skills and also aids development of the underpinning skills of self-awareness, assertiveness, confidence, and personal development. Reflection is acknowledged as a key component in helping the practitioner to change perspective and develop new insights; reflection on practice leads to action and change (Johns, 1995). But it is also a skill in itself that needs development and leads to 'reflection as a way of being' (Johns, 2005: 6). We can distinguish between reflection as a tool and as a skill by considering:

- reflection on practice—learning from practice experiences (reflection on action);
- reflection in practice—applying reflective skills during practice (reflection in action).

Reflection on practice (reflection on action)

Reflection on practice aids the nurse to consider actions, decisions, and dilemmas arising from practice experience and consider them through analysis and evaluation. There are a host of reflective practice tools and methods that can be used for this purpose, which extend from directive guidance for the novice reflector, to internal insight and self-directed reflection for the expert reflector (Morgan and Johns, 2005). Nurse students may be familiar with some of the more directive methods in the list below.

- **Reflective diary:** facilitates later reflection on thoughts, feelings, and acts written in the context of practice. It communicates the nurse's ability to consider one's practice and seek to improve it.
- **Significant event record:** an account of a specific event reviewed historically for insights on the event.
- **Supervision:** guided refection in dialogue, often using Socratic dialogue from the supervisor to explore meaning of experiences and modify the reflector's thinking and knowledge.
- **Structured reflective models:** such as Gibbs's reflective cycle, Johns's model of structured reflection—two common reflective models that take the reflector through a series of questions to discover new insights on events (see the Online Resource Centre link at the end of this chapter).
- **Intuitive reflection:** sometimes on the spot or later critical thinking without specific tools, sleeping on problems, brainstorming, mind-mapping.

The key aspect of reflection on practice is opening up a personal dialogue with yourself regarding a particular incident, event, or situation that has occurred. This is a form of communication, using tools or mechanisms to engage in thinking.

Reflection in practice (reflection in action)

Reflection *in* practice can be described as the skill of reflection applied in practice (Johns, 1995; Todd, 2005). The practice of reflection on practice develops the nurse's ability to think objectively and form a different perspective about practice and professional development issues. Reflection in practice is putting those reflection skills to use when in a practice situation. In considering communication skills, for example, we may have become aware that, in a multidisciplinary team meeting, we tend to lack assertiveness and need to take opportunities to put our views across. In our next MDT meeting, we are able to assess the situation objectively, find that we have not stated our case well, and therefore act assertively to better present our view to our colleagues.

Figure 16.1 illustrates the difference between reflection on and in practice. This is also illustrated as a cycle that uses reflection on practice to enhance reflection in practice, but also reviews practice historically in order to apply new insights in practice. So, our skills of reflection enhance our skills of practice reflection in situ.

Reflection is an important aspect of personal and professional development for healthcare professionals and has long been seen as a rich avenue towards developing skills in practice (Schon, 1983; Casement, 1985). It is included in this book from the perspective of communication because, without good communication skills, we could not engage in reflection through writing or dialogue if we either were not motivated to engage in reflection or did not have the skills to gain quality learning and development from reflection.

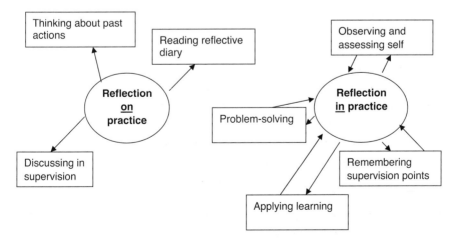

Figure 16.1 Reflecting on practice and reflecting in practice

You will find an illustrated model of Gibbs's reflective cycle and top tips for reflection in Hart (2010).

Post-qualifying personal and professional development

Post-registration education and practice (Prep)

Prep stands for post-registration education and practice (NMC, 2008c) and it is one of ways in which the NMC meets its legal requirements to monitor the professional standards of its registrants. The onus is on the registered nurse to demonstrate both continuing practice and continuing professional development (CPD) when renewing registration.

Currently, a nurse is required to undertake at least 35 hours of learning relevant to practice over a three-year period. In so doing, as a nurse, you will need to maintain a professional profile, or portfolio, of your learning activities. This can be audited by the NMC and you will have to comply with such an audit if asked to do so.

However, there are several ways in which to engage in learning activities and the material in this chapter will attempt to outline those commonly employed by practitioners, outside academic learning and formal training. The NMC outlines basic guidance when considering what is CPD (see Box 16.3).

> ### Box 16.3 NMC guidance on continuing professional development (NMC, 2008c: 12)
>
> - It doesn't have to cost you any money.
> - There is no such thing as an *approved* CPD learning activity.
> - You don't need to collect points or certificates of attendance.
> - There is no approved format for the personal professional profile.
> - It must be relevant to the work you are doing and/or plan to do in the near future.
> - It must help you to provide the highest possible standards of practice and care.

The NMC also provides guidance for recording your learning in a template, and you will find completed examples in the Prep handbook (NMC, 2008c: 12–15): **www.nmc-uk.org/Documents/Standards/nmcPrepHandbook**

- Name of workplace
- Name of organization
- Brief description of role (including direct care, healthcare education, research or management, or not currently working)

- Nature of learning activity: what did you do?
- Date of learning activity
- Briefly describe the learning activity
- How many hours did this take?
- Description of learning activity: of what did it consist?
- Outcome of learning activity: how did it relate to your work?

Importantly, CPD can be demonstrated through non-formal learning activities, as outlined in this chapter.

Professional skills development: continuing professional development on the job

Clinical supervision

The NMC (2008a) describes clinical supervision as an important part of clinical governance, which, in turn, is the mechanism by which all healthcare practitioners will be accountable for maintaining professional standards. Clinical supervision is seen as a formal process of professional support and learning in the workforce by which nurses can take responsibility for their own practice and improve their expertise.

There is seen to be greater need for clinical supervision in modern nursing, as accountability has become more important where nurses are working more autonomously and within a less structured supervisory hierarchy (Butterworth et al., 2008). Models of clinical supervision have been developed from allied professions in counselling and psychotherapy for use in nursing and, arguably, have received greater support and development within mental health nursing (Cutliffe, 2001). However, the NMC now regards it as an important part of clinical governance and states that every registered nurse should have access to clinical supervision (NMC, 2008a).

Clinical supervision can take many forms; in fact, it is recognized that the form it takes should be determined by the field of practice and local circumstances. The principles are, however, that it should:

- be a practice-focused professional relationship between supervisor and supervisee;
- support practice and maintain and develop standards of care;
- be supported by nurses and managers, with local processes that enable open and trusting engagement in a supervision process. It should not, therefore, be used as a management process and, in principle, should be designed to allow open discussion of errors and failings within professional boundaries.

Good clinical supervision requires good skills of communication by supervisor and supervisee and, at the same time, enhances communication skills. Effective supervision needs the supervisor and supervisee to develop a working relationship that encourages discussion. Butterworth et al. (2008) suggest that clinical supervision has many benefits, but also some failings. As a CPD tool, it can increase the supervisee's confidence and self-awareness, reduce their sense of isolation, improve the nurse's work–life balance, and increase personal growth and coping. It facilitates knowledge transfer to less-experienced practitioners and helps to bridge the theory–practice gap.

Butterworth et al. (2008) also point out that effective clinical supervision demands organizational support to overcome problems of tokenism or lack of staff engagement. Poorly practised supervision can create resistance among staff, leading to suspicion, lack of disclosure, and a feeling that it is just a management tool. It could also be destructive by becoming a means with which to air grievances and creating an 'us and them' division between management and staff.

Proctor's model of clinical supervision

Bridgid Proctor (1986) suggested three functional components to clinical supervision:

- **normative**—providing a structure to practice supervision, meeting and addressing professional ethics requirements, and ensuring professional responsibility;
- **restorative**—providing support to staff, enabling personal growth, professionalism, confidence, and problem-solving skills, and producing higher staff morale;
- **formative**—providing educative and skills development among staff, sharing of knowledge and experience, and contributing to the incorporation of theory and practice.

Practice example box 1: Clinical supervision

A nurse brought a concern to her supervisor regarding a palliative care patient with severe dementia. The patient's relatives wanted him to receive communion from the hospital priest. The patient's history suggested that he had lost interest in practising his religion, although the family were practising Catholics. The nurse was unsure for whom she should be an advocate: the relatives or the patient. In discussing this case, the supervisor and supervisee explored the issues of consent and advocacy, and decided that the patient would consent if able as the relatives would be comforted. Additionally, there was no evidence to suggest that he would object and that he might even feel comforted at this stage in his life. The nurse felt confident about deciding to facilitate the communion, and understood more clearly the role of advocate and issues of consent and mental capacity.

Practice example box 1 provides a real-life example of a supervision scenario. First, this formalized supervision provision complies with Proctor's normative component in that supervision was organized and available to the nurse, providing a vehicle for addressing professional ethics and the nurse's accountability. Second, it illustrates Proctor's restorative function of supervision whereby the nurse had moved from having doubts about her practice to feeling confident with her own accountability for the decision made; the nurse had been provided with knowledgeable support and guidance. Third, we can see Proctor's formative component in this example whereby the nurse has developed professionally by extending her knowledge and experience.

Proctor's model provides clarity and boundaries to the relationship of supervisor–supervisee in that it defines the aims of clinical supervision. As outlined earlier, poorly delivered supervision detracts from these functions.

One problem identified by Cutliffe and Proctor (1998) is that supervision relies both on a skilled supervisor and also a supervisee who knows how to use the supervision offered. Lack of understanding of clinical supervision can lead to mistrust and resistance, hence Cutliffe and Proctor (1998) suggest that nurses need to be socialized into receiving and using supervision even during training. Bond and Holland (1998) suggest that the supervisee should understand the supervisee role and needs to be fully engaged and committed to supervision. Supervision cannot meet Proctor's aims, arguably, when the supervision is imposed by management on an unwilling workforce.

Bond and Holland (1998) suggest that the supervisee should:

- have an active part in selecting the supervisor;
- be adequately prepared for the session;
- develop skills in reflective practice;
- identify topics for discussion;
- help to set ground rules.

....

⊕ Learning point 2

Next time you are in a practice placement, find out what clinical supervision processes are in place. There may not be an identified or formal system for clinical supervision, therefore find out how nurses engage in reflection and learning from practice episodes. Do you think these methods meet the requirements of personal and professional development as outlined in the evidence for good practice here? What would improve the engagement in personal and professional development?

....

Suggested answer to Learning point 2

You might have considered whether nurses are engaging in guided reflection, or rely on informal self-directed and insightful reflection. Also, are there any clinical supervision structures in place? If not, how do nurses consider clinical issues from their practice, and are these methods adequate?

Conclusion

Communication skills apply to nursing and nurse training in many ways, as illustrated by this book. This chapter illustrates another, very important, element of nursing that relies on communication skills: continuing personal and professional development. This chapter outlines just two of the many ways in which development can be engaged in and demonstrated for Prep. You will already have experienced reflective practice as a student nurse and may also have been exposed to clinical supervision in practice—at least observing its function among nursing teams. Reflective practices are described as essential tools to support personal and professional development. They aid the nurse to learn from practice (reflection on practice) and to apply reflective skills in practice (reflection in practice). So, like communication skills, reflection is a skill to be developed and understood, and a tool for developing the skills of objectivity and application of learning and experience in practice.

Clinical supervision, on the other hand, is a tool we can use to facilitate personal and professional development and deliver refection on practice. It is a method for developing the underpinning communication skills of self-awareness, assertiveness, confidence, and even self-esteem, and a professional identity. However, both reflection and supervision can be enacted through tokenism—going through the motions—or by quality engagement with professional development. It is the nurse's responsibility not only to demonstrate CPD, but, perhaps morally, also to engage meaningfully with the processes of CPD to enhance practice. Once you have qualified, you will be expected to seek out opportunities and engage in CPD. Learning doesn't stop when you qualify: it could be said that it has only just started!

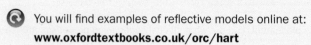 You will find examples of reflective models online at:
www.oxfordtextbooks.co.uk/orc/hart

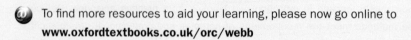 To find more resources to aid your learning, please now go online to
www.oxfordtextbooks.co.uk/orc/webb

Further reading

Johns, C. and Freshwater, D. (2005) *Transforming Nursing through Reflective Practice* (2nd edn). Oxford: Blackwell Publishing.
Nursing and Midwifery Council (2008) *The Prep Handbook*. London: NMC.

References

Bennett, C. (2002) 'Making the Most of Mentorship', *Nursing Standard*, 17(3): 29.

Bishop, V. (2001) 'Professional Development and Clinical Supervision', in V. Bishop and I. Scott (eds) *Challenges in Clinical Practice: Professional Developments in Nursing*. Basingstoke: Palgrave.

Bond, M. and Holland, S. (1998) *Skills of Clinical Supervision for Nurses: A Practical Guide for Supervisees, Clinical Supervisors and Managers*. Buckingham: Open University Press.

Bray, L. and Nettleton, P. (2007) 'Assessor or Mentor? Role Confusion in Professional Education', *Nurse Education Today*, 27: 848–55.

Butterworth, T., Bell, L., Jackson, C., and Pajnkihar, M. (2008) 'Wicked Spell or Magic Bullet? A Review of the Clinical Supervision Literature 2001–2007', *Nurse Education Today*, 28: 264–72.

Casement, P. (1985) *On Learning from the Patient*. New York: Guildford Press.

Cavanagh, M. (2002) 'Being a Mentor', in J. Canham and J. Bennett (eds) *Mentorship in Community Nursing: Challenges and Opportunities*. Oxford: Blackwell Science.

Cutliffe, J. (2001) *Fundamental Themes in Clinical Supervision*. London: Routledge.

—— and Proctor, B. (1998) 'An Alternative Training Approach to Clinical Supervision: 1', *British Journal of Nursing*, 7(5): 280–5.

Department of Health (1998) *Clinical Governance: Quality in the New NHS*. London: DoH.

Hart, S. (2010) *Nursing: Study and Placement Learning Skills*. Oxford: Oxford University Press.

Johns, C. (1995) 'Framing Learning through Reflection within Carper's Ways of Knowing in Nursing', *Journal of Advanced Nursing*, 22: 226–34.

—— (2005) 'Expanding the Gates of Perception', in C. Johns and D. Freshwater (eds) *Transforming Nursing through Reflective Practice* (2nd edn). Oxford: Blackwell Publishing.

Mackintosh, C. (2006) 'Caring: The Socialisation of Pre-registration Student Nurses— A Longitudinal Qualitative Descriptive Study', *International Journal of Nursing Studies*, 43: 953–62.

Morgan, R. and Johns, C. (2005) 'The Beast and the Star: Resolving Contradictions within Everyday Practice', in C. Johns and D. Freshwater (eds) *Transforming Nursing through Reflective Practice* (2nd edn). Oxford: Blackwell Publishing.

Morton-Cooper, A. and Palmer, A. (2000) *Mentoring, Preceptorship and Clinical Supervision: A Guide to Professional Support Roles in Clinical Practice*. Oxford: Blackwell.

Nursing and Midwifery Council (2008a) *Clinical Supervision for Registered Nurses*. London: NMC.

—— (2008b) *The Code: Standards of Conduct, Performance and Ethics for Nurses and Midwives*. London: NMC.

—— (2008c) *The Prep Handbook*. London: NMC.

—— (2010) *Standards for Pre-registration Nursing Education: Draft for Consultation*. London: NMC.

Orland-Barak, L. (2002) 'What's in a Case: What Mentors' Cases Reveal about the Practice of Mentoring', *Journal of Curriculum Studies*, 34(4): 451–68.

Proctor, B. (1986) 'Supervision: A Co-operative Exercise in Accountability', in M. Marken and M. Payne (eds) *Enabling and Ensuring*. Leicester: National Youth Bureau and Council for Education and Training in Youth and Community Work.

Sackett, D., Rosenberg, W., Gray, J., Haynes, R., and Richardson, W. (1996) 'Evidence-based Medicine: What It Is and What It Is Not', *British Medical Journal*, 312: 71–2.

Schon, D. (1983) *Educating the Reflective Practitioner*. London: Jossey Bass.

Scott, I. (2001) 'Clinical Governance: A Framework and Models for Practice', in V. Bishop and I. Scott (eds) *Challenges in Clinical Practice: Professional Developments in Nursing*. Basingstoke: Palgrave.

Todd, G. (2005) 'Reflective Practice and Socratic Dialogue', in C. Johns and D. Freshwater (eds) *Transforming Nursing through Reflective Practice* (2nd edn). Oxford: Blackwell Publishing.

Wilkes, Z. (2006) 'The Student–Mentor Relationship: A Review of the Literature', *Nursing Standard*, 20(37): 42–7.

Glossary

A

Active listening A form of communication that aids the nurse in listening attentively to the patient and shows the patient they are being listened to

Adapted child The controlled child ego state in transactional analysis

Adult ego state The adaptive adult state of interaction in transactional analysis

Ambivalence to change Behaviour change terminology describing mixed motivations to change behaviour

Authenticity Acting with genuineness

Authoritarian leadership Leadership style that directs others with little consultation with team members

Authoritative Positions of superiority in intervention analysis

B

Beneficent Having good intent; intending to do good

Boundaries (in nursing) The limits of behaviour that allow a nurse or midwife to have a professional relationship with the person in his or her care

C

Catalytic Facilitating problem-solving in intervention analysis

Cathartic Producing a release of tension in intervention analysis

Circular questioning Questions that assist in looking at the issue from a different viewpoint

Classical conditioning Behavioural explanation of the learning of physical reactions to external stimuli

Client-centred therapy Form of therapeutic relating developed by Carl Rogers in which the client is empowered to explore and resolve his or her own needs

Clinical intranet systems Computerized system in clinical organization not accessible to people outside; cannot be accessed via the Internet

Clinical supervision Practice of giving and receiving supervision of practice as a form of reflection

Closing down Method for controlling and reducing high expressed emotion and excitability

Cognitive behaviour therapy (CBT) A therapeutic approach focusing on how a person perceives, interprets, and reacts to situations

Conditioning Behavioural understanding of learning

Conformity Adapting our behaviour, attitude, or belief in line with our group identity

Confronting Position of being challenging in intervention analysis

Critical parent The controlling and criticizing parent ego state in transactional analysis

D

Degenerate Destructive communication style in intervention analysis

Democratic leadership Leadership style that facilitates involvement of others but retains a decision-making role

Descriptors (educational) Words in assignments that indicate what the student is expected to do

Diagnostic overshadowing Attributing a symptom to a learning disability and/or mental health problem

Discrepancy Between behaviour and values; outcome sought by motivational interviewers to reveal irrational thinking of person in a state of ambivalence to change

Dyad A protected pattern of communication involving two people within a group

Dysfunctional thinking Thinking styles that are unhelpful and lead to maladaptive behaviour

E

Ego state (parent, adult, child) The attitude of mind a person adopts when communicating with others

Empathy Ability to enter the perceptual world of the other person

Empowerment Strategy or philosophy in which the therapeutic goal is to facilitate another's self-care and self-determination

F

Facilitative Positions of enabling in intervention analysis

G

Game (game-playing) Having an ulterior motive to control others in transactional analysis

Genuineness Being yourself with your patient

H

Heron See Six-category intervention analysis

Humanistic Recognizing human individualism and freedom to choose

I

Informative Positions of information-giving in intervention analysis

L

Laissez-faire leadership Leadership style that permits free access to decision-making by team members

M

Maslow's hierarchy of needs Humanistic model of personal development

Models of care A systematic framework derived from a specific holistic and theoretical model, which is used to underpin the assessment, planning, intervention, and evaluation of care delivered to patients

Mutuality The degree of shared relating between the nurse and the patient

N

Natural child The carefree ego state in transactional analysis

Non-directive An approach to counselling that assumes a relationship of equals

Non-maleficent Having no bad intent; intending no harm

Non-verbal attending Reading body language and vocalizations to listen to another

Nurturing parent The caring parent ego state in transactional analysis

O

Open questions Questions that elicit complex answers

Operant conditioning Behavioural explanation for learnt behaviour

P

Paraphrasing Repeating back to the person what you understand by what they've said

Paternalistic (medical model) Adopting a position of authoritative protection in relation to patients

Position The attitudinal status adopted by one person in relation to another in an interaction

Positive stroke Positive attention-giving interaction in transactional analysis

Prescriptive Giving instruction in intervention analysis

Pro-dromal Relating to the period of pathology that precedes symptom appearance

Proxemics The 'personal space', or proximity, of people to each other and the body zones that are acceptable for touching—or even viewing

R

Reflective practice Applying reflection on past events to problem-solving in present practice

Reinforcement Presentation of stimuli that strengthens reward-oriented behaviour (positive reinforcement) or avoidance behaviour (negative reinforcement)

Rolling with resistance Therapeutic technique used in motivational interviewing that enables the therapist to avoid confrontation

Scapegoat A person blamed for the problems of the group

Self-awareness Being conscious of one's own character

Self-care (in nursing) Patient's ability to provide for own needs

Self-disclosure Technique of sharing experience and improving mutuality

Self-efficacy The belief that one can control one's own environment; a sense of autonomy

Self-statement Outcome elicited in motivational interviewing and brief intervention in which the interviewee verbalizes a key problem

Sequential questioning Often direct and following a sequence of events

Six-category intervention analysis A model for professional interpersonal development, delineating six different styles of interaction

Social identity One's identity as defined by group membership

Socialization The process of developing behaviour, attitudes, and beliefs to adapt to one's social environment

Socratic questioning Pursuing a line of questioning until all of the details are revealed

Strokes Episodes of attention-giving in transactional analysis (positive and negative)

Supportive Encouraging interaction style in intervention analysis

Sympathy Being affected by the same feeling as another

Transaction Interaction between two people in transactional analysis

Transactional analysis (TA) A model of communication marking the 'positions' of the interactors

Triad A protected communication pattern involving a small group within a group (often a subgroup)

Ulterior transaction One position or ego state presenting as another ego state

Unconditional positive regard Humanistic strategy that adopts a non-judgemental approach by encouraging empathy in the therapeutic space

Universality A sense of sharing experiences with others

Vicarious learning Learning behaviour through watching others

Vocal attending Vocal noises and responses we make and the way in which we use our voice

W

5WH Inquiring words: 'when'; 'what'; 'why'; 'who'; 'where'; or 'how'

Index

The page numbers for information in tables appear in italics.